Foundation Hairdressing

Lesley Hatton began her career as an apprentice in a London salon and progressed to management level within six years. She has been involved in film, theatre and photographic work, and feels equally at home with European or Afro hair. She has been a lecturer at the London College of Fashion, City and East London College, and is currently Course Director in Hairdressing at the Selhurst Tertiary Centre of Croydon College. Under her direction the College was selected as an Information Centre for the National Preferred Scheme.

Phillip Hatton BSc(Hons), MIBiol, CBiol, DipEdMan, MIT, MRIPHH, PGCE, was a lecturer for several years at the London College of Fashion. He has been a consultant for several salon chains including Vidal Sassoon's. Phillip is a qualified trichologist and was a Governor of the Institute of Trichologists for several years. He is a senior examiner of the Royal Institute of Public Health and Hygiene and lectures extensively in this country and abroad. His unmatched experience and knowledge is often called upon by the courts in hairdressing litigations. Phillip has been involved in development work for the Hairdressing Training Board and is one of their Trainers. At present he is a Deputy Head of Department at Barking College. Phillip and Lesley regularly write in the trade press and have also featured on radio programmes.

Other books on hairdressing from BSP Professional Books

Colouring — A Salon Handbook
Lesley Hatton, Phillip Hatton and Alisoun Powell
0−632−01922−0

Hygiene — A Salon Handbook
Phillip Hatton
0−632−01921−2

Perming and Straightening — A Salon Handbook
Lesley Hatton and Phillip Hatton
0−632−01865−8

Cutting and Styling — A Salon Handbook
Lesley Hatton and Phillip Hatton
0−632−01851−8

Afro Hair — A Salon Handbook
Phillip Hatton
0−632−02285−X

Hairdressing Business Management — A Salon Handbook
Annette Mieske
0−632−02592−1

FOUNDATION
HAIRDRESSING

Lesley Hatton, *CertEd*
and
Phillip Hatton, *BSc(Hons), MIBiol, CBiol, DipEdMan, MIT, MRIPHH, PGCE*

BSP PROFESSIONAL BOOKS

OXFORD LONDON EDINBURGH

BOSTON MELBOURNE

First published 1990

British Library
Cataloguing in Publication Data
Hatton, Lesley
   Foundation hairdressing.
   1. Hairdressing
   I. Title   II. Hatton, Phillip
   646.7'242

ISBN 0-632-02613-8

BSP Professional Books
A division of Blackwell Scientific
   Publications Ltd
Editorial Offices:
Osney Mead, Oxford OX2 0EL
   (Orders: Tel. 0865 240201)
25 John Street, London WC1N 2BL
23 Ainslie Place, Edinburgh EH3 6AJ
3 Cambridge Center, Suite 208,
   Cambridge, MA 02142, USA
107 Barry Street, Carlton,
   Victoria 3053, Australia

Set by Setrite Typesetters
Printed in Great Britain
at the Alden Press, Oxford

To Silvio Camillo, one of the great hairdressers, who we are honoured to be able to call a friend.

Contents

About This Book

Many people who are just beginning their careers in hairdressing wonder why they need to know so much, when all they really want to do is cut hair. If all there were to hairdressing were picking up a pair of scissors we would all soon be out of business!

Being a success in hairdressing involves skill, artistry, scientific knowledge, personality, communication and commonsense, all in varying amounts. When you start hairdressing it is like being a new-born baby, not knowing anything, until you take those hardest first steps. You cannot expect to develop skills by just copying someone else; there must be a reason for everything you do. Hairdressing is a career that could take off in many directions. Any one of you could develop into the next Vidal Sassoon and become an international household name. For your career to last, however, you will need firm foundations, and this is why we have written *Foundation Hairdressing*.

Those of you following the Foundation Certificate in Hairdressing will need to know everything in this book. It deals with all the subjects incorporated into the syllabus and should equip you to master the basic knowledge that is required to be a competent hairdresser. Every element of knowledge, however, is required for a different reason. Science is not included to make things harder, but because without it you would be a danger not only to your clients, but also to yourself. Although you don't need to be able to make products, it is important to be able to understand why you should use them in certain ways but not in others. When your clients ask why a more expensive product is more suitable for their hair, you should be able to tell them about hair condition and not just profit margin!

Each chapter covers all the activities or elements which go to make up a particular unit. You will find questions throughout the book. These have been designed to test your knowledge of what you have just read. Once you can answer a particular set of questions, you are ready to move on. All you need to know will be in the relevant section, so you can proceed at your own pace. Practical skills are all-important and competence can only be achieved through regular practice. Don't be discouraged if some skills take you longer to acquire than others. Just like learning to drive a car we all proceed at different rates. Practice will make perfect — eventually!

We hope that you enjoy the book and that it encourages you to go on to learn more about hairdressing. If you really enjoy certain aspects of your work and want to learn more about them, try reading the series of 'Salon Handbooks'. Although they are more advanced, they describe everything in the same clear manner as this book. Whenever it is possible, watch other hairdressers working. None of us should ever think that we are so good that we can afford to stop learning. Have a great career!

Lesley and Phillip Hatton
London

Chapter One
Reception

The reception area is the most important part of the salon because it is the focal point for all enquiries and information. A receptionist will deal with a wide range of tasks on an average day: greeting all salon visitors, answering the telephone, making appointments, making financial transactions, recording information for services and sales, selling products and other commodities, gowning clients and possibly being in control of paying in and withdrawing money from the bank. On an unusual day it could involve giving first aid, calling for an ambulance or heaven only knows!

The reception area is the first and last point of contact for *every* client so *each* client must be treated professionally and courteously. Some salons employ a full-time receptionist, but in many salons this is just not possible, so all staff will have to know how to carry out reception duties. The Foundation Certificate is the first hairdressing training scheme really to recognise this fact, so don't treat this part of your training as being unimportant. Always remember that good reception skills are invaluable and people with them are worth their weight in gold. These skills are also transferable to a wide range of other occupations that involve dealing with the public, so put as much effort as you can into learning them.

Making appointments and greeting clients

The first contact clients have with a salon is when they make an appointment. This can either be done by going into the salon or by making a telephone call. First impressions always count. If their initial contact with the salon is not favourable, clients may not honour the appointment that has been made for them. The importance of creating a welcoming and professional atmosphere when you are greeting clients cannot be over-emphasised.

Ideally, a reception area should provide the following:

- a comfortable waiting area;
- magazines, style books, product leaflets and promotional materials;
- refreshments;
- pleasant surroundings;
- sales point;
- retail displays;
- a full list of salon services and prices;
- clear indications of how payment can be made;
- storage for clients' coats and salon gowns;
- information on whether a stylist is running late.

Nothing is more offputting to clients than to walk into any type of business and feeling that they are not welcome. We have all encountered the aloof shop assistant or curt receptionist who has made us feel that we are a nuisance or do not belong in the establishment. These feelings are unpleasant and can produce feelings of anger and hostility. *Every* person that enters your salon is a potential client, from the person who delivers your stock to the child of an existing client. Make sure everybody that walks through your salon door is made to feel welcome.

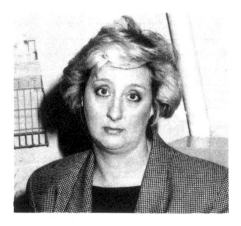

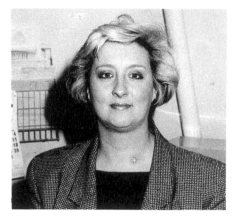

Figure 1.1 (a) How not to present yourself to clients.

(b) That's better!

First, we will look at the importance of the receptionist's appearance. Human nature is such that we all judge people on the way they look. Clients expect receptionists to look smart. After all, what would a receptionist communicate to you about the standard of a salon's work if she were wearing an unpressed overall with holes in her tights? The receptionist, and all salon staff for that matter, needs to promote an image that will attract clients into the salon. That means being well turned out from head to toe, taking notice of clothes, make-up and hair.

Apart from being well groomed, you need to consider the other non-verbal ways in which you are communicating something about yourself. Consider the non-verbal signals you are sending out by the way that you hold or arrange your body (posture). No matter how you talk to clients they will know that you do not really mean what you say if you are draped across your chair rather than being upright and paying them attention. Similarly, use gestures and facial expressions to let others know how you are feeling. Even if you have a violent headache a smile can transmit a welcome signal which is perceived as being more sincere than a cheery sounding welcome with a scowling face. Look at the photographs shown in Figures 1.1(a) and (b). Does the receptionist shown in Figure 1.1(a) look alert, keen to help and interested? Now look at Figure 1.1(b). She would be far more welcoming.

The arrangement of our bodies while at the reception could deter a client from entering the salon in the first place. How can your posture, gestures and facial expressions create the right image?

Set out below are the fundamental dos and don'ts of what you should and shouldn't do while working at reception.

Dos	Don'ts
Do sit up straight and look alert.	**Don't** slouch across the desk.
Do *smile* and show friendliness.	**Don't** act aloof or bored.
Do give each client your undivided attention and look the client in eyes.	**Don't** continue your conversation with a colleague.
Do act in a professional way.	**Don't** chew, smoke, eat or drink at reception.

Once the right image has been created in terms of the reception environment and your overall appearance, the way you use your voice, facial expressions and gestures is what counts. Look clients in the eyes, smile sincerely and greet them in a professional way. Obviously, the greeting used will differ between salons but a simple 'Good morning, may I help you?' would be considered adequate by most employers, and clients! Don't fall into the lazy habit of not greeting the clients properly, by just looking at the client with raised eyebrows as a substitute for a spoken welcome and offer of help.

Once you know the client's name *use* it. Check the appointments book so that if you know that you are expecting a Mrs Smith at 10 AM. you can at least hazard a guess when someone comes in at that time! This will give the client a sense of belonging to your salon and help to develop a relationship that will be of benefit to the salon in developing client loyalty. Make sure you know the correct term for addressing each client as many people are offended if they are called Mrs when they prefer Ms, for example. While we are on the subject of the prefixes that are before people's names, do you know the correct terms of address for a Catholic priest, a nun or even royalty? Listed below are some examples which give the correct terms of address for different people:

'Mr —': a male, regardless of marital status (or, if you don't know the name, 'Sir')
'Mrs —': a female who is currently married or has been married (or 'Madam').
'Miss —': a female who is not married (or 'Madam')
'Ms —': a female who prefers that her marital status is not known — usually because they feel it is irrelevent (or 'Madam')
'Father —': a Catholic priest (or 'Father')
'Reverend —': a Church of England vicar (or 'Vicar')
'Sister —': a nun (or 'Sister')
'Your Royal Highness': a prince or princess

Some members of the aristocracy like to be called Sir or Madam and sometimes even by their first name. Until you know their preference, it is a good idea to use the formal and correct terms of address such as Lord or Lady before their name. Many celebrities *expect* to be recognised and can get quite upset if you don't know who they are! We won't mention any names but we know of instances when famous actors have been called the wrong name when greeted at the salon's reception. It can be very hurtful to be mistaken for someone who is dead! Not a very good beginning to the appointment for the client or the salon!

If, as has happened to us on a number of occasions, you are unsure of the sex of a client, try not to use a specific male or female title until you have got some clues. A high pitched voice is not always going to mean that the client is female!

The important factor to keep at the forefront of your mind is that *every* client is important and should be treated with the same deserved respect. Appearances can be deceptive and the person who looks as though she has spent the last three nights sleeping rough could turn out to be your local MP or someone who could buy your shop a hundred times over!

Once you have greeted the client and offered your assistance ('Good morning, may I help you?') you need to be able to offer the necessary help and information. The potential client could have come into the salon for any of these reasons:

- to make an appointment;
- to cancel an appointment;
- to keep an appointment;
- to enquire about services, prices etc.;
- to purchase products or other commodities;
- to meet somebody who is in the salon;
- to ask directions!

Whatever the reason the potential client has entered your salon for, there should be a reception procedure that you follow. If the client wishes to make an appointment, there are certain questions you will need to ask to be able to carry out this request. For example:

'What day/time would suit you best?'
'Who usually does your hair?'
'What is the appointment for?'
'Can I have your name, please?'
'Could you spell that for me, please?'

Each salon will have its own particular method of making appointments. Some will be using a computer program to enter the bookings while others will be writing the appointments in an appointments register. Whichever method is used, appointments will need to be phased and interlaced. This means allocating the correct amount of time to the stylist according to the service that is to be carried out and, if necessary, booking out the stylist in stages to allow for the time that is 'lost' when a tint is developing or a perm is processed. For example, a salon may employ a person who does all the tinting and perming services. A client making an appointment for a perm may therefore be booked out like this:

10.00 – Booked with stylist for the hair cut.
10.30 – Booked with the perming technician for the perm.
12.00 – Booked with the stylist for completion of style.

Junior stylists might be allocated more time to carry out services than the more experienced stylists. Managers or artistic directors are sometimes given more time, especially if a client is charged more for their services. Additional time may also be necessary if a client has long hair.

Each appointment that is made should be recorded in detail. Notes should be made of the date, time, the client's name, the required service and the name of the stylist(s) attending the client. If this information is recorded into a book it is important that it is written in pencil so that it can be erased if the appointment is cancelled. This allows for another booking to be made in its place. Your writing should be neat and clear

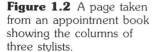

Figure 1.2 A page taken from an appointment book showing the columns of three stylists.

DATE: Monday 18th March

	Steve	Jane	Pauline
8.30 a.m.			
8.45			
9.0	A. Wilson Ⓡ	Mrs Day s/s	Christine
9.15	C BD	Mrs Cane Ⓡ	CBD
9.30	P. Briant*	PW	Mr Shaw R
9.45	C s/s	/////	CBD
10.0	Mrs Shaw*	F. Wilson*	P. Andrews*
10.15	HL (long Hair)	C BD	CBD
10.30	//////	M. Elson*	Mrs Starr s/s
10.45	\\\\\	C s/s	Mrs Mill Cs/s Ⓡ
11.0	Mrs May Ⓡ		/////
11.15	C BD		
11.30	F. Timms R s/s	Mrs Penfold BD	Mrs March *
11.45			Tint

so that others do not have a problem reading it. If you know that your writing is difficult to read, use block letters. Usually, salons will use abbreviations to describe each service and to keep track of the number of new and regular clients. For example:

CBD: cut and blow dry
HL: highlights
PW: permanent wave
* : new client
R : regular client
Rd: recommended client

The last three codes given in the example above can be used to calculate the number of new and regular clients over a specific period of time – especially useful, for instance, if the salon wants to assess the effectiveness of a recent advertising campaign. Usually, depending on the size of the salon, a single page is used for each day. Such a sheet is shown in Figure 1.2.

When making appointments in a book, it is important to remember these points:

- Write in pencil so that the appointment can be erased if it is cancelled.
- Write clearly so that it can be read by anyone who may need to look at the appointment book.
- Concentrate to avoid making mistakes and always check that it has been entered on the correct day at the right time, etc. Don't just open the page at Friday and assume you have the right week.
- Record each appointment in detail and write this information on an appointments card for the client in pen.

When a client comes to the salon to keep an appointment it is common practice to put a tick next to their name to show they have arrived. You will need to inform the stylist that will be attending to the client that they have arrived. You may also need to write the client's name on a 'daily sheet' which records the number of clients an individual stylist has attended during the day. Remember that you will know the client's name so use it when directing them to where they should wait.

Below are a few dos and don'ts of dealing with clients at the reception.

Dos	Don'ts
Do call the client by name.	**Don't** refer to Jane's 10.15 – it sounds like a train!
Do get up and show clients where to sit.	**Don't** remain seated and wave clients in the direction of where they should wait.
Do ask clients if they would like tea, coffee or magazines.	**Don't** leave it to clients to help themselves or go without.
Do apologise for any delay to an appointment.	**Don't** keep clients waiting without giving an explanation.
Do try to resolve problems like double-bookings courteously and patiently.	**Don't** lose your temper – you could lose the client.

If a person comes into your salon to find out the price or other details about a service you should be able to provide this information. You will need to learn all the salon prices, how long each service takes to complete, why some product ranges or services are more expensive than others and the reason for this. Not all services will be suitable for every client's needs nor beneficial to their hair, so having a knowledge of the suitability and benefits of products and services is necessary. For example, one of the benefits of having a permanent tint is that it can effectively cover white hair but would not be suitable for a client who is allergic to the chemicals contained in such colorants.

As an exercise, take a piece of paper and list at the top the following four titles: Service, Timings (Stylist), Timings (Client) and Total Cost. See if you can complete the chart with the services offered in your salon. You need to find out the following information:

- How much time is allocated to the stylist(s) for completing the service and whether the booking is interlaced to allow for the time taken for chemical processing.
- How much time the client will spend in the salon.
- The total cost the client will be charged.

As the reception area is the busiest part of the salon and deals with the greatest flow of client traffic, make the most of this opportunity by displaying products and other commodities such as jewellery and make-up for sale. Selling will be dealt with in Chapter 12 but do remember that there are golden opportunities to make a sale when you are at the reception with a client.

Questions

You could either write down the answers to these questions or get a friend or tutor to question you orally.

1. Who should be the first point of contact that potential clients have with the salon?
2. Why is this first contact so important, even if you think the standard of hairdressing in the salon is high enough to sell the services the salon offers?
3. What things should a reception area ideally provide?
4. Using your own salon as an example, what suggestions could you make to improve the reception area?
5. Why should you always make everyone feel welcome, even if they are not clients?
6. How can a receptionist's appearance attract or put off clients?
7. What does 'non-verbal communication' mean to you?
8. Why can it be as important as what you say or look like?
9. Why is it important to know clients' names when they walk into the salon?
10. Make a list of the correct way of addressing different people and then get someone to test you to see if you know them?
11. How would you talk to a client if you were unsure of their sex? Write down two examples.
12. Why should you treat everyone in the same way?
13. Make a list of reasons why potential clients might come into the salon.
14. What questions would you ask someone who wanted to make an appointment so that you could make it correctly?
15. How long would you book a client in for a perm in your salon?

16. Which member of staff would be booked out for the most time and the least time in your salon?
17. Write down the details you would take from a client when making an appointment.
18. Why and when would you use a pencil?
19. Why and when would you use ink?
20. What abbreviations are used in the appointments book in your salon?
21. How long could clients expect to be in your salon if they were having (a) a perm, (b) a tint, (c) highlights, (d) cut and blow dry?
22. How much would the client be charged for each of these services?
23. Which is the most expensive service that your salon offers and how much does it cost?
24. What should you do to the appointments book if a client cancels a booking?
25. How would you deal with a client that was kept waiting at the reception?
26. What do you say to clients when you greet them in your salon?
27. What information do you write on the client's appointment card in your salon?
28. How should you tell a stylist that their client has arrived?
29. What does it mean to say that reception skills are 'transferable'?

Gowning and protecting clients

A client's clothes must be adequately protected from hair clippings, hairdressing products and water. If clients' clothing is spoilt, they are within their rights to sue the salon for replacement if damaged irreparably, or at least to ask for them to be cleaned at the expense of the salon. Your boss will not be very pleased if this happens because it will cost money and could even cause the loss of a client.

With these facts in mind, you will need to know how to gown and protect every client who comes into your salon, depending on what sort of service they require. Simply putting a gown onto a client may not be enough to give sufficient protection so we will need to look at a range of services and their appropriate means of protection. Although this will vary from salon to salon, we will try to describe what is common practice in most salons, and give the reasons behind different gowning and protection methods.

Gowning

Every client should have a freshly laundered gown, but if this is not possible, the operator should ensure that no part of the gown comes into direct contact with the client's skin. This can be done by placing a disposable piece of tissue or crepe paper between the gown and the skin around the neck area – commonly called a neck strip. This ensures that if an unwashed gown was contaminated by micro-organisms it could not cause the client to get an infection. Gowns should be made of cotton or a mixture containing some cotton (polyester and cotton, etc.) as this will be more comfortable for the client in hot weather. Cotton allows the skin to 'breathe' and also absorbs sweat. Gowns made of nylon do not absorb sweat so may make the client feel uncomfortable if it is warm. Gowns are usually secured at the neck with ties or a velcro strip, or by a tie belt at the waist. Whichever type is used, gowns should be large enough to cover the client's clothing and should not be fastened too tightly at the neck!

A gown should be adequate protection for the client who is simply having a shampoo and blow-dry, or a set, although a disposable plastic cape can be used as additional protection with a towel tucked in around the neck during the shampoo. For cutting, many salons use 'cutting capes' which are draped around clients to protect them from the hair clippings. These capes are usually made of plastic, nylon or rubberised cotton and have the advantage of the clippings not sticking to them as they would to a towel. For chemical treatments such as perms and tints, your salon will probably use tinting capes which can be the same as cutting capes but are usually in dark colours to prevent stains from showing so easily as they would on lighter colours. Salons may use different coloured gowns and towels for particular services. Usually, dark gowns and towels are used when treatments involve the application of tints and other chemicals because of the risk of staining.

Protecting

Because many of the chemicals used in hairdressing are alkaline, they could either burn the skin or cause an allergic reaction. To protect clients' skin either cotton wool or barrier creams are used.

When perming cotton wool is applied in strips around the hairline to prevent drips of chemical running down from the scalp into the eyes or onto the skin (see Figure 1.3). It is applied moistened with water so that

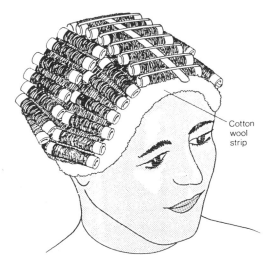

Cotton wool strip

Figure 1.3 Use of cotton wool strips to protect a client's skin during perming.

it is not too absorbent, but should still be replaced regularly as it will absorb some chemical during perming. If it were not replaced the chemical would become more and more concentrated and burn the skin around the hairline. Cotton wool is also used in strips by some hairdressers when drying the hair of a client who has had a semi-permanent applied, so that it does not run down into their eyes.

A barrier-forming product is applied to particular areas to prevent contact between a chemical and the client's skin. Whether the barrier product is in a cream or an oil form it should be carefully applied to avoid it forming an unwanted barrier, for example, by coating the hair that is to be chemically treated so that the chemical cannot penetrate properly. Barrier cream should be applied to the hairline and to the top of the ears before applying perm lotion to a client's hair. In case of accidental drips, the barrier cream will prevent the perm lotion from damaging the client's skin. For tinting and bleaching, barrier cream can also be applied in the same manner which will help stop staining from careless applications (see Figure 1.4).

Apply the barrier cream around the hairline and ears using your index finger or tint brush. Apply the cream by stroking it *away* from the hairline. This should prevent any accidental barrier from being applied to the hair. Use your free hand to hold the hair away from the hairline as you are working. Although barrier creams are produced by the various manufacturers, Vaseline will work as effectively. Remember that in warmer weather the cream will be more 'runny' (less viscous) and will be easier to apply with a tint brush.

Before carrying out some relaxers (chemical hair straighteners) the manufacturer of the product may recommend that the scalp is 'based'. This means carefully sectioning the hair and applying a barrier cream to the whole of the scalp. It is again important not to allow the cream onto the hair or an unwanted barrier will be formed on the hair shaft preventing the relaxer from working efficiently. Figure 1.5 shows how you should section the head of the client into four and then make small partings (0.5 cm) starting at the nape, working up towards the crown and front hairline. This helps you to cover and protect the entire scalp.

Always make sure that the jewellery and clothing worn by the client are not causing an obstruction to your work. High-necked sweaters and large pieces of jewellery that could get in your way should be removed. Politely ask your client to go to the toilet to take these off if necessary. Be careful not to get the gown caught on a necklace clasp — there are few sights or sounds as embarrassing as beads from a necklace falling onto a floor and shooting off in all directions!

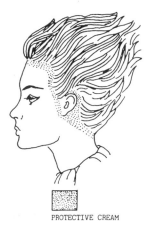

PROTECTIVE CREAM

Figure 1.4 Application of protective cream to the hairline.

Figure 1.5 Sections for applying protective cream to the scalp before a relaxer application.

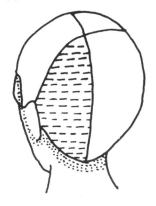

Questions

Rather than start you with a list of questions for this particular section we have suggested that you try completing the following exercises first:

1. Make a list (in the correct order) of how you would gown clients in your salon for these services: (a) perm; (b) tint; (c) shampoo and haircut; (d) shampoo and blow-dry.

2. Find out what happens in your salon if a client's clothing should become spoilt and a claim is made against the salon.
3. Compare the quality and costs of a range of gowns, capes, towels, etc. and divide your findings under the following headings:
   - cost;
   - availability (supplier and address);
   - advantages/disadvantages;
   - suitability and use.
4. Describe how you would deal with a client whose clothes are wet after their hair has been shampooed.
5. What would you do if you had run out of fresh gowns to protect the skin of a client?
6. How would you use cotton wool to protect the skin of a client?
7. Why is cotton wool moistened with water before being applied?
8. Why must it be replaced regularly?
9. List the reasons why you would apply barrier cream to the skin of a client.
10. Describe how you would apply the barrier cream.
11. What is 'basing'?
12. How and when should you base?
13. When should you ask a client to remove jewellery or clothing before a service?

Telephone technique

We probably all use the telephone in our personal lives for making and receiving calls to and from friends and family – after all, there are approximately 28½ million telephones in Britain today even though the population is only just over 50 million! People have telephones fitted into their cars and even carry portable ones around in their bags!

When you are using the telephone at work, it is for a different purpose than at home, and it is necessary that all employees use the telephone in the same way when answering, etc. When you speak on the telephone in the salon, you are representing the salon that employs you. The person on the other end of the line will judge the salon on the way that *you* speak and the way that *you* handle the conversation. If they have not used the salon before they have only this initial contact to judge it by.

In the salon, you will be using the telephone in a range of hairdressing situations. You will receive calls from clients wanting to make or cancel appointments, or making enquiries about the services offered in your salon and how much each costs. You may also deal with enquiries from people responding to special salon promotions or job advertisements that they may have seen in the press. Also, the representatives ('reps') from manufacturers and other businesses will probably be in contact with the salon by telephone to make appointments with the salon to sell products or to give information about orders.

If you are ever put in the position of not being able to offer the assistance or information the caller requires, always try to pass the caller onto somebody who can help. If this is not possible, take a detailed message and phone them back when you have found it out for yourself. Nothing is more irritating for a caller than feeling the person at the other end of the line is either not prepared to help or cannot put you into contact with someone who can. The caller will get frustrated and may never call your salon again.

You will usually find that salons have rules about staff accepting personal calls from friends while they are at work, especially if the caller wants to speak with a stylist who is attending a client. Find out the rules concerning this for your salon to save you making an embarrassing mistake. There may be a pay phone or card phone in your salon for use by clients and staff. This is a good idea because not only does it avoid the need to ask the person to pay for the call but also leaves the salon line open to accept incoming calls – something that the selfish hairdresser often forgets! If a potential client was phoning around different salons to get an urgent appointment this could lead to an unknown loss of business.

Telephone services

Emergency services

999 is probably the best known telephone number in the UK and has remained unchanged since its introduction in 1937. The 999 emergency service is available 24 hours a day from any telephone, including public call boxes, and is free (at home no charge is made while in a call box you do not have to use coins or a phonecard).

The role of the operator is to connect the 999 call to the appropriate emergency authority as quickly as possible. Currently, Fire, Police and Ambulance authorities are served by the UK emergency switchboards. Where other emergency services request it, exchanges serving appropriate areas connect calls for Lifeboat, Coastguard and (as ancillaries to the Police) Mountain Rescue and Cave Rescue.

The procedure for an operator answering an emergency call has remained unchanged since the introduction of the service. The answering of 999 calls is given top priority at any time of the day or night and the operator will ask which emergency service is required and the caller's number. The operator asks for the caller's number in case there should be a break in the line so that they can ring you back. If a caller collapses without giving a number the operator can find out where the call came from by the exchange staff tracing the call.

Once the operator knows which service is required, the call is connected to the control room of the appropriate emergency authority but the operator will monitor the call in case there is a break in the line. In a recent move to further improve the service, all emergency calls are now being recorded to help in sorting out any problems that may occur later. If an exchange is evacuated (due to fire, etc.) or if there is an exchange failure due to malfunction of machinery, 999 calls are immediately switched to be taken by a nearby exchange.

The UK emergency service is one of the best in the world and has progressed enormously from the days when you would have to summon help by sending someone in search of a policeman, doctor or street fire

Figure 1.6 Making a 999 call. (Courtesy British Telecom.)

- Lift the telephone handset and call the operator by dialling '999'.

- Tell the operator the emergency service you want and your telephone number.

- Wait until the Emergency authority answers.

- Then give them the full address where help is needed and any other important information.

REMEMBER

All emergency calls are free.

You can make a call from:—

- Your own home telephone.
- A public telephone kiosk.

Remember to rotate the 9 to the finger stop and remove your finger to allow the dial to return freely. With push button phones push the 9 button firmly. Do this three times.

Remember to **keep calm** and **speak clearly** when making an emergency call. **Listen carefully** to what the operator asks.

Never make a false call. This could risk the lives of others who really need the help of an emergency service, it is also breaking the law.

When you have finished the call, remember to replace the handset on the telephone rest.

alarm. (A street fire alarm would be found on the corner of a street and was a glass fronted box with a lever inside. When the lever was pulled an alarm sounded in the local fire station.) It was the Belgrave Committee that was set up by Parliament which designed the 999 emergency service. The 999 number was chosen because it is an easy number to remember and is simple to dial in the dark or a smoke-filled room. Although 111 may be the obvious number that many would choose because it would be easy to find and quick to dial, this was not used because there was a danger of false calls being made due to the wind or trees causing the overhead wires to touch and give three false single pulses! Most places were served by overhead cables at the time of making this decision, whereas today most cables are underground.

Operator services

There are other important telephone numbers that you may need to use. These are set out below for your information and convenience:

Number	Contact	Service
100	Operator	The operator is there to help you if you have difficulty making a call or if you wish to use the special call services. These include: alarm calls, advice of duration and charge, credit card calls, freephone calls, personal calls, transferred charge calls, subcriber-controlled transfer.
142	Operator	Directory enquiries for callers in London for central London numbers.
192	Operator	UK and Irish Republic directory enquiries outside the London postal area.

Charges

Telephone charge rates will vary according to four conditions: (a) the time of day you are calling, (b) the day of the week or if it is a Public or Bank Holiday, (c) the distance of the call, and (d) the destination of the call.

If you want to make a call when everybody else does, that is between 09.00 and 13.00, then this is the most expensive time. Calls can be made more cheaply by calling at other times. The charge rate is made up of units and it is the unit charge that you will see on your telephone bill. The more time you get for each unit, the cheaper the cost of your call. There are three local call rates which relate to different times of the day and week. These are shown in Figure 1.7.

Figure 1.7 Local telephone call rates.

Peak rate	9 AM — 1 PM Monday to Friday
Standard rate	8 AM — 9 AM and 1 PM — 6 PM Monday to Friday
Cheap rate	6 PM — 8 AM Monday to Friday and all day and all night at weekends and Public Holidays

In Figure 1.8 the cost of calls is shown in diagrammatic form.

There are two types of call for which no charge is made. These are any number beginning with 0800 and Freephone numbers which are connected by telephoning the operator. When dialling an 0800 number, always dial the full number — 0800 followed by six digits.

Beware of making calls where you can listen to a recorded message

Figure 1.8 Cost of telephone calls. (Courtesy British Telecom.)

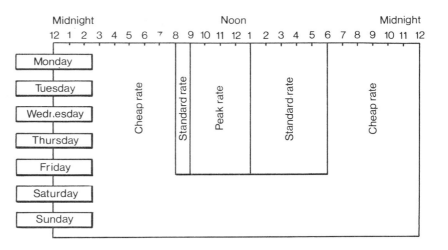

from a pop star or favourite record, as these often have very high charge rates. Often a call to listen to a number one record will cost as much as buying it! So next time you see one of those advertisements for such a service, have a look at the charge rates per minute!

Dialling codes

Telephone calls are also categorised according to the distance of the call and if the call is made on a heavily used route. These call rates are classified as follows:

'l' rate – Local area rate
'a' rate – Up to 56 km (35 miles)
'b' rate – Over 56 km
'bl' rate – Some of the frequently used routes over 56 km
'm' rate – Dialled calls to mobile telephones

There are three different types of dialling code:

- Local codes
- National codes
- International codes

Local calls are those made in your area and a map showing this area will be in the front of your British Telecom code book. You will not need to dial the local code if you are making the call from within your local area.

National codes are fixed and apply from almost anywhere in the UK. Here are some examples of national codes:

071 – Inner London } (Previously 01–)
081 – Outer London
021 – Birmingham
031 – Edinburgh

041 – Glasgow
051 – Liverpool
061 – Manchester

In May 1990 the traditional 01 for London numbers was changed to 071 for Central London and 081 for outer London. This decision was made because of the ever increasing number of telephones in use in London.

If you are making a call from Manchester to Liverpool you would need to dial 051 and then the number after the hyphen. However, not all numbers are in all-figure form which means some may have exchange names associated with the number. For numbers which are not in all-figure form, you will need to dial a code to reach the exchange and this code can be found in your dialling code booklet. For example, the telephone number found on a letterhead could be Aberdeen (0224) 34344. This gives you the area code in brackets. Some people do not bother to do this so it would be necessary to look up Aberdeen in your dialling code book. When you record the telephone number of a client, always try and record the dialling code at the same time.

International codes apply to countries outside the British Isles. Currently, over 98 per cent of international calls made from the UK are dialled direct, which means you do not need to make the call through the operator. When using International Direct Dialling (IDD) there are four steps to follow when dialling:

- Step one – dial the international code
- Step two – dial the country code
- Step three – dial the area code
- Step four – dial the number you want

As an example, imagine that you need to make a call to Brussels in Belgium from the UK. You would need to dial the following figures:

010 – the international dialling code (this is always 010 when phoning from the UK)
 32 – the country code
  2 – the area code
1234 – the customer's number

Therefore the number you would dial would be this: 010 32 2 1234. On International Direct Dialling (IDD) calls you pay only for the length of time you are connected and the cost will vary according to the 'charge band' the country is in and the time of day you make your call. To find out which countries fall into the various charge bands and their relative costs, telephone the international operator on 155 or check in a recent telephone charges guide.

Tones

There are a number of standard phone tones which are provided to tell you that the line you have called is busy, that you have a line to make your call, that the number you have dialled is ringing or that it is unobtainable. New phone systems are becoming sophisticated and you will hear voices telling you that you have dialled incorrectly or that lines are busy! In Figure 1.9 the different tones are set out to tell you how each tone sounds and their meanings.

Figure 1.9 What the different telephone tones tell you. (Courtesy British Telecom.)

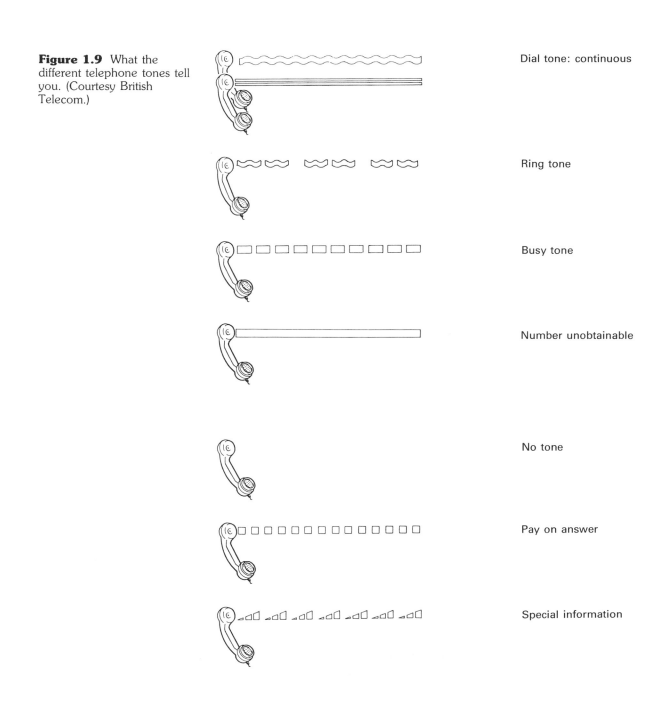

Dial tone: continuous

Ring tone

Busy tone

Number unobtainable

No tone

Pay on answer

Special information

Directories

Telephone directories are issued free for a customer's own area. They contain other people's telephone numbers so are used to find numbers when you do not know them.

All entries in telephone books are listed in strict alphabetical order from A–Z. You will find that all entries are set out in this order: surname or business name, the initial letter of the first name, the address.
For example:

Brown A. 128 Morland Road
Brown B. 1a Fitz Square
Brown D. 17 Langdon Street
Brown D. 123 The Parade

As you can see from the example there could be a large number of people who share the same surname, but they may be identified by having different initials for their first names. Where both surname and first name are the same you may be able to identify the required number by the different addresses listed.

When double-barrelled names are entered they are alphabetically listed according to the initial letter of the first word. For example, Smith-Jones would be listed under 'S' in the directory and not 'J'. This also applies to business names such as Trevor Sorbie, Joshua Galvin and John Freida. For example:

John Freida
John-Freidman

If you are not sure of the spelling of the name you are looking for in the directory, try to look for alternative spellings for similar sounding names, e.g. Hatton, Hatten. However, if you cannot find someone's number, it doesn't necessarily mean that they don't have a telephone. They could be ex-directory which means they prefer not to be listed in the telephone book. If you do not specify that you wish to be ex-directory, your number will be automatically listed.

The Yellow Pages directory lists all business subscribers under their respective trade, profession or services that they offer in the area covered by your copy of the directory. The exact boundaries of your area will be shown on a map in the front of the book. If you should require Yellow Pages for different areas outside your own, they can be ordered by completing the form at the back of the book. The cost of any ordered Yellow Pages will be added to your telephone bill. If you have a telephone line or group of lines rented at the business rate, British Telecom will give you a free entry in Yellow Pages which will comprise your business name, address and telephone number in light print. Larger and bolder entries with local or national coverage are made through the Yellow Pages Sales Ltd department for which there is a charge.

Entries in Yellow Pages are classified under headings which describe either the goods supplied by a company or a statement which tells you the type of service they offer. At the front of the book there is an index which lists all these headings. For example, in the H section, you will find a number of headings relating to hairdressing, classified according to whether they are ladies' salons, men's salons, hairdressing schools, hairdressing suppliers, etc.

Telephone techniques

When you need to show your telephone number, like on a letterhead or appointment card for the salon, always write your number in full to help callers who may contact you from outside your area by including the national code (the number before the hyphen or the exchange name), e.g. 051-246807.

If you deal with correspondents abroad, you should also include the international code, e.g. +44 51 246807. The + symbol tells callers to dial their own international prefix, which will vary from country to country. 44 is the 'country code' to reach the UK. You will notice that the '0' at the beginning of the national code is not dialled by those calling from abroad.

When making a telephone call, make sure you know the number you want and, when necessary, the dialling code. If you are in doubt, check them in the telephone directory and dialling code booklet. If you have to call Directory Enquiries, have a pen and paper ready to make a note of the number. Figure 1.10 shows the correct procedure for making a call.

When answering the telephone, always answer it promptly and announce the name of the salon (obviously, at home you would give your

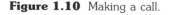

Figure 1.10 Making a call.

- To dial a call, first lift the receiver and listen for dial tone – continuous purring or high pitched hum.

- Dial the code, if required, followed by the number. Dial carefully taking the dial right round to the finger stop and letting it return freely. If you have a press-button telephone, press each button carefully to its full extent making sure that you do not let your finger slip nor press two buttons at the same time.

- If you make a mistake while dialling replace the receiver for a moment or two, and then start again. After you have dialled there may be a pause before you hear a tone: hold on for up to 15 seconds (up to 60 seconds on international calls) to allow the equipment time to connect your call.

- When your call is answered say to whom you want to talk and then say who you are. If you know the number you are calling has a switchboard, give the extension number you require. If you do not know it, enquire and make a note of it for future use.

number). If you are answering an extension telephone (as might be the case for a salon within a department store) announce the name of your department or your name, whichever would be most helpful. Have a pencil and paper at hand so you can write down any messages and if you take a message, repeat it back to the caller to make sure you have taken it down correctly. Make sure you have all the necessary details like the caller's name and telephone number. Try to pass the message to the intended person as soon as possible. You may need to leave the telephone to make an enquiry or to collect information. If so, tell the caller how long you expect to be and tell them that you will call them back.

Here are a few tips on telephone technique:

- It is better not to shout on the telephone; talk quietly but distinctly into the mouthpiece.
- If you can't be heard by the other person, try changing the pitch of your voice and speak more slowly.
- Replace the receiver carefully but firmly after each call. If you fail to do this you will be unable to receive calls and your line may be temporarily disconnected. If you made the call, and the receiver were not replaced properly, the charge for the call would continue until the receiver is replaced. This could be an expensive error if a line were open all night!
- If you are cut off on an incoming call, replace your handset and wait for the other person to call you again. If you made the call, replace your handset for a few moments and dial again.

Figure 1.11 Tips for talking on the telephone. (Courtesy British Telecom.)

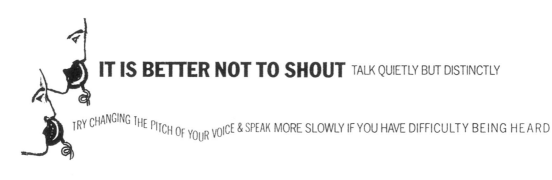

IT IS BETTER NOT TO SHOUT TALK QUIETLY BUT DISTINCTLY

TRY CHANGING THE PITCH OF YOUR VOICE & SPEAK MORE SLOWLY IF YOU HAVE DIFFICULTY BEING HEARD

When speaking on the telephone, clear and careful pronunciation prevents errors and helps you work more quickly and efficiently. When spelling out words, using a 'telephone alphabet' like the one shown in Fig. 1.12, can be of help.

Apart from words being misunderstood over the telephone, numbers can also be confused. Figure 1.13 is a guide on how to pronounce them over the telephone.

When giving telephone numbers over the phone, group the numbers together in whatever way seems natural to you. Usually, groups of two

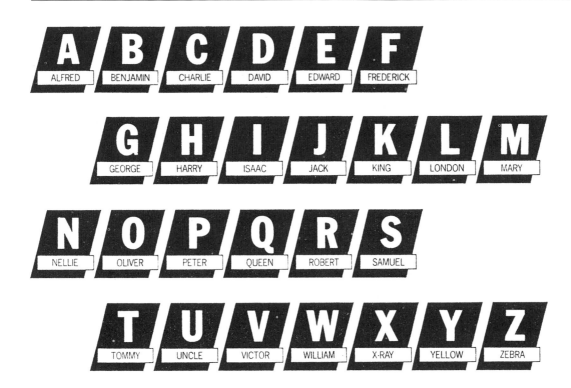

Figure 1.12 Telephone alphabet. (Courtesy British Telecom.)

Figure 1.13 Number pronunciation. (Courtesy British Telecom.)

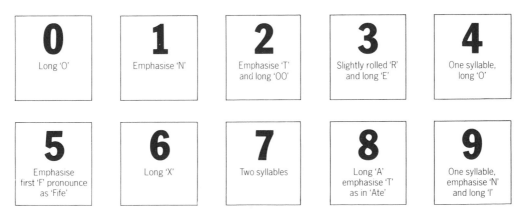

or three numbers come most naturally. Try never to exceed four numbers at a time as this can be confusing for the person listening.

If you cannot understand someone on the other end of the line, possibly because of a strong accent, do not tell them that you cannot understand them! Use tactics such as 'This is a very bad line on my end, could you repeat that slowly'.

Unfortunately, there are a few people around that make 'nuisance calls'. It is a criminal offence to use the telephone service to make menacing, offensive or indecent phone calls. Offenders may be prosecuted and denied the use of the telephone service. If you should receive a nuisance call *hang up immediately*. *Never* give your name or address and if the calls continue, contact the police.

Questions

You could either write down the answers to these questions or ask a friend or tutor to question you orally.

1. How many telephones are there in the UK?
2. Why is it important that all salon staff answer the telephone in the same way?
3. Who might you deal with on the telephone and for what reasons?
4. What should you do if you cannot answer a question from a telephone caller?
5. What happens in your salon if someone wants to speak to a stylist about a personal matter?
6. How do you go about making a personal call in your salon?
7. How could the salon lose out if the business line is used by salon staff for making personal calls?
8. What is the best known telephone number in the UK?
9. How much does it cost to use this number?
10. What are the three main services that most people would ask for?
11. What other services could be asked for?
12. Why should you give your number to the operator?
13. Why was '111' not chosen as the emergency number?
14. Make a list of numbers that you would use to find out different information.
15. What time would be the cheapest to make a local telephone call on a Monday? When would be the most expensive time?
16. What are the three call charge rates called which refer to different times of the day and week?
17. What is the *full* telephone number for your salon?
18. What numbers would you dial to reach the following? (a) Operator. (b) Directory Enquiries for a number outside the London postal area. (c) The emergency services.
19. What does the 'number unobtainable' tone sound like?
20. How does the 'busy tone' sound?
21. If you make a call and you are cut off, who should redial, you or the person you were connected to?

22. How are entries classified in the Yellow Pages?
23. How are entries listed in telephone directories?
24. If a person is having difficulty hearing you, what can you do to your voice and the way you speak to improve this?
25. Why is it important to replace the receiver properly after a call?
26. What should you have near at hand when you are answering the phone or calling Directory Enquiries?
27. What do the initials IDD stand for?
28. What is the International code for calls made from the UK?
29. What should you do if you receive a nuisance call?
30. What does ex-directory mean?
31. What are the four things which determine the charge of a telephone call?
32. Describe what a 'telephone alphabet' is and how its use can avoid misunderstandings over the phone.
33. If you cannot understand someone what would you say to get them to repeat what they had just said?

Cash transactions in the salon

In this section of the Reception unit, we will be looking at the method of handling cash in the salon, as opposed to dealing with cheques, credit cards and other forms of monetary transactions. These other methods of payment will be dealt with in the following section.

What is currency?

We all handle money every day of our lives and have learnt through this use to recognise the various coins and notes that make up our currency. The currency of the UK is called *sterling* and if you look in any bank, travel agency or Bureau de Change you will see how much of any foreign currency would be exchanged for £1 sterling. This rate is not fixed as it is dependent on exchange rates that can alter from day-to-day as they are set according to the economy of individual countries.

The currency of any country is made up of coins or notes that have different denominations or values. Sterling bank notes are of different colours and the higher their value, the larger their size. Bank notes are issued in the following denominations: £50 (the largest of the notes), £20, £10 and £5. All sterling bank notes have a water mark and silver thread passing through it to prove that it is genuine tender. You may have seen cashiers in shops or supermarkets holding notes up to the light to check the note has the water mark and silver thread. When forged money is in circulation, local businesses are usually informed by the police and rewards are given to alert cashiers who recognise a forgery which can lead to a conviction. Incidentally, if you are unlucky and are unknowingly passed a forged note, it is totally worthless.

Coins are available in different sizes, colours and thicknesses:

- The one pound coin − this coin is the thickest of all the coins and has a serrated edge. It is very similar in size to the five pence coin which also has a serrated edge. Blind people have had to learn to distinguish between these two coins by the thickness. Sighted people can distinguish between these coins more easily because the pound coin is a bronze colour and the five pence is silver in colour.
- The fifty pence coin is the largest and has seven sides which are not serrated; it is silver in colour.
- The twenty pence coin is smaller than the five pence coin but slightly larger than the penny. It has seven sides which are not serrated, and is also silver in colour like the fifty pence.
- The ten pence coin is similar in size to the fifty pence coin but is round and not as heavy. The edge is serrated and it is silver in colour. It is about to be replaced by a new smaller version.
- The five pence coin is silver in colour and round with a serrated edge which is also about to be replaced by a new version.
- The two pence coin is round and does not have a serrated edge. It is larger than the five pence but smaller than the ten pence coin. This coin is copper in colour.
- The one penny coin is the smallest of the coins and is round with a non-serrated edge. It is the only other copper-coloured coin.

Note: There is a two pound coin in existence which is rarely seen in the normal money circulation because it was minted to mark the Commonwealth Games. A new two pound coin has also just been minted. There are 'crowns' minted for special occasions which are worth twenty-five pence (see below).

The only consistent marks on each coin in sterling currency are that of the Queen's head facing to the right, the date the coin was issued and the value of the coin. There are many coins that are issued to commemorate famous people, special occasions and events such as royal weddings, Winston Churchill's death and anniversaries of a monarch's reign. On the side of the coin which does not show the monarch's head in profile view, you will see a variety of designs ranging from a portcullis to a lion. As these will vary according to the time the coins are minted (made at the Royal Mint) we have avoided describing them in detail. You may be wondering however why the term 'new pence' is embossed on the coins. This is because the UK's monetary system became decimalised in 1971 and all coins minted from that time bear these words to show they were the new pence coins. New coins introduced since that year do not bear these words, e.g. the pound coin and twenty pence coin.

Coins that are still in circulation and were minted before decimalisation include the five pence. You may have noticed that such coins have 'one shilling' on them which was their value before decimalisation. Many of the old coins are now collectors' items and certain years and commemorative coins are particularly valuable. It is not strange that our vocabulary has changed because of the decimalisation. Gone are the expressions like 'a bob' and 'half a crown' which were terms used to describe a shilling and a coin worth two shillings and six pence.

'Legal tender' is the term used to describe the notes and coins that will be accepted in any given country. If a particular coin or bank note is withdrawn from circulation by the Bank of England, sufficient notice is given to the public. However, there are certain coins or notes that are accepted by the Bank of England although they originate from other countries. An example of such are the coins and notes of Jersey (an island belonging to the UK which is close to France). Jersey money holds the same value as other UK currency so is deemed as legal tender. Depending on what part of the country you are in you may find Scottish money which is exactly the same value and is treated as legal tender. Beware of money from the Irish Republic as much of the coinage is the same size and colour, but not the same value! Coins or notes from countries outside the UK are usually not accepted as legal tender because of the fluctuating exchange rates between countries. Banks will often not exchange foreign coins although you should have no problems with notes. As transaction charges are made for this service you could find it costing you money to accept foreign currency in small amounts. Because of this an extra charge should be made.

When handling cash in the salon, it is obviously important to check that the coins and notes that you receive and give as change are legal tender. Even when you instantly recognise a bank note as sterling, remember to check for the water mark and silver thread if it has a high value and you have received warning of forgeries in your area. If you do accept an Irish coin by mistake, don't try to pass it to the next customer in change to get rid of it, they may notice and think that you were doing it on purpose!

Taking cash in the salon

Most salons will have either an electronic cash register (a till) or a facility on the reception computer to register sales, etc. At the minimum level there will be some sort of drawer or box which will serve as the place where cash will be placed. The advantages of using an electronic cash register or computer with a cash till facility are that all the cash transactions are recorded in varying detail, it can usually supply a receipt and can calculate the amount of change that is given to the client. If your salon has neither of these, you will probably be required to record the sales and services for which payment is given by writing this information on some sort of daily takings sheet. Most of these sheets will require you to display this information in a particular format which will show at a glance which stylist has performed the most services and what these services included. If using either of the more sophisticated methods, there is the normal facility of being able to allocate particular codes to individual employees that will classify sales and takings accordingly, dispensing with the need to record this laboriously by hand. Electronic cash registers save time when taking cash and also at the end of the day when the total sales and takings are calculated.

Whichever system your salon uses, there are four steps to any cash transaction in the salon. These are:

- Step one − Calculate the bill for the client and inform them of the final amount. Whenever possible this bill should be presented in writing or rung up, item by item, on a cash till. Also, try to approximate bills as a double check to prevent overcharging. If there were four items that the client was to be charged for, you could approximate by rounding each up or down to the nearest pound, then add these together to get an approximation of the final bill.

Amount to be charged	Rounded up or down to nearest pound
£6.49	£6
£10.95	£11
£1.99	£2
£1.25	£1
Totals £20.68	£20

Thus the approximated bill is fairly close to the real bill. If you had made a mistake with the real bill your approximation would have made you suspect something was wrong!
- Step two − Check that the cash offered to you by the client in payment is legal tender. Count out the money the client has given to you if it involves a number of notes or coins so that you are aware of any shortfall before placing it in the till or cash box. If you had counted it straight into the till the client cannot be sure you did not make a mistake in doing so once it is mixed with other coins. If the client has paid with a large note, keep it on top of the till in sight of both yourself and the customer.
- Step three − Take out the change you or the cash register has calculated and count it into the hand of the client. Give the client a receipt and thank him/her.
- Step four − Once this is over place the money into either the till or cash box and close it.

If anyone has ever tried to shortchange you in a shop or a bar, you will know how indignant you will have felt, whether it was an accident or done on purpose. If carried out correctly, the four steps should prevent this from happening. There are always mistakes made in any organisation, but if a client thinks you have done it on purpose they may not come back. As you cannot always bank on the honesty of a client, this should also rule out any cheating on their behalf. It is important to concentrate when taking cash in the salon. If a mistake does occur and a dispute arises, a great deal of time can be taken up with completely checking the entire contents of the till to resolve the situation. Concentrate on the matter in hand and don't try to do two things at once.

When working with cash, your employer will be entrusting you with a responsibility which should not be spoilt by the stupid idea that he or she will not notice the odd pound or two missing from the till. We are by no means insinuating that anybody reading this would be foolish enough to steal in this way, but it has been known. The usual action of the employer in such circumstances is to dismiss the thief instantly. We know of cases where a client has been asked to pay with marked money which eventually was found in a hairdresser's handbag. The person in question not only lost her job but practised hairdressing behind bars!

The float

Because the salon will be accepting cash and giving change, it is necessary to have a float in the till. A float is an amount of money which is made up from various denominations and is necessary to be able to give change to clients. The float is usually a small amount when compared to the average salon's takings and is often left in the till overnight. Depending on the size of the salon and the amount of takings generated in a single day the float will vary. However, whatever its size it is important that it is made up of different value notes and coins. It would be of no use, for example, if you opened the till in the morning to give a client change from a twenty pound note to find nothing but twenty pence pieces! Many salons with expensive cash tills leave them unlocked overnight because it would be far more inconvenient to have the till damaged in a burglary than to lose a few pounds.

Cashing up

At the end of the day the total takings for that day will be calculated and checked against the takings in the till. Remember that the float is not part of the takings and should be separated out for the next day. On most cash registers the 'cashing up' (calculating the day's takings and organising the float) is made easier by the sophisticated machines. As was previously mentioned, cash registers are available which will classify takings according to each operator or service, identify retail sales and even tell you if a client failed to pay! All this is done for you by the simple action of pressing a few keys for each command. If you are not working with such equipment the cashing up is going to take considerably longer as you will have to check that the amount in the till (less the float) corresponds to the amount of money on the till roll. If the takings are over (too much money for the number of recorded sales) or under (not enough money for the recorded number of sales) it can take a very long time crosschecking each transaction against the appointments register and record of sales. If it is *approved* practice for staff to be allowed to take a 'loan' from the till, an IOU should be placed in the till for the amount and only tear it up once it has been honoured. When the daily takings are balanced at the end of the day, the type of sheet that could be used is set out in Figure 1.14. Ask someone in your salon to go through the system used with you.

Some salons make regular or unscheduled till checks throughout the day to deter theft and assess when it is necessary to clear large amounts of money for security reasons. If the salon is having a particularly busy day, the security-conscious employer may remove some of the cash and

DAY	Anne	Jo	Wilson	Sarah	Jean				Sales
MON									
TUE	96.65	40.60	108.40	134.70					18.30
WED	100.20			140.20					20.00
THUR	90.80	46.20	100.20						22.30
FRI	120.30	60.80	150.00	170.20	125.00				28.90
SAT	135.00	65.80	168.00	161.30	108.60				34.40
SUN			206.60	180.40					28.00
TOTALS	542.95	213.40	733.20	786.80	233.60				151.90
WEEK ENDING Sun 16th June					WEEKLY TOTAL £ 2661—85				

Figure 1.14 Weekly record of takings.

either put it into a safe or have it banked. Alternatively, regular till checks also help prevent the awful situation of running out of change after the banks have closed. In such a case the responsible person will need to estimate the amount of change that will be required based upon an approximation of the number of clients that could require change. This estimation would be done by checking the appointments register for the number of clients booked.

Questions

1. What is the currency of the UK called?
2. What notes of currency are used in the UK?
3. What does the term 'legal tender' mean?
4. How would you know that a bank note was legal tender?
5. Describe the different coins available as legal tender in the UK?
6. What do all of these coins have on them?
7. Why do some coins have 'new pence' inscribed on them?
8. When did decimalisation occur?
9. Why would most salons charge more to accept foreign currency?
10. Why would you never accept foreign coins although you might accept notes?
11. What do you do with money accepted as payment in your salon?
12. How are financial transactions recorded in your salon?
13. What advantage do electronic tills give a salon?
14. What are the four steps to a cash transaction?
15. Why should large notes be kept out in sight of both yourself and the customer until a cash transaction is completed?

16. What is a 'float' and how should it be made up?
17. Is the float included as part of the daily takings?
18. If someone has a small 'loan' from the till how should this be recorded to avoid mistakes in the daily takings?
19. Why do some salons make till checks during the day?

Verifying and receipting non-cash payments

Not all clients will pay for their service or other purchases with cash. In the United States there are places such as car hire offices that will actually refuse to take cash because of the risk of robbery. The use of cheques, credit cards, charge cards and the newest method of directly debiting a person's bank account, by an electronic funds transfer card, are becoming increasingly popular in this country as well. As salons will receive payment by some or all of these methods, you need to have an understanding of the basic principles of how each method works and what you will need to do to ensure each transaction is properly verified and receipted.

Cheques

Quite simply, a cheque is a written instruction to a bank, telling them to pay money either to the account holder (in cash) or to someone else that has been named on the cheque. There are a number of details to be written on the cheque by the account holder and it is important that these are verified by the person accepting the payment. The details to be entered are the date, the name of the person (or company, etc.) to be paid, the amount that is to be paid (in figures and words) and the signature of the account holder. Below is an example of a cheque which shows how these details are entered.

If the person writing the cheque should make a minor error, in the date for example, it is still valid as long as the correction made is initialled by the account holder as in example Figure 1.16.

A cheque guarantee card is a card issued by a bank or building society which tells the person being paid by cheque that the bank guarantees the payment up to a certain amount. Most of these cards will guarantee payment up to fifty pounds while some may go up to one hundred pounds. It is unwise for any business to accept payment by cheques which are not supported by such cards because there is no guarantee from the bank that they will honour the payment. You cannot be certain that the person paying for the service is the person named on the cheque, so be careful to check that the signatures on the cheque and cheque guarantee card match (see Figure 1.17). If you are unsure ask them to sign again on the back of the cheque. Never accept a cheque if it is not signed in front of you. When verifying payment by cheque, you

Figure 1.15 Example of a cheque.

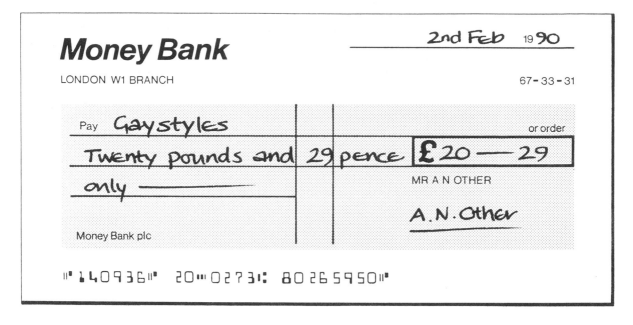

Figure 1.16 Initialing of a correction on a cheque so it remains valid.

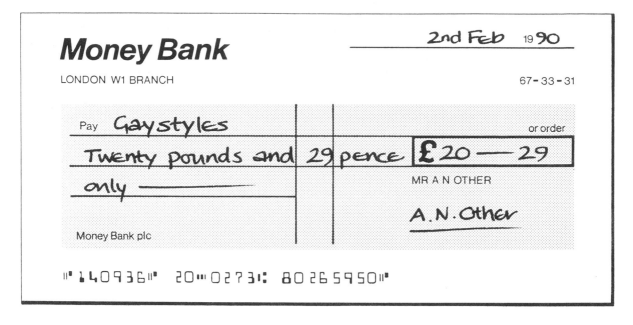

will need to ensure that you carry out the following simple rules:

- Check all the details are entered correctly in words or figures as appropriate.
- Check that the account number on the guarantee card and cheque correspond – this is the last group of numbers on the bottom right hand side of the cheque.
- Check the expiry date of the guarantee card and only accept it if it is still in date.
- Check for the similarity between the signatures on the guarantee card and cheque.
- Write the number of the guarantee card on the reverse of the cheque – this guarantees that payment will be made by the bank.

Figure 1.17 The NatWest Servicecard which can act as a cheque guarantee card and an electronic funds transfer card. (Courtesy National Westminster Bank PLC.)

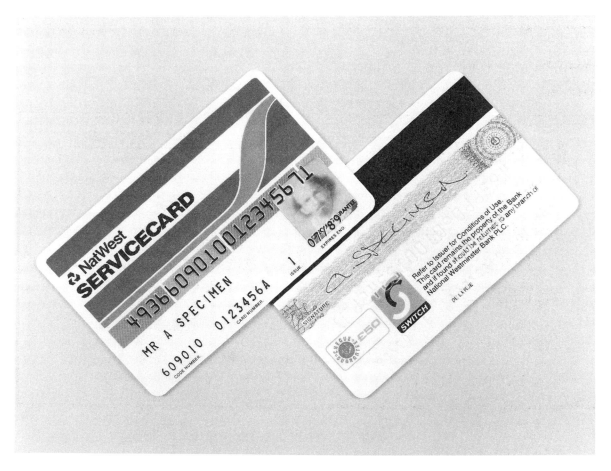

Credit cards

Credit cards are an easy way of making payment and do not restrict the holder to the limitations of the amounts guaranteed by cheque cards. Each individual who applies for a credit card will have the credit limit set at different amounts depending on the individual's income. The largest credit card companies in this country are Access and Visa. Many stores also operate their own credit cards. Credit cards can be used to provide free credit if they are paid up as required by the conditions of use of a particular card. This can give several weeks of free credit for the card-holder. However, if the account is not settled within the specified time limit the amount of money that is still outstanding attracts a comparatively high rate of monthly interest. This is usually around 2 per cent per month, which means a payment of £2 interest on every £100 borrowed. As an annual percentage rate this is commonly near 30 per cent.

Your salon can only accept payment by credit card if your management has an agreement to do so. Not all salons will want to accept payment by credit card as part of the agreement with the credit company will be to pay around five per cent of each credit card transaction to the company. It needs to be determined if credit cards will bring in extra business to pay for this transaction charge. If your salon does accept payment in this form, there will no doubt be a sticker on the window or reception desk advertising this fact. There may be more than one credit card accepted by your salon in which case several stickers will advertise this point.

When accepting payment by credit card, it is the person receiving payment that does most of the writing – all the card holder has to do is write his or her signature. Usually what happens is the card is placed in a special device which presses the numbers of the card and the name and address of the business onto a receipt which has three carbon copies – one to be given to the customer as a receipt, one is retained by the salon and the other is used to inform the credit company of the transaction. The person accepting the payment will need to enter the following information onto the carboned receipt booklet using a ball point pen:

- the date;
- brief details of purchase (hairdressing service);
- the amount that is to be charged.

You must check the expiry date on the credit card has not been reached otherwise the card is not valid and any payment taken is not supported by the card so is lost. The customer will then be asked to sign the receipt as agreement to the transaction. The top copy is given to the customer as their receipt, and the carbon paper is discarded before placing the bottom two carboned copies into the cash till or drawer. It is important that the salon checks that any writing has gone through to the bottom copy of the receipt as without a signature the transaction will be void and the salon will be unable to prove that the customer has agreed to the payment. The signature should be closely checked to make sure of similarity to that on the credit card, in case the card was stolen. If the signature was very different the credit card company would be justified in not paying because of your negligence. Lists of stolen credit cards are issued regularly so that you should be aware of names on stolen cards. As a general rule, check the cards of clients who are unknown to you.

Some modern systems do not require this to be done as credit notes are electronically printed, although the customer must still sign as proof of agreement to the transaction. Often a telephone call is made to check that the client has enough credit to pay for a service; the credit card company then issues an authorisation code which is noted down in much the same way as a cheque card number is to guarantee the payment.

Charge cards

Charge cards work in exactly the same way as credit cards in the way sales transactions are undertaken between salon and client. They are different because the client is expected to pay the full sum that is 'spent' back to the charge card company at the end of each charge period, rather than have the facility to pay interest for the credit obtained. Some stores have charge cards that can only be used in their particular stores, but there are also cards such as American Express which can be used in a vast number of outlets.

Electronic funds transfer cards

These are the most recent innovation on the money scene. They are now offered by the major banks to operate with current bank accounts and often work as a cheque guarantee card and service card at the same time. An example of such a card is shown in Figure 1.17. The 'switch' symbol refers to the electronic funds transfer operated by the National Westminster Bank. The card can be used by the client to obtain cash from service tills and to guarantee cheques up to £50.

These cards are simply a way of debiting a current account electronically, without having to write a cheque. The card is 'swiped' through a special terminal which stores the details of the transaction. A voucher is provided which is signed by the client to confirm the transaction. It has two parts, one retained by the client as a record of the debit, while the other part is placed in the till as a paper record of the electronic transfer of funds. It is important that you check the signature of the client carefully against the signature on the back of the card. The information is passed to the bank the salon banks with either on tape or via telecommunication links so that the appropriate credits can be made, while the client's account will be debited. Just like normal cheques, three working days should be allowed for bank clearance. The advantage of such cards, which banks refer to as EFT cards (see heading above), is that the usual £50 limit placed on cheques can be exceeded because the amount of money in the client's account can be checked at the time of use.

Questions

1. Why do you think some establishments prefer payment to be made without cash changing hands?
2. What does a cheque tell the bank it is drawn on to do?
3. What should you ask clients to do to a cheque if they make an error, so that the cheque still remains valid?
4. How should you check that a cheque is written out correctly?
5. How do you guarantee that a bank will honour the cheque?
6. What is a credit card?
7. What credit cards, if any, does your salon accept?
8. How do you validate a credit card transaction in your salon?
9. Is there a limit that your salon will accept on a credit card without having to obtain an authorisation from the credit company? You may need to ask the salon manager/owner about this.
10. Why do you need to pay particular attention to matching signatures on the credit card and sales voucher?
11. What would you do if you were unsure of signatures matching on the credit card and sales voucher?
12. How do you check for the possibility of a credit card being stolen in your salon?
13. What is the difference between credit and charge cards?
14. What is an electronic funds transfer card?
15. What is the main advantage of such cards over cheques?

Paying in and withdrawing money from bank accounts

Many of you using this book will already have your own current bank account so will be familiar with what you need to know about banking procedure. Most banks are keen to get you as a customer, while many jobs that you have will pay you by cheque or by direct credit transfer into your account. This eliminates the risks of collecting large amounts of cash to pay employees at the end of each week or month. When you pay money into an account the bank refers to this as a *credit*, while when you withdraw money from an account this is referred to as a *debit*.

Paying money into an account

Money to be paid into an account can be in the form of cash or cheques. To pay money into a particular account you will need to know a number of things about that account:

- the bank name and branch;
- the six figure sorting code number for the bank and branch;
- the account number (usually an eight figure number);
- the name(s) that the account is in.

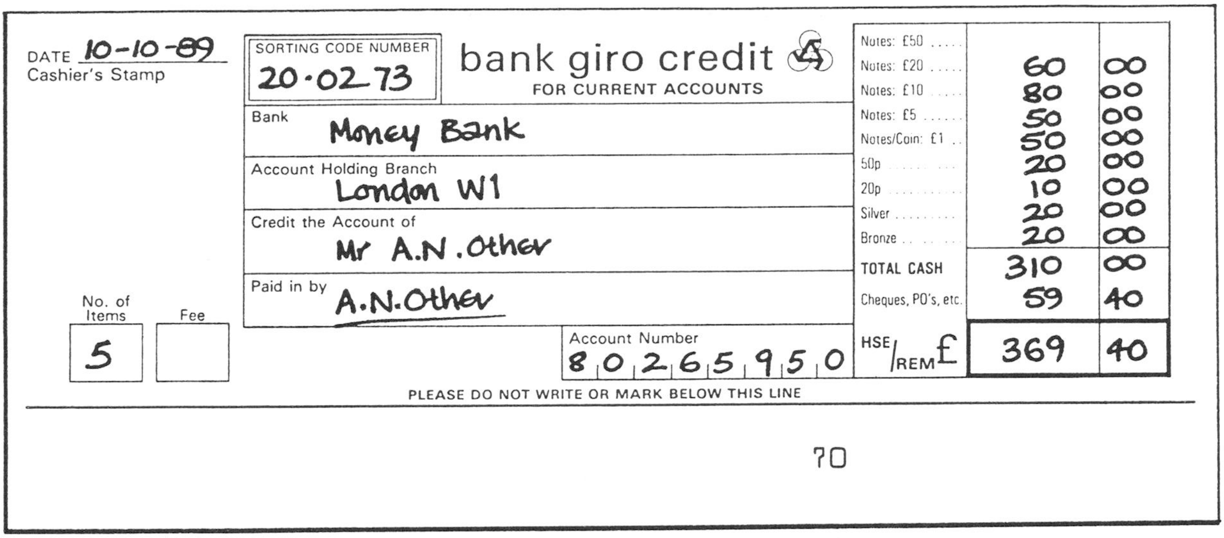
DATE 10-10-89
Cashier's Stamp

SORTING CODE NUMBER 20·02·73

bank giro credit
FOR CURRENT ACCOUNTS

Bank Money Bank

Account Holding Branch London W1

Credit the Account of Mr A.N.Other

Paid in by A.N.Other

No. of Items 5

Fee

Account Number 8 0 2 6 5 9 5 0

	£	p
Notes: £50		
Notes: £20	60	00
Notes: £10	80	00
Notes: £5	50	00
Notes/Coin: £1	50	00
50p	20	00
20p	10	00
Silver	20	00
Bronze	20	00
TOTAL CASH	310	00
Cheques, PO's, etc.	59	40
HSE/REM £	369	40

PLEASE DO NOT WRITE OR MARK BELOW THIS LINE

70

Figure 1.18 Bank paying in (bank giro credit) slip which has been filled in for the paying in of cash and cheques.

This is often already printed on a paying in slip. In the example slip shown in Figure 1.18 you can see that the bank is the Money Bank, London W1 Branch. The six figure code for this is shown as 67–33–31. The account number shown at the bottom of the slip is 80265950. The account is in the name of A.N. Other. If it is not printed on the slip you will need to know these details to pay in any money. The reason it is called a bank giro credit is that you can pay money into any bank account in the UK if you know these details, from a branch of any bank. As a general rule no fee is charged for this if it is paid in at a branch of the same bank that the account is held in. However, some banks will make a charge to cover their costs if an account is held by a different bank. In the example given there would be no charge made at any branch of Money Bank although there might be if it were paid in at a Barclays Bank branch.

When you wish to pay in money to an account you will need to separate the money into cash and cheques. A list of the amounts on individual cheques is then made on the back of the paying in slip, which are then added up to give a total for the amount of money in cheques (see Figure 1.19). In this example there are five different cheques which add up to £59.40. Note that the names of the customers have been included, just in case the cheques become separated from the paying in slip (something which is very rare). It is a good idea to keep a list of names yourself, together with the amounts on each of their cheques.

The amount of money that you have in cash then needs to be broken down to show how much of it is in different notes or coins. Coins should be placed in coin bags which are available from banks. Thus on the example given in Figure 1.18 there is £10 in 20p coins; these would be placed in a separate bag so that when they were paid in they can be

Figure 1.19 The reverse side of the paying in slip showing the individual cheques and final total for these cheques.

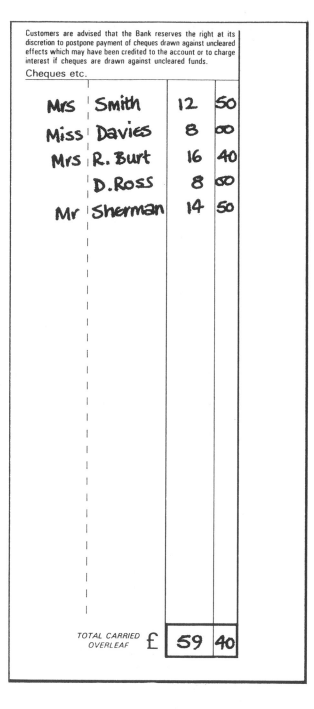

Customers are advised that the Bank reserves the right at its discretion to postpone payment of cheques drawn against uncleared effects which may have been credited to the account or to charge interest if cheques are drawn against uncleared funds.

Cheques etc.

Mrs	Smith	12	50
Miss	Davies	8	00
Mrs	R. Burt	16	40
	D. Ross	8	00
Mr	Sherman	14	50

TOTAL CARRIED OVERLEAF £ | 59 | 40 |

weighed to see if there is the right amount of coins (counting would be far too slow!). Thus, although there is a separate total for bronze (£20 in the example), you would be expected to divide your 1p and 2p coins into different bags for paying in. The total in cash in the example is £310.00. The total cash is then added to the total for cheques to arrive at the amount of money that is to be paid in. In the example this is £369.40. You will note that the credit is dated (10−10−89) and signed by the person who has paid in the money, and a note has been made that five cheques were paid in. The bank cashier will take all the money together with the paying in slip, stamp the slip and also a credit acknowledgement so that you have a record of the total paid in, the date it happened and the branch of the bank where it happened. After three normal working days the amount paid in should appear on the account (it can sometimes take longer and remember that Saturday and Sunday do not count as working days). You can find out how much is in the account by asking at your branch, or by using a service till. You can also request a statement which will detail credits and debits on your account. These can be requested when required, but many banks send them on a monthly basis.

Withdrawing money from an account

If you wish to withdraw money from an account you must first be sure how much money there is in the account. Banks are run as a business and they do not like you to take out more than you have! If this happens you will go overdrawn or into 'the red' (when you are in 'the black' you are in credit). If this should happen to you the bank will then charge you for every transaction that you make, usually over a six-month period, which can be very expensive! Most bank managers will allow an overdraft if you ask them, fixing the maximum amount that you can go overdrawn according to your means of paying it back.

The easiest way to withdraw money from an account at any bank is with a personal cheque supported by a cheque card (see Fig. 1.17). This is usually limited to £50 by the cheque card guarantee limit but there can be problems trying to withdraw more than this unless it is being done at your own branch. If you were to try and withdraw £200 from a bank that was not your branch there would need to be telephone calls made to your branch, extra means of identification provided (driver's licence is usual), as well as a wait in the bank for all this to happen! The cheque in Fig. 1.20 is made out for cash and will be honoured at any bank with a cheque card to support it. If it were presented at the actual branch shown on the cheque they would not require the cheque card. If you wanted to pay for a service or goods you would simply write the payee's name instead of cash, and write your cheque card number on the back of the cheque. If you require cash from your own bank branch and have run out of cheques you can ask for a debit slip which will act as a cheque if you fill in your account number. When you write cheques it is worth keeping a note of the amount, date and to whom it was payable on the cheque stub. This helps you to keep track of your money and also gives you a record should a cheque be lost in the post.

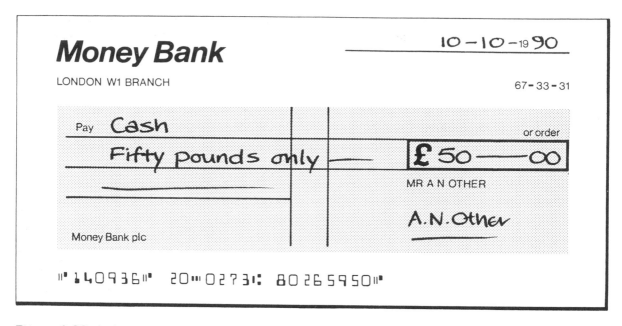

Figure 1.20 A cheque made out to cash for the sum of £50.

Most of us who have current accounts also have a cash or service card which enables us to withdraw money from an ATM (Automated Teller Machine) outside of normal banking hours. The card is inserted into the machine which requests you to punch in a four figure number to verify that you are the user of your own card. (This acts as an electronic signature; if your card was lost it should be useless to the finder as only you should know the number.) You are usually set a weekly withdrawal limit depending on your earnings which cannot be exceeded. These machines allow you to order statements, new cheque books and also instantly to find out the balance of your account.

If you were ever asked to pay in or withdraw money for your salon you would need the correct paying in books and withdrawal slips. This would not normally be required of a trainee, but it is worthwhile simulating in the salon the way it should be done. This will familiarise you with salon documentation for recording such information. During your training you could go along to a local bank and collect some paying in and withdrawal slips to practise on.

Questions
1. How would you list the money to be paid into a bank if it were made up of cheques and cash (make up some figures and do this on a paying in slip, then get someone to check that you have done it correctly)? A calculator should be used to check that your addition is correct.
2. When answering question 1, write down the bank sorting code, the account number and the name of the account.

3. Make out a cheque to obtain £30 cash for yourself from your own bank branch. Get someone to check you have done it correctly.
4. If the cheque was presented at another branch what would you need to write on the back?
5. How else can you get money from your account?
6. What does being 'overdrawn' mean?
7. Why does being overdrawn cost you money?

Recording information

Many people who work in salons do not like filling in record cards because they think that their memory is good enough to recall the different chemicals that they have used on their clients! Even if this were true, what happens if they leave the salon, are on holiday or are even ill for a day? It is essential that records are kept of services that each client has received. There are a number of reasons which we have just touched on:

- You may not remember what products were used or how and when you used them.
- This could be particular shades of colorant, peroxide strengths, perm lotion strengths or relaxer strengths.
- You may hold a number of product ranges as well, so how can you be sure which one you last used?
- With different colouring techniques you may have used more than one colour.
- When you next see the client how can you check on the product performance?
- How will you know when the client last visited the salon and what service was given?
- If you are ill, there will be no guess-work involved for your colleague attending to your client.
- Clients will be aware that they are being professionally treated if records are consulted before the service.

There are two ways of recording such information:

(1) writing the information on a card;
(2) entering the data onto a computer.

Record cards

Record cards are an efficient and economical method for recording and storing information. Usually, salons will file the record cards in alphabetical order, according to the surnames of the clients. They are stored in either filing box or a cabinet. Cards should be filled in and refiled after use, making it easy to retrieve the card in the future. Because others will rely on you to refile the cards in the correct alphabetical order, do make sure that you can do this. If you are at all unsure of what alphabetical order actually means, go back for a detailed explanation and examples (the alphabet was shown in Figure 1.12). A great deal of time can be wasted looking for misfiled record cards.

There is a great deal of information that can be recorded on such a card. Many salons buy preprinted cards whilst others design their own card layout according to their requirements. You may find that some salons separate the cards into different boxes for particular services (e.g. separate boxes for tints, perms, treatments, etc.), while others will use the same box or cabinet for storing all the informatfon. This will depend upon the size of the salon's clientele. The information that should be recorded will vary between salons; below is a list of the things that most salons include on their record cards, together with reasons for their inclusion:

- *Client's name* − Include surname and forename, or initials, also their title (Mr, Mrs, Ms, Dr, etc.). This will help to avoid any confusion between client record cards.
- *Address* − You will be able to check this with the client to ensure you have the correct card. It will enable the salon to mail clients details of special offers or changes in services offered.
- *Telephone numbers* − These should include home number and work number, so that you could contact the client in the event of staff illness or other problems.
- *Date of appointment* − This enables you to see when the client last visited the salon.
- *Stylist* − This tells the salon which stylist attended the client. This information is extremely important if the client finds the service to be unsatisfactory.
- *Scalp condition* − The condition of the scalp should be recorded to note any abnormalities or changes. Some scalp conditions may indicate that certain salon services should not be given.
- *Hair condition* − This gives details of the hair in terms of whether it is porous, resistant, damaged, etc. − all vital information to the stylist.
- *Technique* − Records the type of service, for example, conditioning treatment, highlights, perm, fashion colouring such as touch-colour. This gives the stylist a clear and concise 'hair history' for each client.
- *Products* − Sets outs quantities, strengths and types of products used. If you are checking product performance, you will need to know which products were used.
- *Development time* − If this is appropriate to the service given (many services require a product to stay on the hair for a specified time). This should indicate not only the time that the product was left on the hair but also if a machine was used to accelerate the development time.
- *Result* − If the result was not satisfactory − that means the client was not completely happy with it − the reason for this should be recorded. If the result was good, then record why it was good, e.g. target colour achieved, improvement to scalp condition, perm result soft as requested, etc.

Figure 1.21 A client record card.

NAME						SPECIAL INFORMATION	
ADDRESS							
DAYTIME TELEPHONE NO.							

DATE	STYLIST	SCALP	HAIR	TECHNIQUE	PRODUCTS	DEVELOPMENT	RESULT

Figure 1.21 is an example of a typical record card used in a salon.

Due to the fact that record cards limit you in how much you can write on them because of their size, your salon may find it more efficient to use a kind of shorthand. This must be written in such a way that all the salon staff can interpret and understand the meaning, not just the person who has written it. For example, instead of writing the name of the tint on the card, use the numerical colour code. Instead of writing 'thirty volume hydrogen peroxide' put 30 vol H_2O_2, or 9 per cent H_2O_2 if your salon uses peroxide measured in percentage strength. Also, you could abbreviate words such as highlights and permanent wave to H/L and P/W respectively.

Computers

Many larger salons use computers to record this kind of information. Computing requires one of two things to occur to really work. The first is to train all staff to use the computer, while the second is to employ someone to feed in the information from hand-written cards. You will have to be shown the way the system operates in your particular salon. Every computer is operated by a program which is referred to as the 'software' ('hardware' being the actual computer). This program tells the machine the functions it is to perform and not all programs are suitable for all computers. The type of program used for classifying, storing and retrieving information is called a database. A few database programs have been designed with the needs of the salon in mind. Before buying a computer, seek expert advice about the machine's memory capacity and facilities. Computers with small memories are cheaper but a powerful one can react quickly to commands, saving valuable minutes in the salon. Do remember though, that a computer will store the information given to it — it does not have the capacity of knowing that a client's name has been wrongly spelt or that the wrong product name has been entered. With a little in-salon training, all staff would be able to master the use of a computer in a short while.

Apart from storing data about clients, a database could also be used to monitor stock control and to record takings, sales and salaries. It would, in fact, be able to help with all the mundane tasks that looking after a business involves and would save valuable time, storage space and too many headaches! The computer could tell you how much money the salon took over a particular period and might even be able to classify these figures into retail sales, perms, colours, etc. It could keep records of staff holidays, salaries, sick pay, courses attended, commission and anything else an employer may need to know at a moment's notice. The information that is called up from the computer's memory will be displayed on the monitor or screen. To get a 'hard copy' or, in other words, this information on a piece of paper, it is necessary to have a printer. The command is given to the computer to 'print' and the document will be set out on paper for you. How easy it would be to issue salaries in this way instead of typing the same details out for each employee!

If the thought of using a computer in the salon fills you with horror, do consider seeing a demonstration on how they can make the business run more efficiently before dismissing the idea. Also, there are many places that offer short courses in the use of computers and many of the companies that have developed programs for salon use offer training for the salon's staff at very competitive prices.

The alternative to using a computer is to perform the tasks outlined earlier by hand and store the information in books or files. A calculator is an invaluable help when a great deal of figure work has to be done and most people have used one before. Put simply, a calculator is a device that does sums for the user. Calculators vary in complexity and will be more expensive if you want them to do complicated calculations. For salon purposes a basic function calculator should be adequate. Do remember, however, that the bigger the number keys are, the less likely you are to hit the wrong button accidentally!

Daily and weekly takings

The main types of calculations that a hairdresser might need to do are those regarding the totalling of daily and weekly takings. Calculating salaries and profit margins would be the task of the salon manager/ owner so will not be dealt with in this book. Because many salons calculate wages on the amount of money each worker earns for the salon, it is important that a concise and accurate record is kept to work out the commissions earned. At the end of each working day the contents of the till (less the float) is totalled and divided up to show how much each worker has earned for the salon. As we said before, sophisticated electronic cash registers or computers can save a lot of time because each worker has a key code which is pressed to tell the machine that the money put into the till has been earned by a particular person. A command is given to the machine (usually the pressing of a single key) and it will total the day's takings and separate it so that it shows how much each person has taken for the salon. If required, the machine may also have the facility of separating retail sales from monies taken for particular salon services. If you do not have this facility, it will be a matter of getting out the calculator and record books and beginning to check the individual tear-off tickets that are written out each time a money transaction takes place. These tear-off tickets are commonly called 'dockets' and are simply numbered sheets of coloured paper that tear off rather like a raffle ticket. Each stylist would be allocated a particular colour and every time a client paid for a service carried out by the stylist, one of the tickets would be completed. As they come already printed there is only the need to tick the service that is being paid for and enter the costs. The total cost is calculated and written in the box at the bottom of the ticket. The total must also be written on the stub that will be left once the ticket is torn off. When totalling up these tickets, it is a quick task to separate the different coloured paper allocated to each worker. The consecutive numbers on each ticket and the stub help when cross-checking the figures, especially if the till is suspiciously 'under' − in other words, does not have the amount in it that the tickets say it should.

Figure 1.22 shows an example of a typical ticket that would be used to record individual stylist's takings. Notice the list of services on the left hand side which only need to be ticked to show the service or services that were given.

Figure 1.23 shows an example of the type of record sheet that could be used for daily takings. Notice that the takings are divided for each stylist and that a separate column has been made for retail sales which, for this particular salon, earn a different rate of commission to salon services.

The amounts entered into each column are totalled at the end of the day showing how much work each worker has carried out. These totals are then added together to show a grand total for the day. This grand total should, of course, match the amount of money in the till.

It is usual to identify whether a payment was made by cash, cheque, credit card or charge card. If your salon is part of a large organisation, gift vouchers may also be accepted by your salon. These details would normally be recorded at the time the payment is made, by noting this on the ticket or entering the data into the computer or cash register. Whichever method of payment is used the salon may wish to know how much money was received from these different sources so that they can be categorised. Credit and charge card payments have to be claimed from the finance company (using the carboned receipts) and cheques need to be paid into the salon's bank account. Money from gift vouchers is recouped in a similar way to credit and charge cards.

The way in which money is paid into a bank account is dealt with earlier. You should be able to tabulate information such as the methods by which payments have been made (by cash, cheque or credit card) to find out what is the most popular way of settling a bill for the clients in your salon.

Figure 1.22 A sales docket or ticket used in the salon.

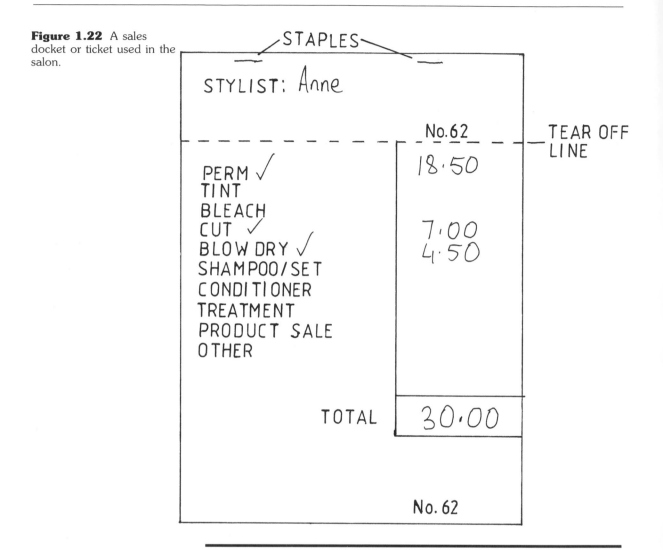

STAPLES

STYLIST: Anne

No. 62 — TEAR OFF LINE

PERM ✓	18·50
TINT	
BLEACH	
CUT ✓	7·00
BLOW DRY ✓	4·50
SHAMPOO/SET	
CONDITIONER	
TREATMENT	
PRODUCT SALE	
OTHER	
TOTAL	30·00

No. 62

Questions
1. Why should information about clients be recorded?
2. Give reasons why such information could be useful.
3. Where are record cards stored in your salon?
4. How do you find the card of a particular client?
5. How do you replace the client's card in the right place in the filing system?
6. What information is on the record cards used in your salon?
7. Give some examples of 'shorthand' used in your salon.
8. What advantages do computers have for storing client records?
9. Can you think of any disadvantages?
10. What electronic machine can be used to help with figure-work?
11. When are mistakes most likely to be made with such a machine?
12. What does the till 'being under' refer to?
13. Collect examples of salon documentation used in your salon.

Figure 1.23 A daily takings record sheet used in the salon.

TUESDAY 11th June									Reception Sales
Anne	Jo	Wilson	Sarah						
3.85	6.50	30.00	3.85						2.40
6.50	6.50	3.85	3.85						2.40
3.85	3.85	3.85	30.00						3.25
6.50	5.50	6.50	30.00						1.99
30.00	18.25	15.95	15.95						2.40
15.95		18.25	15.95						1.99
30.00		30.00	6.50						3.95
			6.50						
			3.85						
			18.25						
96.65	40.60	108.40	134.70						18.38

	DAILY TOTAL	398.73

Additional information — first aid

It is extremely important that anyone who deals with the general public have some knowledge of first aid, especially as you are offering a service where accidents could happen.

First aid is the first action that should be taken to minimise damage in the case of an accident or sudden illness. It is discussed fully, with reasons for the actions taken, in *Hygiene — A Salon Handbook* but here is a quick reference for the more common things that you might encounter in the salon.

Bleeding

In the event of a minor cut apply pressure until bleeding stops. Because of infectious diseases such as AIDS and hepatitis B, direct contact with blood should be avoided. Whenever possible, get clients to use a piece of cotton wool to apply pressure themselves, and ask them to throw the cotton wool into a plastic bag or bin afterwards. Use alum powder in men's hairdressing rather than the styptic pencil which could spread infection. If there is a large loss of blood apply pressure using clean towels or hands (which should be in rubber gloves if possible), and phone for an ambulance as quickly as possible. In the case of a nose bleed tell the client to pinch the bottom of the nostrils, so that their blood can clot. They should lean with their head forward and not blow their nose for sometime afterwards. Any blood spillages on tiled or vinyl surfaces should be mopped up with a cloth and some household bleach. Always wear rubber or disposable gloves if you are dealing with blood. Rinse blood off gloves before you remove them. If blood should spill onto fabric, wash it off with disinfectant or hot soapy water. Obviously, care must be taken not to ruin furniture.

Burns

Whether burns are dry or wet (scalds) cool the skin immediately by immersing in cold running water. This should be done until the pain goes or for twenty minutes. It removes heat from the burn so that it does not cause as much damage to the skin. If you cannot get a client to water, hold a soaking wet towel against the damaged area. Seek medical advice if the burn is large. A large burn can be covered with sterile gauze until medical help is received. If a chemical burn occurs flood the area with water to dilute and remove the chemical. For the eye it is best to use flowing water rather than an eye bath, as this removes the chemical rather than simply diluting it. Seek medical advice if necessary.

Fainting

Fainting is caused by a lack of oxygen to the brain and any first aid given should improve oxygen supply. If a client feels faint put the head down between the knees and loosen tight clothing. If a client has fainted raise the legs on a cushion so that they are higher than the head. Using smelling salts will shock someone out of a faint but do nothing to alleviate the cause. Similarly, placing someone in front of an open window will cool him or her down but does nothing to improve the oxygen supply to the brain.

Hysterical fit

This occurs when someone has lost control of their emotions. They may begin to laugh or cry, scream and shout, or even roll about on the floor. This has been known to occur in salons as a result of shock after a change in hair colour, style or hair length. It should be treated by getting the person alone (away from an audience), being firm and not expressing any sympathy. After the hysteria has died away do not express sympathy (but don't be unpleasant!) as the client may start again, thinking that she has just cause to be upset!

Epileptic fit

Many people who suffer from epilepsy are on medication which reduces the chance of fits occurring. If a fit does occur, however, the client will fall unconscious to the floor. After a short time the limbs will begin to jerk uncontrollably. When this happens make sure that objects that could cause injury are removed, or simply stand in front of fixed objects that the sufferer might collide against. After the fit, lay the client in the recovery position (on one side) so that it is impossible to choke or smother on vomit. It is usual to phone for an ambulance if it is someone you do not know in case it is their first fit. They may take some time to become conscious again.

Breathing stops

For whatever reason this occurs, check the airways to see if they are blocked. If they are tilt the head back to unblock them. Now begin mouth-to-mouth resuscitation by covering the mouth with yours, and while squeezing the nostrils together blow into the mouth. The chest will rise and then fall. Repeat until breathing resumes and ask someone else to phone for an ambulance (you are preventing possible brain damage which can occur within four minutes if the brain is totally starved of oxygen).

Heart attack

The client may complain of chest pains and the skin may go blue. In this case keep the client upright and loosen clothing. Allowing the client to lie down would put an extra load on the heart to pump the blood around the body and could cause a heart attack. If the client is on the floor support the back on cushions. This makes breathing less difficult. If the heart stops place the client onto his/her back and begin mouth-to-mouth resuscitation. Alternate this with cardiac massage (press firmly down once on the breastbone using both your hands and your body weight to apply the force). Do one push to approximately six to eight breaths. Keep checking for a pulse and get someone else to phone for an ambulance.

Electric shock

If someone is being electrocuted do not touch the body as you may be electrocuted yourself, but immediately turn off the electricity. Do this by unplugging at the mains or by turning switches off. If the heart stops begin mouth-to-mouth resuscitation and cardiac massage until the patient recovers. Get someone else to phone for an ambulance.

Fractures

Keep the patient still if you suspect a broken bone (a leg or arm may be at a peculiar angle). Phone for an ambulance.

Sprained ankle

Bandage the ankle with a wet crepe bandage. The bandage will support the sprain while the cold water will help reduce swelling.

Never give alcohol to anyone who is feeling ill or who has been hurt in case they should need anaesthetic on entry to hospital. If you do, they will have to wait longer for treatment.

The first aid box

All salons should have a first aid box which is available in case of accident. This requirement varies with the number of people on the premises and is governed by the Health and Safety (First Aid) Regulations of 1982. Many first aid boxes are marked with a red cross on a white background or a white cross on a red background. However, the most modern first aid boxes are *green* with a *white cross*. The box should close tightly so that it is dust- and moisture-free. It should be put in a place that all employees are aware of. The following are minimum amounts of items if the number of employees is between (A) 1−10, or (B) 11−50.

Item in first aid box	Number of items	(A)	(B)
First aid guidance card		1	1
Individual sterile plasters		20	40
Medium sterile dressings		2	4
Large sterile dressings		2	4
Extra large sterile dressings		2	4
Sterile eye pads/bandage		2	4
Triangular bandages/slings		2	4
Sterilised wound coverings		2	4
Safety pins		6	12

These are the minimum recommended contents. Because of the risk of AIDS and hepatitis B several pairs of disposable rubber or plastic gloves should be kept in all salon first aid boxes. This is not a scare tactic; Government health statistics show that hepatitis B is at present three to four times more common in hairdressers than it is in nurses. It is also useful to have some cotton wool and tissues; surgical adhesive tape; a crepe bandage for a strain and a bowl for pouring water. The first thing to run out in a first aid box is plasters. As it makes sense to keep cuts covered have a supply of waterproof ones for protection. If you want to learn more about first aid phone your local St John's Ambulance who regularly run courses.

Questions

1. What is the purpose of first aid?
2. What is the first aid for bleeding?
3. Why should you be careful not to get blood onto your skin when giving first aid?
4. What is the first aid for a nosebleed?
5. How should a spillage of blood be dealt with?
6. What is the first aid for a burn?
7. Why is flowing water better to use than an eye bath when a chemical enters the eye?
8. Give the first aid for when a client feels faint or has fainted.
9. What is the first aid for an hysterical fit?
10. What action would you take in the event of a client having an epileptic fit?
11. What is the first aid if someone should stop breathing?
12. Why should you start the first aid immediately rather than phone for an ambulance first?
13. If someone has a heart attack, what should you do?
14. If someone is being electrocuted why should you not touch them?
15. If a client fell and you suspected a fracture, what action would you take?
16. What is the first aid for a sprained ankle?
17. What items should be found in every first aid box?
18. In your own salon, what items are missing from the first aid box or are extra compared with this list?

19. Describe the first aid box found in your salon and say why a first aid box should be easy to identify.
20. What items are likely to run out first from a first aid box?
21. Why have rubber gloves become an item which should be found in the first aid box?

Chapter Two
Consultation and Diagnostics

Every client who walks into your salon is different. They wear different clothes and makeup; are of different heights, weights and shapes; have different skin and hair colours, hair textures and hair lengths; come from different social backgrounds; are of different ages and sexes, and may have a variety of things wrong with their hair or scalps. This is why you must spend time on every client to ask questions and make professional observations, so that you can match what each client says they want with what is really possible. If something goes wrong in the salon it is you who are at fault and not the client! As one well-known hairdressing presenter is fond of saying: 'fail to prepare, prepare to fail'. If a client comes into your salon and asks for a 'bob', how do you know exactly what they mean by that term? It is too late to confirm what they mean once you have cut off their hair!

The experience gained by working in the salon for years may eventually mean that you do not have to spend so much time on this area in the future, but until you have gained that experience, stick to basics and learn!

Basic facts about the hair and skin

The first thing any hairdresser needs to know about is the hair that they will be handling every day of their lives. Every head of hair you handle will both look and feel different. Hair can range from being straight to tightly curled, with a remarkable range of colours, whether real or unnatural, to match. Some hair will feel fine and silky while some will be coarse and feel like straw. In short, even without the services of the hairdresser, every head is different. Clients think that the hairdresser is the font of all knowledge about their hair, even if it is your first day in a salon! This first section will cover some of the more important facts about hair and skin which you should really know about from day one!

What is hair made from?

Hair is made from a type of protein, called keratin, which is different from other proteins because it contains sulphur. It is this sulphur that allows us to perm and straighten hair (see Chapter 8 and Chapter 9 for more information). If you have ever burnt your hair you will know how strongly the sulphur in it smells. When you cut hair clients do not scream out in pain! This tells you something else about the hair, that it is dead. Keratin also makes up our skin and nails, and this is why hairdressing chemicals affect them as well as the hair for which they were designed. Always protect your hands when using hairdressing products which are designed to change the hair, as they can damage the skin and nails. Some more sensitive individuals have had to leave hairdressing because their skin has developed an allergic reaction that is usually referred to as dermatitis. The word 'dermatitis' literally means red or inflamed skin. (Don't panic if you already have dermatitis, as the majority of hairdressers get over it, especially when they get away from the shampoo basin! It is dealt with in Chapter 4.)

Is there only one type of hair?

No, you know this from the hair on your own body. Scientists have classified hair into 3 main types: *lanugo*, *vellus* and *terminal* (although for reasons which will become apparent we only really deal with one type).

- *Lanugo hair* is found on the human foetus before birth, usually as an unpigmented coat of fine, soft hair. It is shed between the seventh and eighth month of the pregnancy – so we can forget about it as far as hairdressing is concerned!
- *Vellus hair* is the fine downy hair found on the body and it may also be seen on the scalp, especially on the balding heads of men. Because it is so fine it is of no importance to the hairdresser. It can, however, be a nuisance if it is dark or becomes coarser, as most women consider this masculine. There are a number of ways of correcting this which range from the painful pulling out of the hair (plucking, waxing, sugaring, or using an epilady), to shaving, sanding, bleaching or electrolysis. Many women on the continent are glad to be hairy, as men there often prefer it. On holiday you may notice many more hairy legs and underarms!
- *Terminal hair* is coarser and is found on the scalp, on men's faces, under the arms, and on the pubic regions. Its growth is under the influence of male hormones (even females produce a little male hormone). This is the hair that we, the hairdressers, are concerned with.

What is the structure of a hair like?

Figure 2.1 shows a simplified diagram of the structure of a hair showing its three layers. Figure 2.2 shows the outer surface of a highly magnified hair. The photograph was taken with an electron microscope and what you are seeing is a hair magnified over one thousand times. The scales that you can see are one of several layers (about seven in European hair, and up to eleven in Chinese hair). This outer layer is known as the cuticle. There are more cuticle layers around the hair shaft near the base of the hair than there are towards the older tip of the hair, purely because of wear and tear. If you look at the end of the section on hair

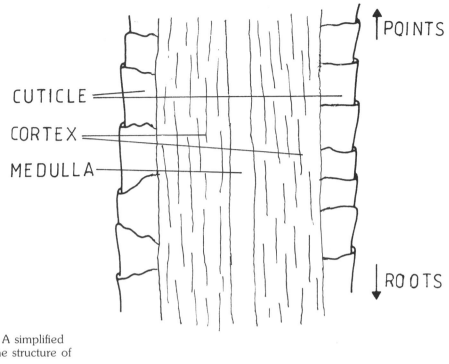

CUTICLE
CORTEX
MEDULLA
POINTS
ROOTS

Figure 2.1 A simplified diagram of the structure of the hair.

Figure 2.2 The outer surface of a highly magnified hair, showing the cuticle.

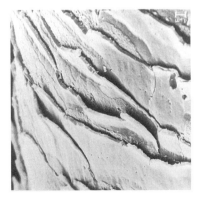

growth, the oldest part of the hair will be the points. Because it is older it will have been brushed more, exposed to more weather, heat and possibly chemical treatment.

The cuticle is the protective layer of the hair and prevents things from entering the layers below. Physically, it is rather like the layer of tiles on a roof which protect a house from the weather. But unlike a roof, there are several layers. The free ends of the overlapping scales (called imbrications) point upwards in the direction of the hair growth, that is, towards the tip. This can be clearly seen in Figure 2.2. If you take a hair between the finger and thumb and gently rub it up and down the hair, you will find it feels smooth from root to point, but rough from point to root. This is because the tips of the cuticle scales cause resistance. Because the cuticle scales are translucent (something translucent allows *some* light to pass through whereas something transparent allows *all* light to pass through) we can see the colour of the hair pigment in the layer below.

If the cuticle is damaged by excessive physical or chemical treatment, the second layer of the hair, the cortex, may be exposed to injury. This second layer forms the bulk of the hair and it is in this part that the chemical changes of bleaching, tinting, perming and straightening take place. Figure 2.3 is a highly magnified picture of a hair to show the structure of the cortex. It is the most important layer of the hair and makes up between 75 per cent to 90 per cent of the hair's bulk. Many of the physical properties of hair are dependent on the cortex. These include:

- Tensile strength (amount of pressure needed to break a hair);
- Elasticity (ability to stretch and return to original length);
- Direction and type of growth (straight, curly);
- Diameter of hair shaft (whether it is fine or coarse).

Figure 2.3 Highly magnified picture of a hair to show the structure of the cortex.

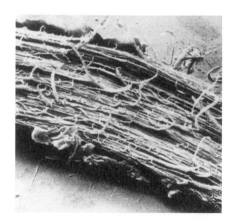

Put simply, the cortex has a structure made up of a number of long fibres, which resemble a bunch of straws, held together by a series of different bonds (see Chapter 8 for details of bonds). Individual fibres have a structure rather like that of a spring, enabling them to be stretched, yet still spring back to their original lengths. Keratin in its normal un-stretched state is called alpha keratin. When stretched it forms beta keratin, which should spring back to alpha keratin once pressure is taken off the hair (see Chapter 7 for further information on this). Granules of colour pigment (either melanin or pheomelanin) are found throughout the cortex (see Chapter 10 for further information on this). The centre of the hair is the medulla, which is basically an air space which may contain melanin. Some people have a medulla throughout the length of each hair, some have one only in parts of each hair, and some have none at all — while others have two! As it serves no useful purpose, ignore it!

What is the skin?

First the easy part! Skin is the outside covering of the body, with an average area of 1.6 square metres (18 square feet) and an average weight of 3 kilograms (6 pounds). It is remarkably complex, and will only be looked at here in outline so that we can understand its relationship to hairdressing. Figure 2.4 shows a generalised vertical section of skin. This is a diagram that includes all relevant skin structures, although some would not be found on particular parts of the body. Have you got hair on the palms of your hands, for example?

Figure 2.4 A generalised vertical section of the skin.

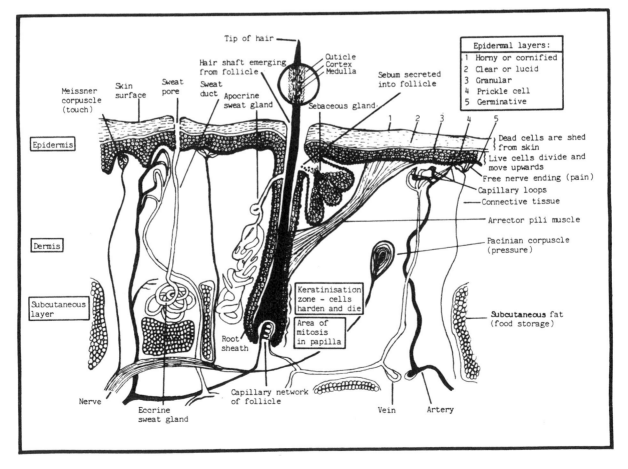

What do the different parts of the skin do?

Briefly, the skin is a protective layer with numerous nerve endings to tell us about our surroundings. They can respond to heat, cold, pain, pressure and touch. If we get either too hot or too cold it can help us reach normal body temperature again. It can also show when we are embarrassed (blushing red) or shocked (white with fear). It stores food in the form of fat (something that many of us know to our cost!), and can manufacture vitamin D (needed to absorb calcium from our food for healthy bones and teeth) and melanin (needed to protect live skin cells from being burnt by the sun's ultra violet rays, which could result in scarring or even cancer).

Hair follicles are found almost everywhere (but not on the palms of hands, soles of feet or the lips). The sebaceous glands, which are attached to the follicle, secrete an oily liquid called sebum. This helps to waterproof and lubricate the skin, as well as helping to prevent fungal infections such as ringworm. The hair is also coated with sebum and this helps to maintain moisture in the cortex of the hair. Sebaceous glands are under the control of hormones (particularly male androgen hormones) which make the glands enlarge and secrete more at puberty. Acne and greasy skin are directly related to this. On the hairs of the underarms, the follicles also have a special type of sweat gland, the apocrine sweat gland. These secrete a sweat which is mostly water, but which also contains fatty acids. These fatty acids cause body odour when they are broken down by bacteria. Antiperspirants reduce the size of the sweat pores so that we sweat less, while deodorants inhibit the growth of the bacteria which break down the sweat. Washing on a daily basis will remove stale sweat and bacteria. Personal hygiene is essential to the hairdresser as clients will not come back to you if you have an odour problem!

The hair follicle also has an arrector pili muscle which makes the hair stand on end. This is supposed to trap an insulating layer of warm air in the hairs around the body but would only be really effective on extremely hairy people.

The normal sweat gland (eccrine sweat gland) produces sweat which is mostly water (98 per cent), with a little salt (2 per cent). This sweat cools the skin when it evaporates, as it requires energy in the form of heat to turn sweat into water vapour. This can be demonstrated by wrapping some cotton wool around the base of a thermometer. Note the temperature and then add a few drops of ether (if you have no ether try some methylated spirits); the temperature begins to drop as the liquid evaporates. The sweat glands are under the control of the nerves, as most of us have found when we have been nervous and had sweaty palms. In hot climates loss of sweat without drinking can result in dehydration. Even on a cool day the body loses about a litre of sweat, with several times more being lost in dry heat.

The epidermis is the top layer of the skin and is itself made up of five layers, as shown in Figure 2.4. The lower cells are alive, dividing by mitosis (this is the type of cell division where a cell splits in two and produces two exact smaller copies of itself). They then push upwards where they become full of keratin and die. When this process happens too quickly, dandruff or psoriasis can result (see later). In normal skin it takes about thirty days for a cell to pass from the bottom to the top of the epidermis. Melanocytes are found in the germinating layer and produce the pigment melanin to help protect the skin from ultra violet radiation in sunlight. When you tan the pigment absorbs the ultra violet light so that it does not damage the skin. If you do not tan, the ultra violet reaches live cells and you burn! The epidermis forms a protective barrier against physical injury, and contains no nerve endings or blood vessels. Without the top horny layer, which is made of dead scales of keratin, water loss would be increased by twenty times, which would mean possible death by dehydration. The hair follicles and sweat glands are actually part of the epidermis, which has downgrowths into the dermis. If you look closely at Figure 2.4 you will see that the germinative layer of the epidermis is continuous around the follicle and glands.

Because the sebum and sweat produced onto the skin's surface have an acid pH, we say that the skin has an 'acid mantle'. This pH of between 4.5 and 5.5 discourages the growth of bacteria on the skin as it is antiseptic. We refer to hairdressing products being 'pH-balanced' if they have the same pH as the hair and skin. pH is discussed fully in Chapter 8.

Questions
1. What is hair made from?
2. Why is this different from other proteins?
3. Why should you protect your hands when using many hairdressing products?
4. What is dermatitis?
5. What are the three different types of hair?
6. Why is lanugo hair not considered important?
7. Where do you find vellus hair?
8. Where do you find terminal hair?
9. What are the three layers of the hair from the outside to the inside?
10. How many cuticle layers does a European hair have?
11. How many can a Chinese hair have?
12. Where on a hair are there most layers of cuticle?
13. Why?
14. Using your fingers, how could you tell if you were running them from root to point or point to root on a hair?
15. What is the purpose of the cuticle?
16. What does the cuticle being translucent mean?
17. Where do chemical changes take place in the hair?
18. What properties of the hair are dependent on the cortex?
19. Describe the structure of the cortex.
20. What is the difference between alpha and beta keratin?
21. Why is the medulla not important in hairdressing?
22. What is the average area of the skin?
23. What can the nerve endings of the skin respond to?

24. How can the colour of the skin show our feelings?
25. How does the skin store food?
26. What is the purpose of vitamin D?
27. What is the purpose of melanin?
28. On what parts of the body are there no hair follicles?
29. What are the sebaceous glands controlled by?
30. What is the link between sweating and body odour?
31. How can you prevent body odour?
32. What does the arrector pili muscle do?
33. What are the two major components of sweat?
34. What is the function of sweat?
35. What is the epidermis?
36. How are new cells produced in the epidermis?
37. If this occurs too quickly, what happens?
38. Why does the epidermis produce melanin?
39. Why is the horny layer important?
40. What is the pH of your skin?
41. What would the pH of an acid balanced product be?

Recognising abnormal hair and scalp conditions commonly seen in the salon

Many clients who come into your salon will have different hair and scalp conditions. Clients may not realise that there is anything wrong with their hair or scalp, but they will expect *you* to know what that something is and what can be done about it!

Such conditions can be roughly broken up into two main groupings, infectious and non-infectious. If something is infectious it can be 'caught' by coming into contact with it, either directly (by touching it) or indirectly (by using towels, brushes, etc. which have been in contact with the infected client). If something is non-infectious it cannot be caught, but can still cause clients a lot of concern about their appearance. Some non-infectious conditions may look 'nasty' in appearance, so it is important that you make judgements on fact and not on feelings! If you tell clients with a non-infectious scalp condition that you cannot work on them they will not be very happy, while if you do not recognise an infectious condition and catch it yourself or spread it to other clients this would be equally unprofessional.

Questions
1. How are skin and scalp conditions divided up?
2. What is the difference between this division you have described?
3. Why is it important that you make judgements on knowledge rather than feelings?

Infectious conditions

Infectious conditions are caused by tiny micro-organisms which cannot be seen without the aid of a microscope. There are three main types of micro-organism which cause infectious scalp conditions: bacteria, fungi and viruses. You may also come across clients who have an infestation of tiny insects called head lice. These are infectious so will be considered here along with another infestation of the skin, scabies.

Impetigo

This is an infection of the skin caused by bacteria. It is commonly seen on the face and the scalp. The bacteria invade the top layer of the skin, the epidermis, causing small blisters filled with clear liquid to occur. The liquid thickens and a yellow crusty scab appears. It is highly infectious and can be spread directly by touch or indirectly on tools or towels. On the scalp you may simply see tiny yellow pustules. See head lice below. *No service should be given.*

Warts

These are flesh-coloured raised areas of skin, which can be smooth or rough and are commonly seen on the hands or on the scalp. They are caused by a virus in the epidermis and will usually last for at least two years if not treated. They are infectious when damaged, as could happen if they were not noticed during hairdressing! A service can be given if care is taken *not* to damage the warts. Hairdressers with warts on their hands would be well advised to have them removed (usually by freezing at your local hospital) as everyone cuts their hands at some time!

Ringworm of the scalp

Also called Tinea capitis, this infection is most commonly seen in children and is caused by a fungus which digests the protein keratin — the protein that our epidermis, hair and nails are made of. It can be recognised by the presence of circular bald patches with redness, greyish scaling and brittle short hair stumps in the patches. Ringworm can be caught directly by touch or indirectly by contact with infected pieces of hair that could be on brushes or towels. *No service should be given.*

Head lice

Also called Pediculosis capitis, this infection is most commonly seen in children. The lice are tiny insects. They cling to individual hairs with their claws, which resemble those of a crab (see Figure 2.5). The lice lay eggs, called nits, directly onto the hair shaft. They are cemented onto

Figure 2.5 The head
louse. (Courtesy Napp
Laboratories Ltd.)

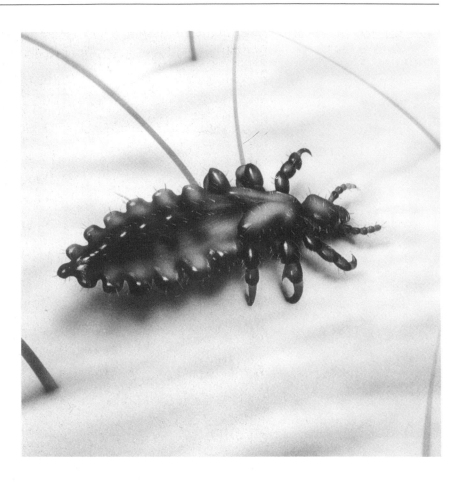

the hairshaft and are similar in colour to the hair of the person with the
infestation (lighter on blonde hair and darker on black hair). Thus they
are difficult to spot. Nits are shown attached to a hair in Figure 2.6. The
lice feed on blood by biting the scalp, and it is the bite marks which you
are likely to see on the scalp of the client. If ever a client has scratch
marks on their scalp, check for the presence of nits, no matter how old
the client is. The worst case of head lice seen by us was in an old lady
who had been to her doctor with it but, because of her age, he had
diagnosed eczema! Lice are found in the nape region of the head and
this is where you will see the bite marks along with scratch marks (the
client develops an allergic reaction to the bites and begins to itch).
Closer examination of such scalps will reveal the nits which will stay
attached to the hair if you try to comb them out. We have known many
hairdressers confuse nits with dandruff so it is worth using a comb to see
if the 'nits' move − if they do it is dandruff! Lice are spread by direct
contact and the lice walk from one head to another. Head lice infestations
are at their height in September and October, as children go back to

Figure 2.6 Nits attached to a hair. (Courtesy Napp Laboratories Ltd.)

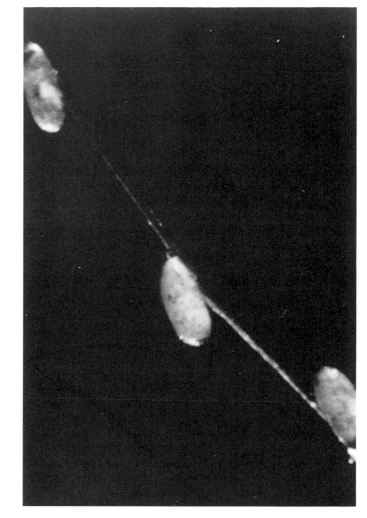

school and give the lice plenty of fresh heads to go onto! *No service should be given*, but you must be aware of what happens in *your* salon if a client has lice. It would be normal for a senior stylist to inform the client that something is wrong as tactful handling will ensure that the client is not too embarrassed to come back again. The best treatment for head lice is insecticidal lotions which are much more effective than shampoos. Figure 2.7 represents the lifecycle of a head louse in a very memorable form.

Note: Impetigo is often seen on scalps alongside head lice infestations when the damaged skin, due to scratching the bite marks, becomes infected. It is referred to as a 'secondary' infection because it would not have occurred without the headlice.

Figure 2.7 The life cycle of the louse. (Courtesy Napp Laboratories Ltd.)

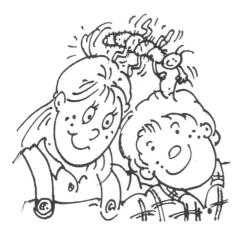

(1) Transfer
The head louse spends its day wandering around from head to head, feeding where it wants to.

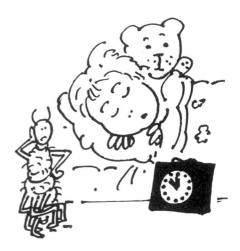

(2) Lays eggs
The female lays eggs. It's an intricate task, glueing an egg to a hair, very near to or touching the scalp to keep warm. She usually does it at night, when her host is still. She tries to make it blend with the surroundings, and will lay 7 or 8 each night.

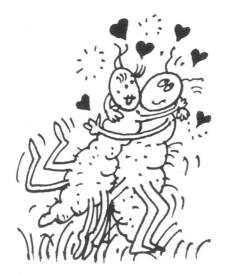

(3) Mating
The female usually mates between laying each egg. As females outnumber males about 4 to 1, father louse's night work is at least as demanding!

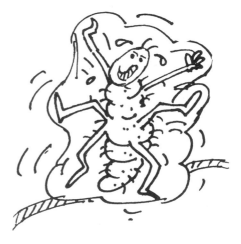

(4) Hatching
Each egg takes 7–10 days to hatch. When the louse is ready to hatch, the plug at the end of the egg is too small, when removed, for the louse to get out. So it gulps in air, passes it through the body until the louse, under pressure, 'pops' out of the egg. The empty egg shell (the nit) is left on the hair and is now gleaming white.

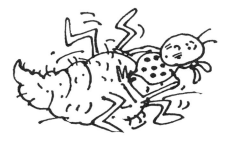

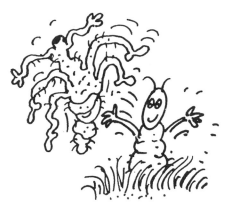

(5) First Drink

The newly hatched, colourless, louse has its first feed and its body can be seen filling up with blood. It pierces the skin with its mouthparts and couples up to a capillary, meanwhile pumping in a local anaesthetic and anti-coagulant. The louse feeds five times a day.

(6) Moulting

The young louse moults three times before becoming adult (and will then be just under match-head size).

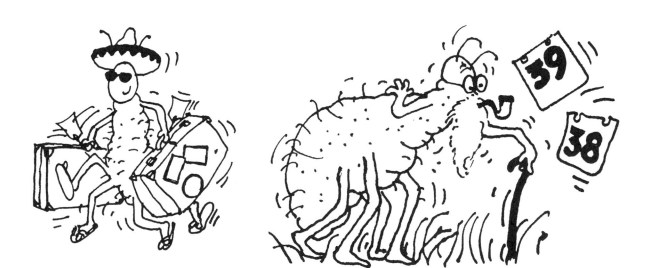

(7) Opportunity

Now an adult all the louse wants to do is travel (from head to head) and have a good time with the opposite sex, never missing a chance to change heads or partners, and doing its bit for the louse population.

(8) Old age

If it lives that long, it will die of old age at about forty days.

Scabies

Scabies is an infestation of the skin caused by the itch mite, which burrows into the epidermis. It is not seen on the face or scalp but can be found on skin anywhere else on the body. It is highly infectious and could be caught by touching a client with the infestation. The burrows can be seen as tiny raised red lines on the skin, and as sufferers get very itchy skin scratch marks and impetigo could be present. *No service should be given as you could put other clients at risk.*

Questions

1. What are the causes of infectious conditions?
2. Which of these is the cause of impetigo?
3. How would you recognise impetigo?
4. Give examples of how impetigo could be spread.
5. Should a service be given to someone with impetigo on their scalp?
6. How would you recognise warts?
7. What causes warts?
8. How long do warts last without treatment?
9. When are warts infectious?
10. What should you do if you had warts on your hands?
11. What is the other name for scalp ringworm?
12. What causes ringworm?
13. What does this digest?
14. Why can you suffer from ringworm on the skin, hair or nails?
15. How would you recognise scalp ringworm?
16. Give examples of how ringworm of the scalp could be caught from an infected client in the salon.
17. Should a service be given?
18. What is the other name for head lice?
19. Who is most likely to suffer from head lice?
20. How do lice cling to hairs?
21. What are nits?
22. Where would you find nits?
23. Why are nits difficult to spot on the hair?
24. What do lice feed on?
25. Where are you most likely to find the lice or nits?
26. What can nits be confused with?
27. How would you tell the difference?
28. How are lice spread?
29. What time of the year are there most cases of head lice?
30. Should a service be given to a client with lice?
31. Why might you suspect that a client had head lice in the salon?
32. What is the procedure if you spot head lice on a client in your salon?
33. Why is great tact required if a client has head lice?
34. Using Figure 2.7, briefly describe the life cycle of a head louse.
35. Why is impetigo often seen along with head louse infestations?
36. Why is it then referred to as a 'secondary' infection?

37. What causes scabies?
38. Where would you find the burrows?
39. How would you recognise these burrows?
40. What bacterial infection might be present alongside scabies?
41. Would you give a client a service who had scabies?

Why is hygiene important in the salon?

Hygiene is important because following certain routines will help prevent possible spread of infection between clients, or between clients and hairdressers. Never before have hairdressers been so concerned about the risk of spreading infection during their work. This concern has much to do with the arrival on the scene of the HIV virus that causes AIDS. The correct routine for dealing with cuts was given in the additional information at the end of Chapter 1 and if you have forgotten it, go back and check it again.

Of course, for years it has been possible to contract other diseases from a visit to the hairdresser, but these were not killers.

It is important that the industry is seen to be doing its fair share to protect clients from AIDS. Many salons do not know what to do, so we will make some suggestions for guidelines. Although the public are most concerned about AIDS, these guidelines will also help to prevent other diseases such as hepatitis, impetigo, and ringworm. Hepatitis, which can be spread by blood if you were to cut an infected client, is four times more common in hairdressers than nurses, and it can kill.

Is the client in any danger from the hairdresser?

The simple answer is 'yes', but only if the hairdresser has an infectious disease. The golden rule should be that you do not touch a client if you have some kind of infectious skin condition yourself, unless this is on the body and is covered by clothes. If you have something wrong with you, ask your doctor if it is necessary to take precautions to stop it spreading.

How can dangers be minimised for the client?

- You should wash your hands if you have been to the toilet, sneezed, blown your nose, or eaten something.
- Always use sterile tools on each client, including fresh towels.
- Where possible use disposable neck strips, etc.
- Check the head of *every* client before you shampoo them. Check for possible infections, or infestations of lice. Be suspicious if the skin is at all red or scratched. Working on a client with an infectious condition puts other clients at risk.
- Wash down salon surfaces as a regular routine.
- Keep bins covered, use pedal type if possible.

What methods are suitable to sterilise tools in the salon?

The words 'sterilise' and 'disinfect' have slightly differing meanings. If you sterilise anything, it becomes completely free of all living organisms. Disinfectants will kill germs if used long enough, and strong enough. Many people will not carry this out correctly, and it is possible that some resistant spores will survive (a spore is a bacterium or fungus that has a tough coating protecting itself; they are usually the last things to die during sterilisation). In salons it is important always to clean a piece of equipment before any method of sterilisation is carried out. You cannot sterilise dirty equipment, so before using any of the methods described below, wash your equipment in hot soapy water.

Moist heat sterilisation

This involves boiling water, so is only suitable for equipment that can withstand heat or which will not rust. Towels should be washed between every client, and the hot wash cycle of most washing machines should be suitable for this. It is designated as wash cycle 1 and should reach 95° C. Boiling water can be used to sterilise some heat-resistant plastics but the problems associated with steam and condensation must be thought of. It is possible to cause electrical safety hazards if there is excessive condensation, and it is always irritating if mirrors steam up. One of the most effective methods of sterilisation is with an autoclave, a sophisticated type of pressure cooker. By trapping steam inside a sealed vessel so that there is a build-up of pressure (usually 15 pounds per square inch), the boiling point of water can be increased from 100°C to 121°C, ensuring sterilisation. This is illustrated in Figure 2.8. Some manufacturers have developed electrically operated autoclaves that can be bought for a few hundred pounds and operated without danger in salons. One is illustrated in Figure 2.9: tools are placed in an internal tray. Check that your tools can withstand the heat before placing your favourite brushes in the autoclave. Between 20 and 30 minutes is

Figure 2.8 Water boiling (a) in an open container and (b) in a pressure cooker.

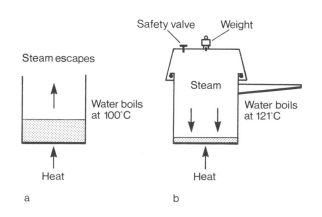

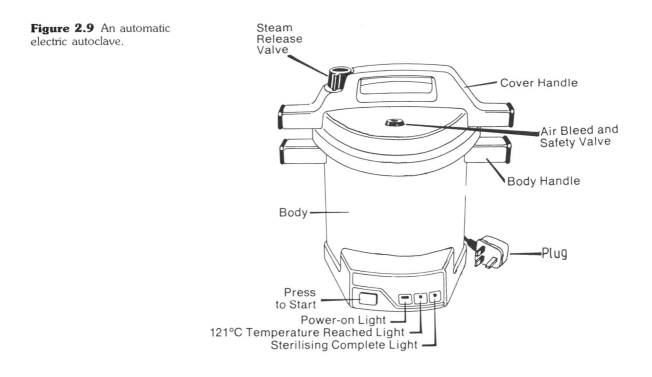

Figure 2.9 An automatic electric autoclave.

required for moist heat (simple boiling) to be effective and the cycle for most autoclaves is also about 30 minutes.

Chemical vapour

This method involves the use of a cabinet that allows equipment to be surrounded by a sterilising vapour. The vapour used in the past was formaldehyde, which is produced by placing some liquid formalin in a dish above an electrically operated heater. Once the formalin is heated it gives off the formaldehyde vapour. The cabinet has perforated metal shelving for equipment to be placed on. A diagram of a cabinet is shown in Figure 2.10. It is particularly useful for hair nets and sponges, as the vapour will penetrate them. It is not recommended for metal tools as it attacks the surface and can cause pitting. Use for 20 minutes.

There have been scares about formaldehyde causing cancer, but if used as directed a cabinet should be safe. Alternative liquids to formalin have been produced recently so that this is both an effective and utterly safe method of sterilisation.

Ultra violet

This type of radiation is used in many salons in sterilising cabinets. It is so common because it does not produce smells and looks modern. It is

Figure 2.10 Vapour
sterilising cabinet.

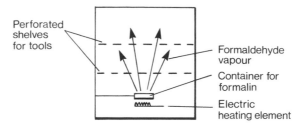

only effective on the surfaces that the ultra violet rays touch, so is not
suitable for equipment that needs more than surface sterilisation. Tools
must be turned because the mercury vapour lamp that produces the
ultra violet light is situated at the top of the cabinet, as shown in Figure
2.11. The cabinets are a good place to keep tools which have been
sterilised by other methods until they are ready for use and this would
be our recommendation for the salon.

Figure 2.11 Ultra violet
sterilising cabinet.

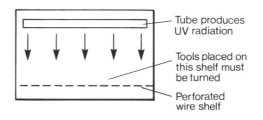

Disinfectants

There is a variety of disinfectants on the market and manufacturers are
marketing ones specifically for use in salons. Because your tools are in
constant use disinfecting jars such as the ones produced by Barbicide
are particularly useful. Tools can be stored in the disinfectant, in this
case a quaternary ammonium compound, in between clients. (Barbicide
was first patented in America by a chemist who had picked up ringworm
while at the hairdresser!) Figure 2.12 shows jars in two sizes. The one on
the left is designed for manicure equipment, while the one on the left is
for hairdressing tools. This particular solution will not cause rusting so is
particularly suitable for scissors, razors, clipper blades, brushes and combs.
The tools can be removed from the Barbicide jar by raising the lid as
shown in the jar on the right.

Figure 2.12 Barbicide disinfecting jars being used on a variety of tools. (Courtesy of Renscene Ltd, Surrey.)

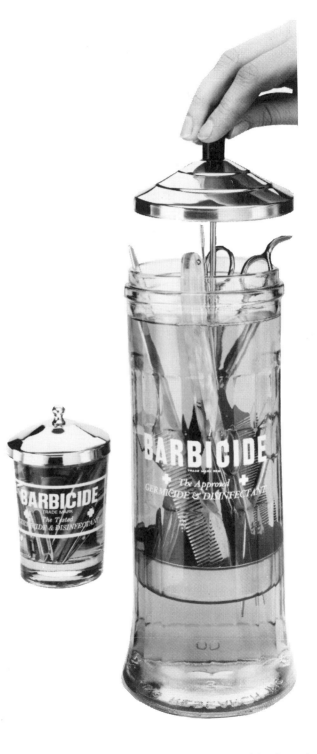

There are some other suitable disinfectants available, based on compounds such as glutaraldehyde which are equally effective. Recently this has become available in an aerosol spray form so that it can be used on clippers. Alcohol can also be used to sterilise your tools, but remember that it is flammable and should never be used near a naked flame. Once alcohol disinfectants have been used they should be poured down a sink with plenty of running water to dilute them. The most important thing about using disinfectants is to make up solutions freshly as directed by the manufacturer. Clean your tools before immersing them in the solution, leave them in for the *required time* and change the solution as directed by the manufacturer. Check with the manufacturer about rusting of metal tools before you commit your salon to using a particular brand. Remember to also wash down worksurfaces daily, with hot soapy water and disinfectant. Never use abrasive cleaners for cleaning surfaces (including basins) as these will cause tiny scratch marks where germs can multiply.

> After sterilisation is complete (by whatever method), equipment will only remain sterile until it comes into contact with the air in the salon. Keep it in a sterilisation cabinet until its next use and place onto paper towel rather than directly onto work surfaces. Do not place tools in pockets or hold clips in the mouth.

Questions

1. Why is hygiene so important in the salon?
2. Can the client be in any danger of catching infection from the hairdresser?
3. List six points of salon hygiene that will minimise the dangers of spreading infection.
4. What is the difference between sterilisation and disinfection?
5. What is the last thing to die during sterilisation?
6. What should be done to tools before they are sterilised?
7. What are the two main methods of sterilisation using moist heat?
8. What kind of tools should not be sterilised using moist heat?
9. Why does water in an autoclave boil at a higher temperature than normal?
10. Why is formalin not used as much as it used to be in vapour cabinets?
11. What kinds of salon equipment can be effectively sterilised in a vapour cabinet?
12. Would you use an ultra violet cabinet as your only method of sterilisation in the salon?
13. For what other purpose can you use an ultra violet cabinet in the salon?
14. List the three main points that you should observe to use disinfectants properly?
15. Why should abrasive cleaners not be used on work surfaces?
16. How long does equipment remain sterile?

17. Should you sterilise tools between clients even if they do not have an infectious condition?

Non-infectious conditions

Dandruff (also called Pityriasis capitis)

This is one of the most common scalp conditions seen in the salon, with about half the population being sufferers. There are usually patches of small dry greyish-white scales on the scalp. This is caused by abnormal shedding of the top lay of the epidermis and, when severe, the scales are seen on the clothing of the sufferer. Normal services can be given and your salon should carry products to treat the condition. It is simply an over-production of epidermal skin cells, and may be seen on skin anywhere on the body.

Psoriasis

This is recognised by the presence of red patches covered by silvery-white scales. Each individual patch of psoriasis may be fairly thick and raised above skin level, with red edges. It is caused by a rapid increase in cell division in the epidermis and appears to run in families. Two per cent of the population are affected by psoriasis. On the scalp psoriasis is usually seen in patches which may protrude onto the forehead or neck. This is illustrated in Figure 2.13. Sufferers often have attacks linked with emotional stress, but there is nothing psychologically or mentally wrong with them! Normal services can be given as long as the scalp is not damaged.

Figure 2.13 Psoriasis scales on the front hair margin.

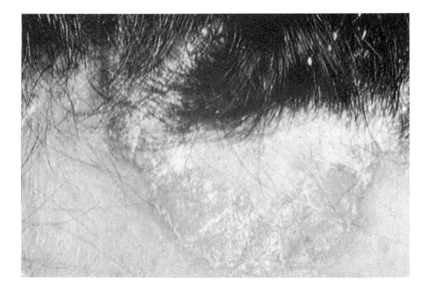

Seborrhoea

Put simply this is excessive production of sebum caused by overactivity of the sebaceous glands. This is a condition which is diagnosed by the client, as it is very much a personal opinion whether or not you think you have excessively greasy hair. It is more common in males than females as sebaceous gland activity is linked to sensitivity to male hormones. Because it is linked with male hormones (called androgens) it begins at puberty. By 16 years of age males usually are producing higher amounts of sebum than females. The female hormone oestrogen inhibits sebum production so many women have problems once they reach the 'change of life'. Someone with true seborrhoea, rather than slightly greasy hair, will have lank hair which is difficult to style because of the amount of sebum produced. Sufferers usually also have problems with acne. Although normal services can be given refer to the next section for tips on management of the condition.

Seborrhoeic dermatitis

This is a condition which is most common amongst those of us with Celtic ancestry (Irish, Scottish and Welsh). It resembles a cross between dandruff and psoriasis, being recognised by redness and patches of scale. It will be worse than dandruff but the scaling is not usually as thick as that seen with psoriasis. Although the name implies a connection with sebum the skin is usually dry. Old names die hard, however! It is commonly seen near the ears and along the hairline and outbreaks in sufferers are often linked with stress. Normal services can be given.

Sebaceous cysts

These can be recognised as hard lumps which vary in size from that of a pea to an egg. This is caused by a blockage of the sebaceous gland and such cysts can often give the hairdresser a shock. Sometimes a fatty excretion can be squeezed from the cyst. Normal services can be given, although care should be taken not to damage the skin.

Alopecia

This is a general term which means 'baldness', but there are several types that you should be able to recognise. *Androgenic alopecia* or male pattern baldness – the common baldness of the ageing male – has a characteristic pattern of development, even if it starts in the late teens! The earliest change is a slight recession of the front hairline, usually followed by thinning on the crown. If the condition develops fully, there is complete loss of

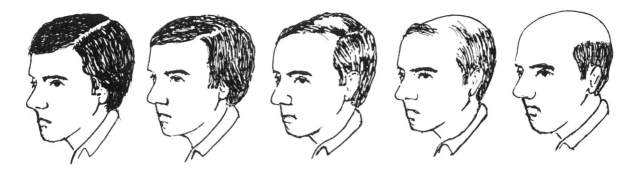

Figure 2.14 The progression of male pattern baldness.

the hair on the top of the head. See Figure 2.14 for diagrams of the progression of the baldness.

The condition is caused by a sensitivity to the male hormones (androgens) and there is usually an obvious family history (like father, like son). This type of baldness develops in many women after the menopause when female hormone levels drop, and it can sometimes be difficult to distinguish between the sexes in geriatric wards. Normal services can be given. Figure 2.15 shows male pattern baldness in a 30 year old man, in this particular individual the hair loss began at 19 years of age.

Diffuse alopecia — a gradual thinning of the hair rather than a straightforward bald patch — is the most common cause of hair loss in women. The causes are varied, ranging from a lack of iron (anaemia), to thyroid

Figure 2.15 Male pattern baldness in a thirty-year-old man.

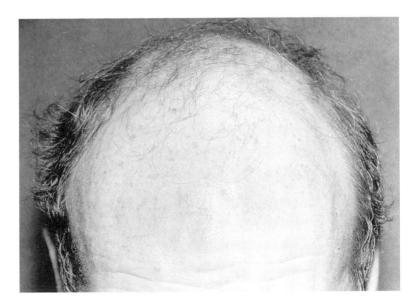

problems, tumours, severe illness or following the birth of a child! Many women have problems after they stop taking the oral contraceptive pill. Normal services can be given.

Alopecia areata is a type of baldness which starts as small circular bald patches. The skin in the patches is normal (look back at ringworm of the scalp and compare this), although there may be some short hairs on the edges of the patches. The patches enlarge in size and begin to join up, forming larger bald areas. The condition appears to run in families and is often brought on by shock or stress. Basically all the follicles in the bald patch have gone into the resting stage of the hair growth cycle (see the end of this section) at the same time, so the condition should last about four months before the hair regrows (this regrowth is often white at first). In some cases the baldness may spread to produce total loss of scalp hair, but you are unlikely to see clients like this because they will not require your services. Normal salon services can be given.

Cicatricial alopecia is baldness caused by scarring. The scarred skin contains no hair follicles so no hair can grow. Scarring could be due to physical damage to the skin, burning by chemicals or heat, or as the result of infection (commonly seen with boils on necks or small bald areas on scalps caused by chicken pox scars). If you examine the bald area carefully there will be no sign of a hair follicle opening on the skin surface. Normal services can be given, although the baldness will be permanent because the hair follicles have been destroyed. An example of cicatricial alopecia is shown in Figure 2.16.

Figure 2.16 Cicatricial alopecia due to the scars left by bacterial infection.

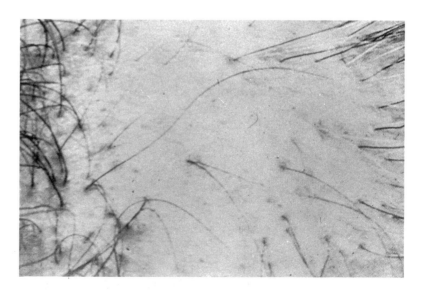

Traction alopecia is a loss of hair due to constant pressure being placed on the hair, such as would occur from a tight pony tail. The loss of hair would be at the front hairline. It is also seen in plaiting and Sikhs commonly suffer from it. Normal services can be given. Some people, usually children, pull out their own hair (called trichotillomania); students studying for exams often 'twiddle' their hair as they read!

Figure 2.17 Split ends.

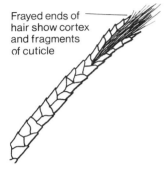

Frayed ends of hair show cortex and fragments of cuticle

Split ends (also called Fragilitis crinium)

This condition refers to the splitting of a hair at its ends, although the splitting may occur along the hair shaft. The hair is dry and brittle, the cause being misuse of chemicals and too much physical abuse (heat, brushing, sun). It is common on long hair, because the hair is older at the ends and has taken more abuse. The splits may be short in length or may eventually 'run' to affect greater lengths (see Figure 2.17). Although normal salon services can be given the results will not be as good as they would if the hair was not damaged.

Trichorrhexis nodosa

This is the term given for the condition where nodes or swellings appear along the hair shaft and is illustrated in Figure 2.18. The node is produced when the cuticle of the hair is damaged and is a swelling of the cortex outwards. The condition is normally caused by either physical or chemical damage to the hair, but there are also some rare genetic and metabolic disorders which produce it. Those who produce nodes when very little physical trauma has been applied to their hair usually have a disorder in the formation of cortical keratin. The hair of sufferers may show whitish nodules and the hair can be easily broken. There may be short areas of hair because of this on some scalps. Salon services may be limited because of the possibility of hair breakage, depending on how bad the condition is.

Figure 2.18 Trichorrhexis nodosa.

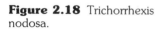
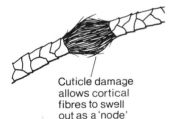

Cuticle damage allows cortical fibres to swell out as a 'node'

Monilethrix

This is a condition of the hair shaft where the hair appears to be 'beaded'. It is caused by an uneven cell division in the dermal papilla of the hair and is hereditary, so may be seen running in families. From the diagram in Figure 2.19 it can be seen how the follicle has produced a hair with wide and narrow zones. No medulla is present where the hair is narrow. You can usually recognise the condition because of the shortness of the hair, which can break with minimal physical damage. There may be alopecia associated with this condition. Luckily, it is a rare condition, and great care should be taken when offering salon services because of the risk of breakage.

Figure 2.19 Monilethrix.

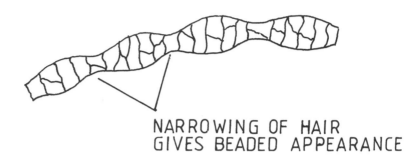

NARROWING OF HAIR
GIVES BEADED APPEARANCE

Trichonodosis

This is simply knotting of hair. It is usually seen in a small number of hairs and may be caused by harsh physical treatment such as brushing. The hair may tangle and is not easy to unknot. Normal services can be given.

Grey hair

Also called canities, this is a mixture of white hair and coloured hair, leading to characteristic greyness. There is no such thing as a single grey hair, it will be either white or coloured. Hairs go white when the melanocytes which produce pigments do not function properly. It can be temporary or permanent and most of us will eventually have some degree of greyness. It is impossible to go white overnight as coloured hairs cannot suddenly lose their colour. However, shock could cause coloured hairs to fall out, leaving the white hairs.

Questions
1. What is the other name for dandruff?
2. How many people suffer from dandruff?
3. How would you recognise dandruff on a client?
4. What causes dandruff?
5. Can it be caught?
6. What shampoos does your salon carry to treat dandruff?
7. Does dandruff only occur on the scalp?
8. How would you recognise psoriasis?
9. What is the cause of psoriasis?
10. How many people suffer from psoriasis?
11. What can attacks of psoriasis be linked with?
12. Can normal services be given?
13. What is seborrhoea?
14. What is the cause of seborrhoea?

15. Who are the most common sufferers from seborrhoea?
16. Can normal salon services be given?
17. How would you recognise seborrhoeic dermatitis?
18. Is there a connection between this condition and sebaceous glands?
19. Where are you likely to see it?
20. Can normal salon services be given?
21. How would you recognise a sebaceous cyst?
22. What causes them?
23. Can normal salon services be given?
24. What should you be careful of?
25. What does the word alopecia mean?
26. What is the other name for androgenic alopecia?
27. How does it usually start?
28. How much of the head can become involved with this type of baldness?
29. What causes the condition?
30. When is it most likely to develop in women?
31. How would you recognise diffuse alopecia?
32. What are the common causes of diffuse alopecia?
33. Who is most likely to suffer from it?
34. How would you recognise alopecia areata?
35. What infectious condition could it easily be mistaken for?
36. How would you tell the difference between the two conditions?
37. What can cause alopecia areata?
38. How long does it take for the lost hair to regrow?
39. What colour can this regrowth be?
40. How bad can alopecia areata become?
41. What is the cause of cicatricial alopecia?
42. How can you recognise it?
43. What are the possible causes?
44. How long does it last?
45. What is traction alopecia caused by?
46. How would you recognise it?
47. What is trichotillomania?
48. What is the other name for split ends?
49. How would you recognise them?
50. What are the possible causes of the condition?
51. Why is it more common on long hair?
52. How would you recognise trichorrhexis nodosa?
53. What can cause the condition?
54. What will limit the service that you can give?
55. How would you recognise monilethrix?
56. What causes the condition?
57. Will a medulla be present in the hair?
58. Can you give a normal salon service?
59. What is trichonodosis?
60. What is the other name for grey hair?
61. Are there single grey hairs?
62. Is greyness permanent?
63. Can a coloured hair turn 'white' overnight?
64. Is there any explanation for someones hair turning white overnight?

Supplementary information on hair growth

How does a hair grow?

A hair grows from a minute pit in the skin called a hair follicle. The hair that we see emerging from the scalp is dead, but at the base of the follicle the hair is alive and actively growing. As the hair we deal with is dead, we cannot alter how it grows by any hairdressing process or treatment. We can, however, alter the physical appearance of the hair once it is visible above the skin, but will always have a problem with regrowth.

All growth in the human body occurs by a process called cell division (technically termed *mitosis*). Basically, an individual cell divides into two, producing two smaller copies of itself. This division of cells occurs at the very bottom of the hair follicle from a group of cells known as the papilla. Figure 2.4 showed a hair in its follicle in the centre of the skin diagram. The blood supply at the base of the follicle is extremely important as it is the blood which supplies the hair with everything it needs to grow. We have already said that hair is made from a protein called keratin. All proteins are made up from a series of tiny building blocks called amino acids, which are linked together in a particular order to make different proteins. The blood supplies the hair follicle with these amino acids so that the hair can grow. All activity requires energy to occur and in the papilla this is provided by the oxidation of glucose. The blood supplies the necessary oxygen and glucose to the papilla. The only way to improve the condition of hair permanently is through the blood supply to the follicle. We get the necessary glucose and amino acids from a balanced diet. As the body cannot store amino acids/protein, we must have it in our diet every day. (This is one of the reasons why the quality of the hair of someone with anorexia becomes very bad and eventually drops out.) As the cells divide and grow in the papilla, they push the older ones upward towards the opening of the follicle at the scalp surface. The dividing cells which are alive at the base of the follicle gradually change shape and develop keratin as they are pushed upwards, becoming dead about two-thirds of the way up the follicle.

Does a hair keep growing forever?

The answer to this is definitely no. Each hair follicle produces hair in cycles. A new hair grows actively for a number of years, it then dies at the base of the follicle and for a few months the follicle rests before a new hair starts to grow. We become aware of this when we brush or comb our hair, as the old hairs are shed. Because this hair growth cycle is in different phases over your whole head you do not go bald! Anyone with pets will know how many of them moult in winter and spring as part of their cycle of hair growth. The growth cycle is explained in Figure 2.20.

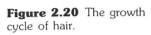

Figure 2.20 The growth cycle of hair.

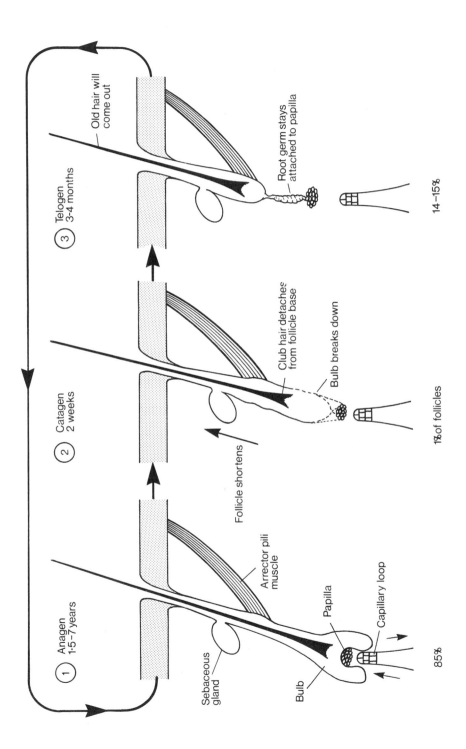

How fast does a hair grow?

The figure quoted in most books is 1.25 cms (half an inch) per month. This is an average figure which can vary from one person to the next depending on a number of factors:

- Hair grows faster in the summer (ultra violet radiation, found in sunlight, speeds up cell division).
- Hair grows faster in the young and slows down with old age (it is at its peak between the age of sixteen and the late twenties).
- It can be slowed down by illness and hormones (including pregnancy and the contraceptive pill).
- New hairs grow fastest; hair growth slows down with increasing length (almost half the original rate when the hair is a metre long).

See Hygiene – A Salon Handbook for more information.

Does cutting hair speed up its growth?

No! Otherwise we would all be having our hair cut short! Cutting does not alter the speed of growth or the diameter of the hair. Thus the story of shaving legs making the hairs grow coarser is untrue. Many young men who shave for the first time are convinced that shaving has made their beards coarser, but it is only because recently shaved stubble feels coarser than if a beard is left to grow (this is because of the length of the hair). So, although it is not true that the hair grows faster it is certainly good for business! Because the lines 'grow out' more quickly on short haircuts clients with such styles will generally visit salons more frequently.

Why does the length people can grow their hair differ?

You should be able to work this one out for yourself from the different information supplied above. If the hair grows about half an inch a month this means it will grow about six inches in a year. People who can grow their hair down to their bottoms must have an active growth of hair (the anagen part of the growth cycle) that lasts for about six years to achieve this kind of length. If someone else can only grow their hair to their shoulders, this will be because the active growth only proceeds for about two or three years (two years would give about twelve inches' growth). So it is the period of active growth, or anagen, which determines final hair length – if scissors do not interfere. The length of time anagen lasts can become shorter as you get older, this accounts for someone who had waist length hair as a child not being able to grow it past their shoulders as an adult.

Questions
1. Where does the hair grow from?

2. Is the hair we see on the scalp alive or dead?
3. Where is a hair alive and actively growing?
4. Why can we not alter the growth of a hair by hairdressing processes or treatments?
5. How does hair growth occur?
6. Where does mitosis occur in the follicle?
7. What supplies the hair with nutrients?
8. What is the hair made from?
9. Why are amino acids required in the blood?
10. Why are glucose and oxygen required?
11. Why should you eat protein every day as part of your diet?
12. Do individual hairs keep growing indefinitely?
13. If hairs die and fall out, why do we not go bald?
14. List the three names given to the parts of the hair growth cycle.
15. How long does each part last?
16. What happens in each part?
17. How fast does a hair grow?
18. What time of the year does hair grow fastest?
19. Why?
20. At what age is hair growth fastest?
21. What can slow hair growth down?
22. Does cutting hair speed up its growth?
23. Does cutting hair make it grow coarser?
24. Why does the length the hair can grow differ from individual to individual?

The action to be taken for different hair and scalp conditions

We have just discussed the common hair and scalp conditions that might be encountered on your clients in the day-to-day working of a salon. Some of these conditions were infectious and therefore should never be treated in the salon. If you were to treat a client with an infectious condition you would be putting both yourself and other clients at risk of the infection. However, you should be able to tell clients the appropriate course of action to take if they have an infectious condition. This could include recommendation of a home treatment available from a chemist without prescription, referral to a doctor or a trichologist (a trichologist is somebody who specialises in the treatment of the hair and scalp). Although the non-infectious conditions cannot be caught it is still very important that you know what action to recommend to a client, as some conditions are caused by serious illness.

Infectious conditions

Impetigo: This will require antibiotics to be taken which the client will need to get from the doctor.

Scalp ringworm: This will require antibiotics to be taken which the client will need to get from the doctor.

Warts: Remember that these are only infectious when damaged. Many people will not want to be bothered with treatment for warts on their scalp if they cannot be seen. Hairdressers with warts on their hands should have them removed as they can easily become damaged and spread. Warts can be burnt off at home over a period of time using chemicals which slowly attack the infected skin. These are available from a chemist without prescription but can take months to work. The quick way to have them removed is to see your own doctor who can then send you to a specialist (dermatologist or skin doctor) at a local hospital. The warts are then burnt off, usually with extreme cold. In the majority of cases this will work first time. The doctors who perform the task are very skilled and leave little in the way of scarring.

Head lice: Any client who has head lice should go to the local chemist and ask for the appropriate lotion. Although shampoos are available they are much weaker and need several applications to work. (If you wanted to kill someone with poison it would be quicker to give one large dose than several small ones! It's the same with lice.) The lotions are available in either an alcohol or a water base. Alcohol should be preferred unless the client has a sensitive scalp (suffers from eczema, etc.). The lotion is applied and left to dry naturally as heat will destroy the action of the chemical. Both lice and nits will be killed by the lotion, but the nits will still be left attached to the hair. Special fine-toothed combs are available to remove these. The alcohol lotions are flammable so great care should be taken with fires and cigarettes. Everyone in a household should be treated at the same time. Many salon workers begin to imagine itchy scalps when they have found head lice, so it is as well to treat yourself if you are really worried! Some useful facts to tell a client with head lice are:

- There are one million cases a year in the UK.
- Head lice prefer clean hair to dirty hair.
- Head lice are not a sign of being dirty or unhygienic.
- Head lice are usually caught from children.
- There is a residual protection from alcohol-based lotions (this means that lice which came onto the scalp a few days later would be killed by the chemical still within the hair) but this can be lost by swimming in chlorinated pools or from having the hair permed.
- Regular combing and brushing of hair (particularly for young school children) helps eliminate head lice as they are damaged by it and eventually die from that damage. Imagine yourself as a head louse for a moment: if you had your arms or legs ripped off you would not feel like having relations with the opposite sex to keep those eggs laying! If lice have only just arrived on a head they might therefore be damaged before they can do anything.

Always try to reassure the client that you are not shocked by it and make them another appointment for after they have treated themselves. Most of us would be embarrassed and you do not want to risk losing a valuable client. Many stylists will offer to check the scalp of the client when they return to the salon — there is no risk if they have been treated!

Scabies: A client with scabies should see their doctor to have the diagnosis confirmed. They will need to obtain a lotion from their chemist which must be painted over the whole body from the neck down. All members of a household are normally treated and bedding and clothing needs to be thoroughly washed.

Questions
1. Why should infectious conditions not be treated in the salon?
2. What are the three main courses of action that you would recommend to a client for treatment of an infectious condition?
3. What would you tell a client with impetigo to do?
4. What would you tell a client with scalp ringworm to do?
5. How can warts be treated?
6. Why should hairdressers have warts removed from their hands?
7. Where would you tell clients to obtain their head lice treatment from?
8. Would you recommend a lotion or a shampoo?
9. Why?
10. What would you tell a client who had eczema?
11. Should clients only treat themselves?
12. How many people in the UK get head lice each year?
13. What kind of hair do the lice prefer?
14. From whom are head lice usually caught?
15. What does the term 'residual protection' mean?
16. Why is brushing and combing of hair useful to help prevent head lice in school children?
17. Why should you make the client another appointment?
18. What should you tell a client with scabies to do?

Non-infectious conditions

Dandruff: Your salon will carry a range of products to treat dandruff so *sell* these to the client. Don't tell them to go down to the chemist and buy one from there! See Chapter 3.

Psoriasis: Some salons will carry coal tar preparations such as shampoos and ointments for treating psoriasis. These can help clients and can be sold to them or treatments can be carried out in the salon. A client with bad psoriasis should be referred to the doctor or trichologist for further treatment. Doctors can use steroids or chemicals which dissolve keratin to clear it or send the client to the local hospital for treatment with ultra violet.

Seborrhoea: Shampoos for greasy hair can be used and a better care routine can be recommended to your client (see Chapter 3). However, if the condition is severe with associated acne that could cause scarring, medical treatment may be necessary and the client should see their doctor for possible specialist referral.

Seborrhoeic dermatitis: This will respond to a number of treatments available in the salon, including those for dandruff and particularly psoriasis. As the condition can be associated with allergies clients should be referred to their doctor for further investigation.

Sebaceous cyst: If any clients have a cyst which they find embarrassing they will need to have it surgically removed and so should see their doctor.

Androgenic alopecia (male pattern baldness): Once someone has it there is little they can do to regain their lost hair. In the salon you could offer massage to help increase blood supply to the scalp. Many men resort to wearing a wig or a weave-on (a wig which is stitched to existing hair to keep it firmly in place). These may look natural at first but, after a few years, may fade in sunlight or the client may turn grey. More drastic measures involve hair being transplanted from the nape to the crown, basically spreading the hair around, or scalp reduction (removal of the bald scalp!). These are all remedies for clients who are really concerned about their baldness, but we would recommend that they see a trichologist before being surgically parted from a large part of their wallets! There are sprays available which will thicken existing hair and therefore increase its covering power.

Diffuse alopecia: As this can have some serious medical causes referral is necessary unless there are more obvious reasons. A woman who has had a baby within a few months has an obvious cause and regrowth should occur with little problem. A woman who has heavy periods and a lack of iron in the diet can improve the situation by eating liver, heart or kidney along with plenty of fresh green vegetables. Although iron tablets can be taken our bodies do not absorb it very easily. Anorexia may also be obvious, and would require specialist medical help. As thyroid problems and tumours may show no other external signs except for the hair loss medical referral is very important.

Alopecia areata: This is a condition that should clear up by itself but in many people the condition gets worse, so medical referral is often necessary. Trichologists also offer a good service for this condition. In the salon massage will help along with anything that stimulates the scalp.

Cicatricial alopecia: As this is caused by scarring little can be done for it. If the scar is very evident you might be able to design a style that makes it less apparent. Some people have hairs transplanted around scars to try and hide them and medical referral would be advisable for this.

Traction alopecia: As this is caused by tension you will need to advise clients about the way that they style their hair so that the amount they use is reduced. Frighten them if necessary by telling them that they will lose more and more hair if they keep applying too much tension!

Split ends: Cutting off split ends is the only permanent treatment but you can recommend a course of conditioning treatments and give advice on haircare to prevent or reduce further problems. Also see Chapter 3.

Trichorrhexis nodosa: This kind of damage is so severe it will not be possible to 'mend' the hair although conditioners will improve the quality and handling characteristics. Advice on haircare to prevent further problems should be given. Also see Chapter 3.

Monilethrix: Little can be done for this condition as it originates at a cellular level and has nothing to do with bad haircare. Conditioning, however, will help improve the strength of the hair. Depending on the extent of the problem you might be able to disguise it with good hairstyling.

Trichonodosis: This knotting of hair can be caused by rough handling so advice on haircare should be given.

Grey hair: This can start in the early twenties, depending on the individual. If it bothers the client the hair can be coloured. Semi-permanents will cover a little grey while tints will be required for a larger amount of greyness. Do advise clients not to use metallic hair colour restorers, which can look very unnatural (they can impart a greenish tinge in certain lights) and prevent a number of further hairdressing processes.

Questions
1. Where should a client get their dandruff treatment from?
2. Has your salon any treatments for psoriasis?
3. To whom would you refer a client with psoriasis?
4. When would you refer clients with seborrhoea to their doctor?
5. What would you advise a client with seborrhoeic dermatitis to do?
6. What can be done for a sebaceous cyst?
7. What can be done for someone who has androgenic alopecia?
8. If someone with this condition was really worried who would you advise them to see?
9. Diffuse alopecia has a number of causes: list four of them and the appropriate actions that should be taken.
10. What action would you recommend for a client with alopecia areata?
11. Can anything be done for cicatricial alopecia?
12. What kind of advice would you give a client who suffered from traction alopecia?
13. What is the only permanent treatment for split ends?
14. Can anything be done to improve the condition of the hair?
15. What can be done for trichorrhexis nodosa?
16. Can anything be done for monilethrix?
17. What advice would you give a client with trichonodosis?
18. What can be done for a client with grey hair?
19. If any clients told you that they were considering using a hair colour restorer what could you say to them to put them off?

Identifying clients' requirements by consultation

Consultation, as defined by dictionaries, will refer to 'a meeting of two or more persons to deliberate and discuss a matter which requires specialist expert knowledge'. In the salon, the hairdresser is the consultant because he or she possesses the expert technical knowledge. The client is given a consultation which will either be to ask the opinion of, or take the advice of the expert.

The terms consultant and consultation are strongly linked to professions that revolve around the process of consultation: the solicitor, doctor, dentist, etc. When we visit the dentist they tell us what should be done to our teeth; they do not ask us how many fillings we would like or whether we want an extraction! However, in many salons it is quite a different story. We have actually witnessed hairdressers *ask* their clients what size of roller they want in their hair! That is certainly neither a professional approach nor a consultation.

A consultation is a *process* which means it requires active participation from all the parties concerned for it to be successful. Although this will be usually just you and the client it could also involve a parent in the case of a younger client. It is not a matter of a hairdresser telling the client what is needed, which is a one-way line of communication. Consultation should be involved with making suggestions, offering expert advice and seeking approval from the client to perform a service at an agreed price. This process obviously takes time and allowances to carry it out properly need to be made in the way the salon arranges appointments. Time spent with the client *before* the service is begun is as important as the time the hairdresser actually spends working on the client's hair. Without the consultation, the hairdresser is reduced to being a menial performing a technical skill as opposed to a professional responding to the needs and requirements of individual clients.

This process can be described as a flow chart:

The consultation process

Client enters salon
↓
Client is greeted and offered a seat
↓
Client is given a consultation by the hairdresser
↓
Agreement is made (by client and hairdresser) on course of action
↓
Service is given or postponed to future date

Finding out exactly what you need to do to clients' hair to make them satisfied can be a lengthy and difficult process. Please notice, that we did not refer to 'what the clients want', because in many cases they do not know and have gone to the hairdressers to be offered advice about what will suit them and their hair type.

All consultations should be carried out before a service begins and when the hair is still dry. You should have checked the condition of the hair and scalp for any signs of disease or damage as described earlier. During the consultation, you will need to ask plenty of open-ended questions to elicit all the necessary information that will assist you and your client in selecting the most appropriate options from those which are available. Please remember that clients may not always be totally honest with the answers they give you because they may fear retribution or that a service might not be given if they tell the truth.

Choosing a hairstyle

Sometimes, clients may have a very clear idea of how they want their hair to look, and often bring pictures with them, cut out of magazines. A particular actress or singer may have a hairstyle that they admire, and they may ask you to make their hair look the same. Don't make the mistake of pretending you know the actress or singer they are talking about if you haven't got a clue who they are, let alone what their hair looks like! Clients will often choose a look that in your professional opinion, is totally unsuitable for them. Unsuitable styles are sometimes chosen by clients because they want to be like the image of the model in the picture. The picture will probably be showing an attractive, youthful female with glowing skin, perfect teeth and an abundance of healthy, shining hair. You look at the client that has handed you the picture and your heart sinks. *Never*, however, make derogatory remarks about a client's request or laugh at their suggestions. Saying things like 'I know I'm good but I can't perform miracles' or 'you can't make a silk purse out of a sow's ear' should only be said in the privacy of the staff room, if they must be said at all! In such an instance, you will need to make alternative suggestions to your client, perhaps based on their original idea, or a new option all together. Always try to say something positive about their unsuitable suggestions so that you respond in a pleasant way while at the same time putting your expert advice across. For example:

- To client with protruding ears who chooses a style which will empha-sise them:
    'The back would look great like that, but if we leave it a little longer at the sides, it will lie a lot better over the ears. What do you think of that idea?'
- To client with a high forehead who wants her hair swept straight back from her face:
    'How do you feel about having a fringe? If we sweep it across like this, it will add softness to the style and will emphasise your nice cheekbones.'
- To client with out of condition hair who wants a perm, which you know will be a disaster:
    'If you have a series of remoisturising treatments, your hair will be in better condition and the perm result will be far better. How do you feel about having your perm in a few weeks' time when your hair is back in condition? You could have the first of the remoisturising treatments today.'

Can you see how, in these examples, the hairdresser puts across suggestions without saying anything derogatory, but at the same time seeks confirmation from the client about the action to be taken?

Many hairdressers find it useful to use visual aids to assist them in discussing ideas and specific looks with clients. Visual aids include style books, photographs around the salon, the hair of colleagues, shade charts, etc.

Finding out about previous treatments

It is always important to establish the previous treatments that the client has had. You will need to question your clients about the number of chemical treatments that they have had done on their hair and how they usually care for their hair between salon visits. In effect, you need to build up a hair history for your clients. Examples of questions you may need to ask are set out below with reasons for asking them. These questions are not in any specific order and they may not all be relevant to every client situation:

Q. When did you last shampoo your hair?' (Helps to diagnose activity of sebaceous glands.)

Q. What shampoo do you use at home?' (Indicates what hair type the client thinks they have and their approach to home hair care.)

Q. 'When did you have this perm? What did you think of the result?' (Tells you what the client expects from a perm.)

Q. 'Have you ever had any form of colorant used on your hair?' (Tells you if the hair colour you are seeing is natural − avoid using words like dye or bleach.)

Q. 'Have you ever had any major colour change?' (Tells you whether the hair has been chemically treated when it is not showing obvious signs of this.)

Q. 'How long ago was your hair last cut?' (Indicates how much the hair has grown since it was cut.)

Q. 'Are you on any medication or have you recently had an operation?' (The general health of hair often deteriorates when a person is taking certain medication, is ill or has undergone anaesthesia.)

While you are asking these questions, it is a good idea to be seated next to your client in a position that encourages intimacy so that they feel 'safe' to answer you honestly, or ask while examining the client's hair. *Never* look at a client's hair with disgust as you examine it. This is both embarrassing and unnecessary. Even if you think the last salon ruined their hair, there is no need to say it. The client wouldn't be sitting in front of you if they thought *That* salon had done a good job. It is unprofessional to criticise the work of another hairdresser and it makes clients feel uncomfortable when you do so. You should not be on an ego trip about your own standards. If a client ever asks you directly 'Do you think they ruined my hair?' a good way of answering is to say something like, 'Well, you obviously aren't happy with it and I think we can improve how it looks'. By responding in this way, you are not drawn into the trap of 'slagging off' another salon. You can never really be sure that the client went to that salon or if she did the damage herself!

Questions

1. What is consultation?
2. Who is the 'expert' in a salon consultation?
3. Who should be involved in the consultation?
4. What is a 'one way' line of communication?
5. Do the clients always know what they want before they come into the salon?
6. Are clients always honest in their answers to questions about their hair?
7. How do clients try to give you a 'picture' of the type of style they want?
8. How should you respond to their suggestions if they are unsuitable?
9. Make up two new examples of client requests and your answers.
10. What do you understand by 'visual aids'?
11. Check to see what is available in your salon.
12. When you are questioning the client how should you be seated in relation to the client?

Diagnosing the condition of a client's hair

We are all born with hair that is in good condition, but it is what we (and others!) do to it that causes it to become damaged. There are two categories of hair damage: physical and chemical. Physical abuse is non-chemical and is caused by the general daily handling of the hair. Examples of physical abuse include:

- excessive heat;
- sea and chlorinated water;
- strong sunlight;
- harsh combing and brushing;
- excessive tension on the hair.

Chemical abuse is caused by the hair being subjected to chemicals such as:

- tints and bleaches;
- perms and relaxers;
- harsh shampoos.

You should be able to recognise when the hair is out of condition and also the reasons for this (see earlier). A client who uses hot tongs every day to style hair will have caused the hair to become dry and brittle. Someone who has a perm on top of bleached hair is also going to cause hair to be in poor condition. You will therefore need to question your clients about previous hairdressing treatments and what they do to their hair between salon visits. You will also need to examine the hair to establish the degree of damage to the outside of the hair (cuticle) and the internal structure (cortex). To determine the degree of damage you will need to carry out two tests: a porosity test for assessing the condition of the cuticle and an elasticity test for the cortex.

Questions
1. What are the two categories of hair damage?
2. Give examples of each.
3. How would you go about establishing the degree of damage to the client's hair?

Identifying hair that has been incorrectly treated

Without doubt, you will encounter clients during your hairdressing career who have damaged hair caused by the incorrect use or application of products or processes. As examples of such mistakes you might encounter any of the following:

- broken hair;
- burnt scalp;
- over-curly hair after perming;
- hair that has gone straight after perming;
- patchy colour results;
- uneven hair cut;
- chemically abused hair;
- physically abused hair.

Often, many of the problems you encounter are very noticeable while others may only be seen once the hair and scalp are examined. Therefore, always part the hair to look closely at the scalp and hair all over the head. While you are doing this you can be asking your client questions that will tell you what has caused this damage.

Questions
List examples of hair and scalp damage which have resulted from incorrect hair treatment.

Styling limitations

During your consultation, while you are examining the hair and discussing options with your client, you should be able to identify any restrictions that you are faced with in terms of future processes or styling that can be offered to the client. Broadly speaking, it is the condition of clients' hair, their hair type or that they are asking for something that will not suit them that are the restricting factors. You will encounter clients who request a perm on top of a recent perm or the client with fine hair who wants a style that will only be successful on hair which is more abundant. There will also be clients who choose a styles that will not suit their face shape or will emphasise, rather than detract from, their less attractive features.

Restrictions caused by the condition of the hair

Hair which is out of condition is more susceptible to further damage because its strength and resistance is already reduced. Having established the degree of damage by doing porosity and elasticity tests, you will be able to determine whether it is advisable to perform certain services or use particular products. Here are some examples of when it would be unwise to carry out chemical treatment, because of the additional damage that would be caused and the poor result:

- perm on bleached hair;
- a relaxer on top of a perm;
- a perm on top of a relaxer;
- a perm on hair that has been treated with henna;
- any chemical service on hair which is showing signs of breakage.

Restrictions caused by the client's hair type

The most frustrating limitation for clients in terms of not being able to have what they have asked for, is being told that their hair is not long enough. Despite being told this, clients will still sometimes repeat their request, saying that they will be satisfied if it is a shorter version of the style. What isn't made clear to clients is that this does not always work. Certain styles rely upon there being sufficient hair in particular areas, and without it the style will just not work.

Having the wrong type of hair for a particular look can be devastating to a client. First, they probably won't believe you and, second, they might think there is another reason why you are suggesting they have something different. Often, hairdressers will treat this situation as a challenge for their skills and will proudly complete the style on a head of hair, forgetting that the client may have tremendous problems maintaining the particular style.

Limitations caused by unsuitable client requests

We have already touched on the problem of clients requesting styles that do nothing to compliment them. One of the first questions you need to ask is 'Why are you asking for this to be done?' There could be the influence of a partner, friend or member of the family that has induced such an unreasonable request, or it could simply be ignorance about what suits them. Try suggesting alternative options and do not ridicule clients. Remember that you are the expert and need to respect your clients' feelings and be sympathetic to their concerns. Obviously, you will need to consider the head and facial characteristics of your clients so that you create a style that suits them.

Questions

1. What do you understand by a styling limitation?
2. What are the restricting factors for a planned style?
3. List examples of restrictions caused by hair condition.
4. List examples of restrictions caused by clients' hair type.
5. List examples of restrictions caused by unsuitable client requests.

Hair growth patterns

The direction of hair growth is very important because nothing a stylist can do will alter how the hair grows naturally. This means that forcing the hair in the opposite direction to its growth can often spell disaster because it will not lie properly and will fight to lie in its natural direction. This is particularly evident if a widow's peak is present on the front hairline, for example.

A widow's peak is a strong, centre forward growing peak of hair found on the front hairline. Trying to style the hair into a full fringe would be difficult because it is going against the direction of the natural growth. The stylist may manage to make the hair look acceptable but the hair would soon separate and lift at the widow's peak and the client may find it very difficult to manage.

A cowlick is also found on the front hairline and is a strong growth of hair which grows in a sworl. Again, fighting the natural hair growth direction is not recommended. It is better to work with the natural lie of the hair.

The nape hairline will have its own unique pattern of growth. It may be low in the neck and grow to one side or be high and grow into the centre. The hair at the nape should not be forced against its natural growth or it may stick out the day after styling. It is not usually recommended to cut above the natural hairline because of this problem, but false hairlines can be created using scissors, razors or clippers.

The crown is usually situated at the top or back of the head and forms the natural hair growth pattern for this area. Occasionally two crowns may be detected, referred to as being a double crown.

A natural parting is where the hair falls and parts naturally from the front hairline to the crown(s).

The true lie of the hair can only truly be seen when the hair is wet because certain hair growth peculiarities may be disguised by the styling

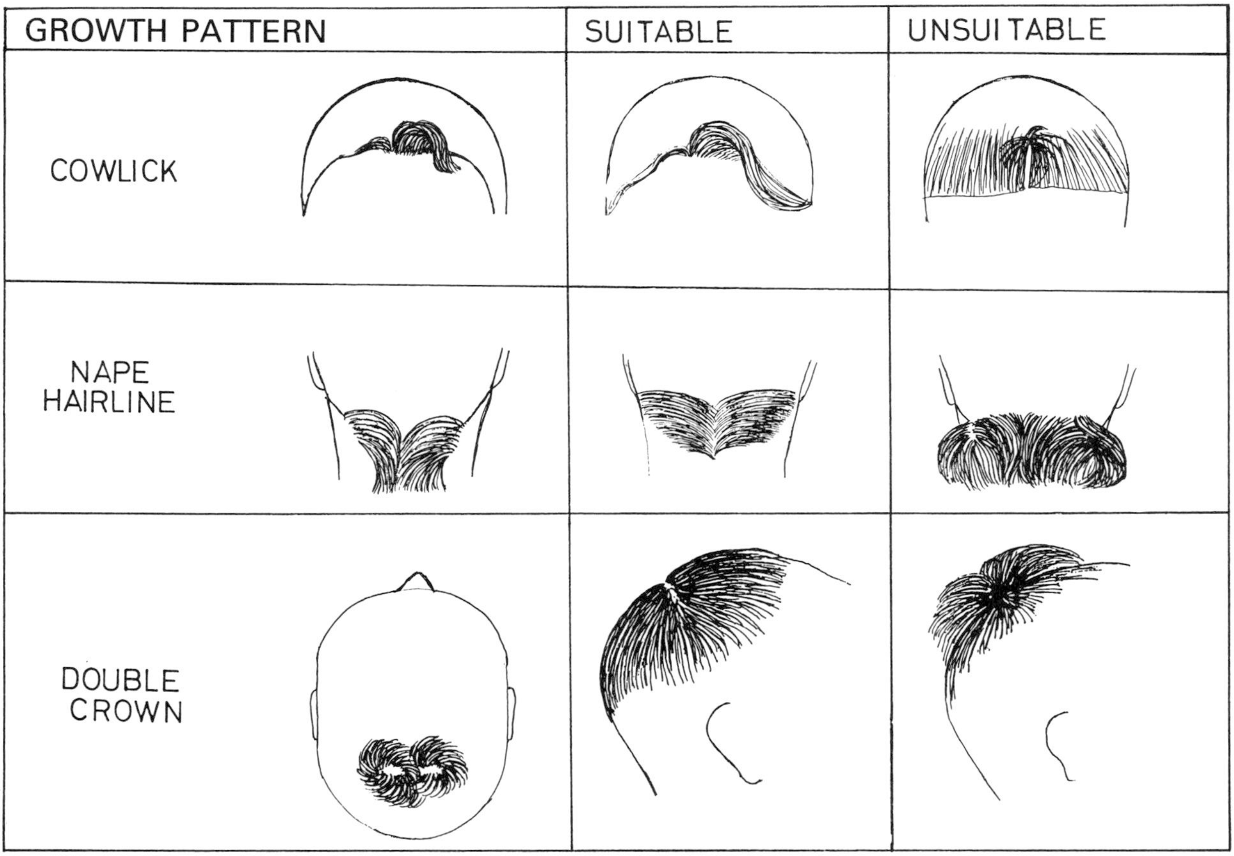

Figure 2.21 Suitable and unsuitable styling techniques for particular hair growth patterns.

technique used previously by the client. The amount of lift at the roots of the hair can also more easily be seen when the hair is wet. Look for unusual root movements and hair growth direction. Words used to describe hair growth include, cowlick, widow's peak, crown, natural parting, root lift, root direction, etc.

In Figure 2.21 are some diagrams which show how different hair growth patterns are more suitable for particular styles than others.

GROWTH PATTERN	SUITABLE	UNSUITABLE
COWLICK		
NAPE HAIRLINE		
DOUBLE CROWN		

Questions
1. Why are hair growth patterns so important to a planned style?
2. What is a widow's peak?
3. What is a cowlick?
4. Look at the nape hairlines of some friends and describe the patterns of growth.
5. What are single and double crowns?
6. What is a natural parting?
7. Why should you wet the hair to see the true lie of the hair?

Explaining hair treatments to clients

When a person goes into hospital for an operation, a doctor will always talk to the patient before the operation to explain what will take place. The doctor will outline the preparation procedures, the operation itself, and how the patient can expect to be feeling afterwards. Things are explained in easy to understand language so that we (the laymen) understand what is being said. Doctors don't use the same language that they would use if they were in conversation with other doctors discussing a similar issue.

When clients come into a hairdressing salon they may be feeling as apprehensive as a person going into hospital for an operation. They will have heard stories about terrible things that can happen to hair and how hairdressers always 'do what they want' and are 'scissor-happy'. They will need reassurance and one way of reducing anxiety is by telling clients what they can expect to happen. It is the unknown that induces fear and anxiety; if clients know, the anxiety is reduced.

In the salon, time should be spent informing clients of the various stages of processing they will be going through for each service. To be able to do this effectively, the hairdresser must be fully informed, so that he or she can speak with confidence and answer any questions that the client may ask. This also means being able to describe things in a clear, concise way and avoiding the use of technical language that can create feelings in the client of ignorance and confusion. For example, if you are explaining to a client the stages of a perming process, there is no need to include words like cystine linkages, ammonium thioglycollate and disulphide bonds. Here is a list of the stages of a perm as we would describe it to a client:

'After your hair has been shampooed and cut, I'll wind the hair on special rollers used for perming. When all the hair is wound up, a special lotion will be applied, and this will be left on the hair for about fifteen minutes. The lotion will then be rinsed out from your hair and another lotion will be applied to the rollers. After about five minutes, all the rollers will be taken out and more lotion is applied. Finally, your hair will be rinsed and conditioned and you'll be ready to have it dried. In all, I expect it will take about three hours to do this, and it will cost you _____.'

It would be a useful exercise for you to practise how you would describe the various treatments offered in your salon. Try doing this with a colleague, who can tell you how well you did. If you are unsure about any of the services you will need to talk about to clients, we suggest that you refer to the necessary chapters to look up the procedures for shampooing, conditioning, perming, neutralising, colouring and relaxing.

Questions
1. Why should you always talk to clients before beginning their hair?
2. What kind of language should be used?

3. Why might clients need reassurance?
4. List, in simple language, the procedures for shampooing, conditioning, tinting and bleaching.

Explaining to clients the limitations caused by previous chemical treatment which was incorrectly carried out

You will remember from previous sections some of the indicators you may encounter which will tell you that the previous chemical treatments the hair has been given have been incorrectly carried out. Not only do you need to be able to identify symptoms of maltreatment but also be able to explain to clients how these symptoms now make their hair unsuitable for certain treatments. For example, a client returns to your salon because a recent perm has completely dropped out and there is no curl left. The client makes the complaint and asks for the perm to be redone. The client's hair is tinted and thus porous. The perm increased its porosity and it now feels very dry and brittle. Although there is no curl present, the hair has been chemically treated and any further perming will make it even drier. It would therefore be unwise to carry out the service of reperming the hair. As an alternative, the client could be offered a course of conditioning treatments (perhaps free of charge in these circumstances) until their hair could be successfully permed.

The causes of unsuccessful or incorrect results can be categorised into ten main areas:

- lack of technical skill and knowledge on the part of the hairdresser;
- under-processing;
- over-processing;
- poor application;
- insufficient product knowledge;
- misinterpretation of client's requirements;
- failure to analyse the client's hair properly and carry out the necessary precautionary diagnostic tests;
- using products which have 'gone off';
- using products which are incompatible with each other;
- failing to follow the correct procedure.

When a client has cause for complaint because of a hairdresser's negligence, it should be remembered that in serious cases, they may try to sue the salon. Please refer to the later section on dealing with clients' complaints.

Questions
1. List the causes of unsuccessful or incorrect results.
2. What could happen if the hairdresser has been negligent in the service that he or she has provided?

Diagnostic hair tests

It is important to remember that clients are not always aware of the products they have used on their hair, or of the significance of answering your questions truthfully. We have all come across clients who have a regrowth but still insist that their hair is natural and has never been bleached or tinted! Unfortunately for the hairdresser, not all products used previously on the hair are as obvious to detect.

Whatever kind of chemical work you are doing to hair, get into good working habits. Eventually you will do things automatically. Tell your clients what you are doing and why. They will appreciate your care and professionalism. An examination of the scalp must be the first thing that you do just in case there is anything wrong with the scalp (as discussed earlier). This examination must be positive and thorough but not embarrassing for the client. It is best carried out during your initial talk with the client, while you discuss the intended style.

Assessing previous chemical treatments

When you analyse a head of hair for any chemical treatment the client may have already had other treatments within the past few months. They may answer your questions about previous chemical treatment, but can you be sure that their answers are totally honest? Clients may feel embarrassed that they had previous treatment at another salon, or attempted to do their own hair at home. Treatments such as perms just may not have lasted so may not be at all obvious.

Why is it important to establish previous chemical treatment?

Once hair has been subjected to chemical processing such as tinting, bleaching, perming or relaxing, its internal structure becomes weaker and prone to further damage. Any further unplanned use of chemicals on the hair could result in a weaker type of hair that will not retain moisture, and will be dry or like 'straw'. The damage may be so extensive that the hair will break off, entitling the client to sue the salon for any damage caused by any new chemical treatment.

How can you establish previous chemical treatment?

Besides questioning the client there are a number of ways by which you can establish previous chemical treatment. Always check the hair near the roots so that you are aware of the natural colour. If the hair has been coloured or lightened you should be able to see this against the natural colour. Previous perming treatments are checked for by a pre-perm test (see later on in this section). First, we will examine the external and internal condition of the hair using porosity and elasticity tests.

Porosity test

A porosity test assesses the hair for external damage, that is, the degree of damage to the outside layer of the hair (the cuticle).

What does porosity mean?

Porosity describes the cuticle's ability to absorb moisture and hairdressing products. Porous hair will obviously allow products to penetrate more easily into the hair than will non-porous hair (see Figure 2.22). It is probably easiest to compare the hair to a sponge: the bigger the holes, the quicker liquid will be soaked up. The porosity of the hair will vary on different parts of the head and also on each individual strand of hair. The older a hair is, the more likely it will be that the ends of the hair are porous; it will have been subjected to more abuse such as chemicals, drying or weathering (sun, sea and wind). This is why people with long

Figure 2.22 (a) Porous and (b) non-porous hair.

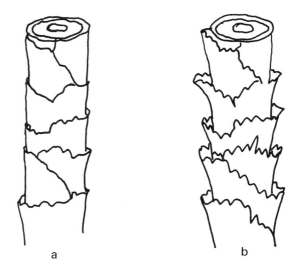

a   b

hair find that the ends of their hair feel drier and rougher compared to the middle lengths or roots. This is what hairdressers mean when they refer to 'uneven porosity'.

What makes hair become porous?

Damage to the cuticle can be caused in two ways: (i) chemically, (ii) physically.

Chemical damage is caused by hairdressing products which are alkaline, as these cause the hair to swell and open up the cuticle (see Chapter 8). This leaves the hair more susceptible to further damage, both internal and external. As so many hairdressing treatments involve alkaline chemicals a certain amount of cuticle damage is unavoidable.

Physical damage can be caused in a number of ways. The regular use of heat is one of the most common. Many people use tongs, heated rollers, crimping irons or excessive heat from a hairdryer every day. Too much sunlight can also affect the cuticle. Backcombing, harsh brushing or the use of elastic bands can also cause damage. The ends of the hair, being the oldest part, will be the most damaged both chemically and physically.

How is a porosity test carried out?

Take a few strands of hair and hold firmly near the points. Slide your fingers down the hair shaft to the roots (against the lie of the cuticle). The rougher the hair feels, the more porous it is (see Figure 2.23). Remember that you may need to test several areas as porosity is never even and will vary over the whole head. The hair at the front hairline will usually be more porous than that at the nape because it receives more physical attention (brushing, etc.) and damage from the weather.

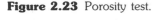

Figure 2.23 Porosity test.

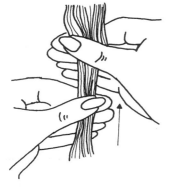

Why should you test for porosity?

If the hair is porous, it means that the cuticle is open or has actually broken off, in varying degrees along the hair's length. As the chemicals for tinting, bleaching, perming and relaxing need to enter the cortex, the chemicals will enter at different rates, depending on the cuticle's porosity. The hair which is most porous will allow penetration most quickly. The hair in such areas will have more air spaces and will therefore absorb more chemical, leading to more rapid chemical processing, and possible severe damage before the rest of the hair is processed. Results will be patchy and uneven with possible breakage in weaker areas.

Can the porosity of the hair be improved?

The simple answer is 'yes', but only temporarily. This is explained in Chapter 3.

Elasticity test

An elasticity test is a method of assessing the degree of damage to the internal hair structure, i.e. to the cortex.

What does 'elasticity' mean?

Elasticity is the ability of hair to be stretched and then return to its original length when the stretching force is removed.

How elastic is the hair?

A hair in good condition can stretch up to an extra third of its length and then return to its original length. The extension of hair is opposed by the weak hydrogen bonds and stronger disulphide bonds (see Chapter 8). The cuticle scales play no part in elasticity and simply slip over each other as the hair is stretched.

If dry hair was extended more than a third of its length it would reach its elastic limit. Beyond this the hair would not return to its original length when the stretching force was removed. As all the hydrogen bonds are broken the coiled structure of the hair collapses and the hair breaks or snaps.

As can be seen from Figure 2.24, wet hair can stretch twice as much as dry hair without being damaged. This is because the amount of moisture present in the cortex allows water to become bound to the hydrogen bonds, allowing them to extend further so that they give less resistance to stretching. Hair which has been dampened with perm lotion overstretches easily because hydrogen bonds are broken by the alkaline lotion. Although it has an elastic limit of 70 per cent the hair structure is damaged (this is why hair is wound without tension in cold waving).

Because of its elastic nature, hair in good condition can withstand relatively great forces without breaking. Hair is stronger than copper wire of the same diameter!

Figure 2.24 Elasticity of hair.

Condition of hair	Elasticity
Dry, normal hair	20–30%
Wet, normal hair	50–60%
Hair, dampened with cold wave lotion	70% (hair damaged)

What makes hair lose its elasticity?

Poor elasticity is due to the cortex of the hair being damaged. It is caused mostly by chemical processing (perming, relaxing, bleaching or tinting) which attacks the disulphide bonds of the cortex. The reduced number of bonds means that the hair stretches more easily but cannot return to its original length. Severe physical abuse such as the use of excessive heat can also cause the hair to lose its elasticity. Little damage is caused to the cortex by combing and brushing.

How do I test the elasticity of hair?

Take a single strand of hair and hold firmly at each end with the thumb and forefinger. Pull gently between the fingers and see how much the hair stretches and springs back. As you will be doing this test (see Figure 2.25) with dry hair, you will not see much stretching if the hair is in good condition. However, if the hair does stretch, or even snaps, it has a weak cortex. Just like an old elastic band, damaged hair will break when stretched as there are not so many bonds present to resist the stretching force.

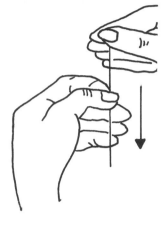

Figure 2.25 An elasticity test.

Why should you test for elasticity?

As has been said above, elasticity is a reflection of the condition of the cortex. Both perming and relaxing affect the bonds of the cortex so it is important to know whether or not the bonds are already damaged. If too many bonds are damaged the resulting chemical treatment will make the hair structure weaker still, making good perm results impossible as the hair will not have the strength to hold the curl. Relaxed hair will be extremely dry and will snap easily.

Can internal hair damage be repaired?

It is impossible permanently to repair the chemical bonds in the cortex once they are damaged but conditioning treatments are available to strengthen the hair (see Chapter 3).

Incompatibility test

An incompatibility test indicates whether or not any products previously used on the hair will react unfavourably with the products that you intend to use. It is specifically to test for the presence of metallic salts which are contained in some hair colour preparations that would have been used by the client at home. They are most commonly found in so-called 'hair colour restorers'. These are products which are used regularly over a period of time to give back colour to grey hair. On each application the hair is coated with metallic salts. These subsequently react with the atmosphere to produce a dark colour. Because the colour takes time to develop it is referred to as a progressive colorant. The best known product is *Grecian 2000*. There are also some henna preparations which contain metallic salts, usually referred to as being 'compound'. Their addition allows henna to have a greater colour range and staying power. Some temporary colours also contain metallic salts. They are usually available as spray colours (aerosols), gels or mousses; often containing metallic glitter. For further information, see *Colouring – A Salon Handbook*.

How can you tell if metallic salts are present on the hair?

The surest way is to carry out an incompatibility test. You might suspect that metallic salts were on the hair because it has a greenish tinge to it, or because it feels unnatural to the touch, even after washing. Don't assume clients will tell you they use it if you ask them, as they may not want people to know they are grey and colour their hair. The advertising used to promote such products makes them sound as if they are natural and undetectable. It is more likely to be the older client who uses them but, if in doubt, carry out the test.

What do you need to carry out an incompatibility test?

You need:

- glass container;
- 20 volume hydrogen peroxide (6 per cent);
- ammonia (0.880 ammonium hydroxide);
- hair samples from client;
- sellotape;
- record card.

How is an incompatibility test carried out?

- Prepare the hair samples by cutting from an unnoticeable area and secure at the root end with sellotape. Make sure your samples are from the areas you estimate to be most affected by the metallic salts. You may need more than one sample.
- Mix together twenty parts of the peroxide with one part of the ammonia in the glass container. If ammonium hydroxide is not available in the salon, substitute perm lotion instead. Ammonia will speed up any reaction that occurs; peroxide alone would be too slow.
- Immerse the sample(s) into the solution. Leave them in the solution for thirty minutes as some hair might be slow to react.
- Check the sample(s) for the presence of bubbles and feel the container to see if it has got any warmer. The hair might also change colour. If any of these occur it is *a positive reaction.*
- A positive reaction means that you cannot use any chemicals on a client that contain hydrogen peroxide, as it will react violently and could damage both the hair and scalp.
- The metallic salts can also combine with the sulphur bonds in the cortex, interfering with perming or relaxing.

Can hair containing metallic salts be permed?

The simple answer is an emphatic 'no' if you use a product containing hydrogen peroxide. Claims have been made that they can be stripped by special treatments, but these have proved unreliable. One firm makes a special neutraliser which can be obtained if you have used their product on your hair. The only way to remove metallic dyes properly and completely is to let them grow out so that they can be cut off.

Pre-perm test for curl

This test is carried out to see the extent to which any previous perm still affects the hair. A previous perm carried out four months ago may not be apparent when the hair is dry, because the hair may have been set or blow dried (which will stretch the hair out). It is therefore necessary to wet the hair to see whether curl is present. Wetting hair will cause set or blow-dried hair (beta keratin) to return to its normal state (alpha keratin). See Chapter 7 for further information on this. If there is any curl remaining only towards the ends of the hair it may be cut off. However, if too much curl remains then permanent waving should not be undertaken because of the risk of damage.

Test curl

A test curl is a precautionary test taken to ascertain whether or not a head of hair will take a perm successfully. It is carried out with different perm lotions so that the result can be achieved with minimum damage being caused to the hair. It is carried out by processing and neutralising one to three meshes of hair wound on rods. By assessing the results of the wound meshes, the hairdresser can establish the following:

- the most suitable rod diameter to achieve the desired curl pattern;
- the appropriate strength and type of perming product;
- the processing time;
- whether the hair can take a perm.

When should the test curl be carried out?

Some salons always carry out a test curl before proceeding with the complete wind to ensure satisfactory results. A few manufacturers recommend that a test curl is done before using their products, so always check the instructions for the product you intend to use. Most often, hairdressers carry out a test curl if they suspect that the hair may not respond well to a perm. In such cases, the hair may already be chemically processed (bleached, tinted or already permed), indicating that further chemical treatment may result in severe damage.

Sometimes the hair may have highlights. Does the hairdresser use a perm lotion suitable for the bleached strands or for the natural hair? The client may be taking medication, which might interfere with the perming process. Pregnant women often find that perm results are unsatisfactory because of changes in their hair structure (due to changed hormone levels and uptake of amino acids from diet into the hair structure being different during pregnancy).

What do I need to take a test curl?

- perm product(s) and matching neutraliser(s);
- curlers of different diameters;
- end papers;
- gloves;
- cotton wool strips;
- applicator bottle(s) for perm products;
- bowl(s) and sponge(s) for neutraliser(s);
- tail comb;
- pre-perm treatment (if hair has uneven porosity);
- plastic cap;
- record card.

How do I carry out the test curl?

1. Prepare hair for perm as directed by product manufacturers.
2. Apply pre-perm treatment if necessary.
3. Make a centre parting from forehead to crown so that the test curl can be positioned at the crown (see Figure 2.26).
4. Wind one to three rods at the crown and damp with the perming product (see Figure 2.26).
5. Position a damp cotton wool strip around the wound rods and cover the head with the plastic cap.

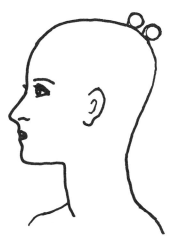

Figure 2.26 Position of rods at crown of head.

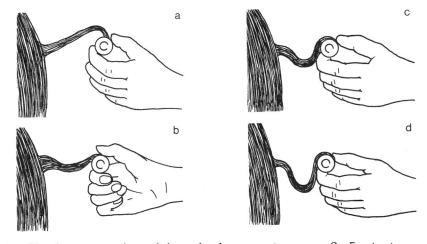

Figure 2.27 Checking curl development in a curl test. (A) Gently unwind your chosen rod without putting any tension on the hair. (B) You can see from the diagram that the rod is carefully unwound without pulling or stretching the hair. (C) The rod is gently nudged forward to the scalp to see if the hair has taken on the new shape determined by the rod size used. (D) The curl test in this example shows that the hair is sufficiently processed because the mesh has taken on the same shape as the rod on which it was wrapped. The 'S' shape will be equivalent to the diameter of the rod.

6. Check your watch, and then check processing every 3–5 minutes. Remember that if the hair is porous it will take up more lotion and therefore process more quickly. Also, the higher the salon temperature, the quicker the hair will process. Figure 2.27 shows how to check curl development.

7. When processing is complete, rinse the rods thoroughly with warm water. Remove excess moisture from the rods by blotting with a towel or cotton wool (excess moisture left in the hair will dilute the neutraliser).

8. Apply the neutraliser as recommended by the manufacturer and leave to process according to instructions.

9. Rinse neutraliser from the hair and apply a conditioner.

10. Check the test curl result(s) and record on the record card.

How do I assess the result of the test curl?

By examining the hair that has been tested you will be able to determine how well the hair responded to chemical processing. This assessment is carried out by answering the following questions:

Curl pattern − has the hair taken on the anticipated degree of movement? If the result is *too weak*, the cause could be related to the following faults:

- The rod used was too big.
- The processing time was too short.
- There was a barrier on the hair so perm lotion did not penetrate properly.
- Insufficient tension was used when winding.
- The perm lotion was too weak for the hair type.
- Neutralising was not carried out properly.

If the result is *too tight*, this is caused by using a curler which is too small.

If the hair is *straight* and *frizzy* it is because the hair is overprocessed. This is due to −

- using too strong a lotion for the hair type;
- allowing the hair to process for too long (often seen on bleached hair because the perming product penetrates through the porous cuticle into the cortex so quickly).

Elasticity − has the elasticity of the hair been weakened by the perming process?

If the hair is now lifeless with no bounce, perming all the hair must be avoided. An elasticity test will indicate the damage that has been done to the cortex.

Processing − how long did the processing take?

If the hair took longer to process than anticipated (according to your initial analysis of the hair and the type of product being used), you may need to use a stronger product to achieve the desired result more quickly.

If the processing occurred very quickly, consider using a weaker product or apply a pre-perm treatment (if you didn't when you carried out the test curl) to act as a buffer, slowing down the chemical reaction.

The warmer the salon is when perming, the quicker the hair processes. If you believe that the hair processed more quickly because of the heat in the salon, process the perm without using the plastic cap (the cap helps trap heat coming from the scalp and accelerates processing).

End papers — did the end papers (used to prevent buckled ends) change in colour?
Sometimes the end papers will show stains of hair colour which are lost from artificially coloured hair during the perming process. However, the end papers may turn pink or purple due to deposits of chemicals from the client's medication which have been taken up into the hair. If this is the case, check the test curl for possible damage and curl pattern. If there is damage, perming may not be possible.

If the test curl is satisfactory, what next?

When the result of a test curl is satisfactory, or you have established what changes need to be made in the light of the test, you may continue with your perm. You will not need to reperm the meshes of hair that were treated by the test curl. Section the test area neatly and wrap in cling film to protect the hair from further chemical treatment. The rest of the hair may be permed using your usual technique.

If the test curl is unsatisfactory, what next?

When the test curl result is unsatisfactory and you have established that changes to the product strength or size of rod will make no significant improvement, you should not perm the rest of the hair. If you were to go ahead with the perm, the result would be no different than the disappointing test curl and your client would be dissatisfied. Instead, explain to your client why a perm should not be carried out and suggest an alternative such as a restyle which does not rely on the support of a curl. The client will value your professionalism once she understands the reasons for not carrying out the perm. If a client is adamant that she wants her hair permed let her have it ruined at another salon!

Once a test curl has been performed a small area at the crown may be curly while the rest of the hair is straight. Suggest a conditioning treatment and stretch out the curl by setting or blow-drying. It is advisable *not* to relax the curl chemically as this would damage the hair.

Curl test

This test is performed during the perming process to check the development of the curl, so that you will know when adequate processing has occurred to prevent unnecessary damage to the client's hair.

If you wound using the pre-damped method (see Chapter 8 for an explanation of the terms used) check the first and last wound rods, while if you use the post-damped method check one rod from the front, crown and nape areas. Follow manufacturer's instructions for when the rods should be checked. As a general guideline there is no need to check for the first ten minutes, but from then on check processing every 3–5 minutes as indicated in Figure 2.27.

> (a) Gently unwind your chosen rod without putting any tension on the hair.
> (b) You can see from the diagram that the rod is carefully unwound without pulling or stretching the hair.
> (c) The rod is gently nudged forward to the scalp to see if the hair has taken on the new shape determined by the rod size used.
> (d) The curl test in this example shows that the hair is sufficiently processed because the mesh has taken on the same shape as the rod on which it was wrapped. The 'S' shape will be equivalent to the diameter of the rod.

Test cutting

This is a way of assessing colour results before the application of the intended product to the entire head of hair. It can be carried out to test the results of temporary, semi-permanent and permanent colours as well as bleaching.

Take test cuttings from unnoticeable areas of the hair and secure them at the root end with either sellotape or cotton. You may need several. Mix your intended products and immerse hair samples into labelled bowls. Process as directed by manufacturer's instructions, rinse off the colour and dry with a hairdryer. Examine the cuttings in natural light. The test cutting will clearly indicate to both you and the client exactly how the hair will respond to the colouring products or method used. Damaged hair has uneven porosity and will result in uneven colour; the test will help you to decide whether the hair can take further chemical treatment, and if it can, what will give you the best results.

Strand test

A strand test is a means of monitoring colour development either at the roots or along the entire length of the hair during processing.

Before a colorant is rinsed from the hair, it is always advisable to do a strand test to ensure it is sufficiently developed. This is done by removing the colorant from a small mesh of hair with a piece of damp cotton wool. By cleaning the colorant off the mesh of hair, the hairdresser can then see if the colour is even along the length of the hair by comparing the points to the root area. If the colour is not even, the hair is given extra development time, but if the choice of colorant was wrong in the first place, it is unlikely that more time will improve the result.

Strand tests are also used during colouring processes to monitor development and to check if a regrowth tint application is ready to be combed through or rinsed off. This is done by either cleaning the tint off a small patch of the roots with damp cotton wool or by gently scraping the tint off the roots with the back of a comb. This procedure is also followed for checking bleach and colour reducer (stripper) development.

Questions

1. Why is it important to establish the previous chemical treatment that has occurred on a head of hair?
2. What can you tell from simply looking at the hair, particularly near the roots?
3. Why should you perform a porosity test?
4. What does porosity mean?
5. Why are the ends of the hair more porous than the roots?
6. How would you carry out a porosity test?
7. Why is porosity important to chemical treatments?
8. What is an elasticity test?
9. What is the difference in elasticity between dry and wet hair?
10. What makes hair lose its elasticity?
11. How would you perform an elasticity test?
12. Why does damaged hair break when stretched?
13. Why should you test for elasticity?
14. What is an incompatibility test?
15. When would you perform one?
16. Describe how you would perform an incompatibility test.
17. What does a positive reaction indicate for subsequent chemical processing?
18. Why would you perform a pre-perm test for curl?
19. How would you perform this test?
20. What is a test curl?
21. Why should it be carried out?
22. How would you carry out a test curl?
23. How would you assess the result of the test curl?
24. What are the reasons for a weak result?
25. What are the reasons for a tight result?
26. What are the reasons for straight or frizzy hair?
27. What could you do if the hair processed too quickly or too slowly?
28. Why might the end papers change colour?
29. What should you do if the test curl is satisfactory?
30. What should you do if the test curl is unsatisfactory?
31. What is a curl test?
32. What rods should be checked if you have pre-damped or post-damped?
33. Describe how you would carry out a curl test.
34. What is a test cutting?
35. When would you use it?
36. Describe how you would carry it out.
37. What is a strand test?
38. When would you perform one?
39. How would you perform one?

Skin tests

Skin tests are performed with small amounts of chemicals to see if a client would develop an allergic reaction. Rather than risk a serious full scale reaction over the whole scalp the client would show a reaction on the skin test area only. Such a positive reaction would indicate that the chemical could not be used on the client. Skin tests are usually carried out before tinting but should also be carried out before application of a number of semi-permanents. This is because they contain either para-phenylenediamine or para-toluenediamine as their active ingredients. An example of a positive reaction to a tint is shown in Figure 2.28. Such allergic reactions are referred to as dermatitis or contact eczema.

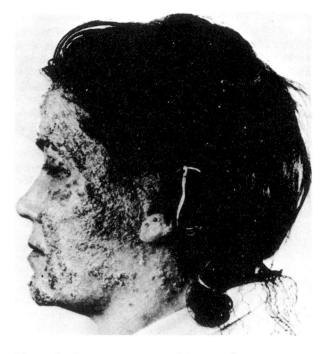

Figure 2.28 An example of an allergic reaction to a tint that could have been prevented by giving a skin test. (From *Practical Dermatology* by I. B. Sneddon and R. E. Church (3rd Edition), Publisher: Edward Arnold.)

How do I carry out a skin test?

The test should be carried out 24—48 hours before the planned application of the tint. The product(s) that you intend to use on the client should be used to carry out the skin test. Giving someone a skin test for a black tint when you intend to use a red one does not make sense as their ingredients are different. It would be like being sick every time you ate an apple and a doctor testing you for allergy to an orange!

- Protect the client with a gown and towel.
- Mix a small amount of tint (i.e. 2 cms or 1 capful) with equal parts of peroxide (use the strength of peroxide that you intend to use on the client).

- Cleanse either the inside of the elbow or behind the ear using cotton wool and spirit (alcohol, which will remove sebum).
- Place a small smear of tint (about the size of a penny) on the cleansed area and allow this to dry naturally or cover with collodion (Nu-skin).
- Advise the client to leave the patch alone until returning to the salon, unless it begins to irritate, when it should be washed off and calamine lotion used to relieve the irritation.
- Record relevant information on your record card.
- Check that there has been no positive reaction when the client returns to the salon. A positive reaction would be redness, swelling, itching or any sign of irritation.
- If there is a positive reaction *under no circumstances* allow tint to come into contact with the client's scalp. Clients could still be offered highlights, lowlights, vegetable colours, bleach, temporary colours and a number of semi-permanents (check that the latter do not contain para-dyes).

About one in twenty-five clients have some form of reaction and product manufacturers recommend a skin test before *every* tint application. Other names for a skin test are patch test, allergy test, hyper-sensitivity test, predisposition test or Sabouraud-Rousseau Test.

Questions
1. Why are skin tests carried out?
2. What does a positive reaction indicate?
3. Why are skin tests carried out particularly before tinting and the application of some semi-permanents?
4. How should you carry out a skin test?
5. What tint would you use for the test?
6. What advice would you give the client following the test?
7. How would you know if the reaction was positive?
8. What would you do in such a case?
9. What other names are there for a skin test?

Design analysis to choose the right hair style

The simplest way of describing design analysis would be to say that it is an evaluation of the clients, their hair and their needs, to determine how the hair should be styled to best enhance their overall appearance.

It is a detailed sequence of discrimination which eventually becomes second nature to the experienced stylist. It is not just a matter of creating a style which is suitable for the shape of the client's face, because the total look includes both the client's lifestyle and the manageability of the style. Ask your clients how they manage their hair at home. Do they blow-dry it or use heated rollers? How do they feel about their hair at this particular moment in time? What do they like or dislike about it?

Figure 2.29 The seven principal face shapes.

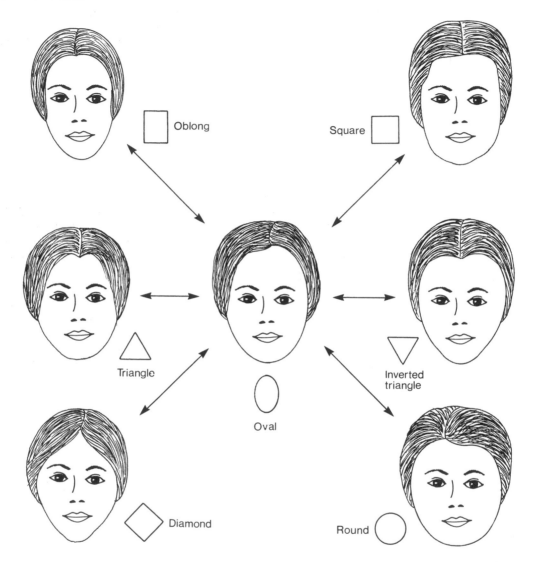

The client may be greatly influenced by partners or friends who might have suggested totally unsuitable styles. If this is the case, try to suggest alternatives (perhaps based on their original idea), backed up by ease of aftercare or fashionability. Never make a derogatory remark about a client to put a point across. We all know someone who would look better with an exceptionally long fringe, but we don't tell them! Design analysis can be broken down into different areas according to the client's needs. What follows is a consideration of these areas.

Face shape in relation to hair design

Whatever the cutting or styling technique used, the one factor that never changes is the importance of creating a style to suit the shape of the face. We can isolate facial form into the seven principal shapes, illustrated in Figure 2.29:

- Oval
- Oblong
- Square
- Triangular
- Inverted triangular (heart)
- Diamond
- Round

The oval face is considered as the ideal shape for which to design a hairstyle. This is because there are no irregular contours or proportions present which will need to be balanced or camouflaged by the hair design. Therefore, it can be said, that when dealing with all of the other face shapes, we are aiming at creating the *illusion* of an oval face by the line and balance of the hairstyle.

When we create the illusion of something being different from what it is, we are controlling the way in which it is to be perceived by others. This concept is demonstrated in Fig. 2.30 which shows how the arrangement of lines and shapes alter our perception of what we are seeing. As hairdressers, we create similar illusions by using the hair to alter the appearance of a person's face and head shape by the way the hair is used to frame it.

Figure 2.30 Perception in hair design. (a) This diagram shows the centre circles to be exactly the same size but they look different because of what has been placed around them. (b) Both of the lines in this diagram are exactly the same but one appears longer than the other because of the way the arrow lines are pointing.

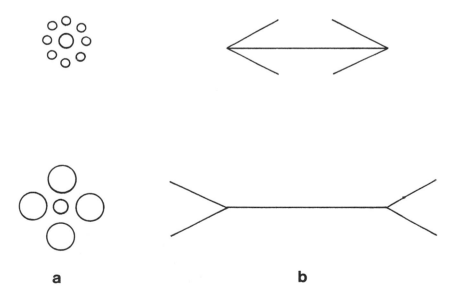

a   b

Figure 2.31 Balancing face shapes.

Face shape   Correction

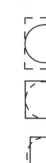

The principle of balancing facial shape can be seen in the series of diagrams in Figure 2.31.

We will now consider the styles that can be used under two headings: positive styles (styles that work to make the face shape appear oval) and negative styles (styles that should be avoided as they do nothing towards making the face appear oval, or emphasise bad features).

Positive styles	Negative styles
Round Styles which add height and are long and narrow through the sides	Styles which accentuate the roundness of the face, such as tight perms, one length cuts and round shapes.
Square Round shapes which soften the angular lines of the face.	Square cut bobs, geometric or angular shapes.
Oblong Asymmetrical shapes which widen the face and add interest.	Styles which are short at the sides and nape and are swept upwards to create height.
Inverted triangle or heart Styles which are full at the bottom to widen the chin and narrow through the top.	Styles which are high and wide through the cheek bone area, as these emphasise the narrow chin.
Triangular Shapes which are wide and full through the top and narrower through the sides. Longer hair will detract from any angular jawline.	Styles which are cut narrow through the top or very short styles as these both emphasise the wide jawline.
Diamond Round shapes which soften the angular lines of the face, which are narrow through the sides and mid-chin length to widen the chin.	Styles which are high, short or full at the sides as these will emphasise the narrow chin and wide cheek bones.

Body shape

Just as there is an ideal face shape there is also an ideal in body proportions. The height of a person should be seven or eight times the size of their head. If someone is short the hairstyle should be designed to give an illusion of extra height, while the opposite would be true for someone who is tall. The hairstyle should balance and harmonise with the height and build of the client. If the head of the client looks small, design a style to make it look bigger, while if it looks large design one to make it look smaller. Remember to take a look at clients while they are walking to gauge their exact height and the way they 'carry' themselves. There are no 'hard and fast' set rules about designing a style to suit body shape as face shape and facial features are so important in reaching correct conclusions.

Head shape

Although our heads all consist of the same bones and conform to a recognisable 'skull' shape, there will be differences of form in some clients to be noted by the stylist. Feel the client's head with your hands. Are there any protrusions? Notable differences in head shape can be felt in the parietal and occipital areas (see Figure 2.32). Some heads are either flatter or rounder here, and you may have to make adjustments in the style so the hair lies as you intend it to. You may also discover warts, cysts or scarring which were not evident from just combing the hair.

Figure 2.32 The main bones of the human skull.

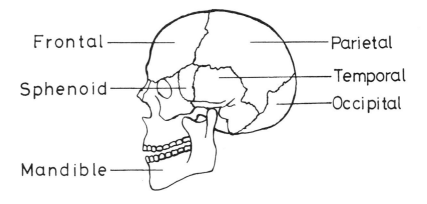

Facial features

Facial features include the eyes, nose and mouth. Styles can be designed which detract from or emphasise facial features. An example of this is when a large prominent nose may be detracted from by dressing the front hair slightly at an angle, rather than symmetrically. Straight fringes will draw attention to wrinkled eyes whereas they will be softened by dressing the hair angled away from the face. A prominent profile will be accentuated by a style swept backwards off the face, so it is better to have the hair softly framing the face.

The neck

A long 'swan' neck will be accentuated if the hair is cut short or upswept at the nape, so the hair should be kept long to disguise the neck. Similarly, a short neck will be lengthened by cutting the hair short in the nape.

The ears

Protruding ears can be disguised by dressing the hair over them. Often, a person's ears are not evenly balanced so that one ear may appear to protrude more than the other or be positioned slightly lower. If there is a very obvious difference, you may need to leave the hair slightly longer on one side than the other to rectify the imbalance or to allow for more protrusion on one side.

Latest developments in hair design

The days of a client going to the hairdressers clutching a photograph of a hair style which may or may not suit them, are definitely numbered. New technology for the hairdressing industry has resulted in the introduction of computerised consultation systems. These systems enable clients to see an image of themselves on a video monitor with a different hair colour, length or shape. This is done by transposing a photograph of the client's face onto the screen and then superimposing different styles onto this image. With this 'photofit' system clients can actually see what they would look like, taking the uncertainty out of 'taking the plunge' to have something different.

Obviously, such equipment is expensive but provides an excellent service for clients. Usually, the cost of this service is about £10 to £15, which is deducted from the client's bill should they go ahead with the new look.

Questions
1. What is design analysis?
2. What type of questions should you ask clients about their hair?
3. Use old magazines to provide you with pictures of examples of the seven principal face shapes.
4. Why is an oval face shape considered as the 'ideal'?
5. Indicate how you would balance the following face shapes:
   (i) round, (ii) square, (iii) oblong, (iv) inverted triangle, (v) triangular, (vi) diamond.
6. What is the ideal body shape?
7. How can head shape affect the design of a hairstyle?
8. Give some examples of facial features that you might want to disguise and how you would go about this.
9. How can long and short necks be disguised?
10. How could prominent ears be disguised?
11. How can new technology help you to show the client different styles?

Advising, persuading and inducing clients to modify their original requirements

If a client resists your professional advice, there are only three possible courses of action that could be taken. Please note that option three is *not* recommended!

- To carry out the client's wishes no matter how much you disagree with the idea, providing the hair or scalp will not become damaged.
- To refuse to carry out the client's wishes, even if this results in the client going to a competitive salon.
- Ignore the client's requests and protestations and carry out your own idea (*not* recommended).

It takes time, patience, consideration, skill and knowledge to convince and persuade many clients that their proposed idea is not suitable. Sometimes, when a hairdresser is lacking in the necessary powers of persuasion to reconcile such situations, both parties can become upset as communication breaks down. This can then result in stress for both parties.

We have already mentioned in this chapter how we communicate with each other both verbally and non-verbally, and the effect this can have on promoting good human relations. In this kind of situation you have to 'win the client over' with your idea at the expense of the client's sacrificing the original request. As you will appreciate, this is more difficult to do with some people than others but we have made a list of guidelines to be considered when involved in persuasive communication.

Guidelines for persuasive communication	
Dos	Don'ts
Actively listen to your client.	Appear to be uninterested or butt in as they speak.
Maintain eye contact to build trust.	Avoid eye contact.
Position you and your client so that you are in close proximity, e.g. sitting next to each other.	Place a barrier between you like a reception desk or be on different levels, e.g. with you standing and the client sitting on a chair.
Use easy to understand language.	Use technical language that can confuse your client or make them feel ignorant.
Use visual aids and the mirrors to explain and emphasise your advice.	Over-tax the client's imagination.
Reassure the client and show concern and understanding.	Be unsympathetic and lack consideration for their feelings.
Respond positively, politely and confidently.	Ridicule the suggestions of the client, be rude or aggressive.
Suggest options (based on their original idea).	Rule out *everything* they have suggested.

The sequence of persuasive communication can be broken down into four steps:

Step 1 – Establishing a relationship with the client.
Step 2 – Asking questions and responding to what you hear.
Step 3 – Offering alternatives and explaining options.
Step 4 – Gaining agreement on course of action.

(1) Establishing a relationship with the client

Greet the client so that they feel welcomed and comfortable. *Use the client's name.* Smile and show friendliness without being over-familiar. Position your client so that you are sitting next to each other in a place that has a degree of privacy so that the client will not feel that everyone is listening to what is being said. Make sure that both seats are of the same height; if you are sitting higher than your client they can feel inferior to you. Sit so that your body is slightly turned towards your client which shows interest. Hold eye contact with your client and by tilting your head slightly to one side this will signal (non-verbally) that you are attentively listening to what is being said. The occasional nod will also confirm that you are listening and that you understand what they are saying.

(2) Asking questions and responding to what you hear

There are many different types of questioning techniques and the ones which are suggested can be distinguished as follows:

(a) Open
(b) Closed
(c) Probing

Open questions are most useful because they require the person being questioned to give information. Open questions begin with the words what, which, when, how. For example:

Q. 'When did you have this perm?'
A. 'Around Christmas time, I guess.'

Closed questions are questions that have a 'yes' or a 'no' answer. They are useful for confirming points that have been raised. For example:

Q. 'So you had the perm about a month ago?'
A. 'Yes.'

Probing questions are used to investigate certain points in greater detail. For example:

Q. 'Tell me why you are not happy with your perm?'
A. 'Well, . . .'

You can see from the above examples that it is useful to question in this sequence:

OPEN
↓
CLOSED
↓
PROBE

(3) *Offering alternatives and explaining options*

It is important that you sustain the trust and confidence the client has developed in your expert opinion. These feelings of respect and security will be instantaneously and totally destroyed if you ridicule the client's suggestions. It is hard for most of us to take criticism at the best of times, even if it is constructive and the person means well. For clients that could be feeling apprehensive about their visit to the salon, having ideas laughed at can be devastating to morale and self-confidence. If this happens, the client will probably become defensive and unwilling or unable to participate in the consultation process. It is very hard to reconcile this situation if it occurs so avoidance of this happening is the best solution. When you disagree with suggestions or requests that your clients have made, try to respond in a way that respects their personal feelings. Often it is better to respond to an unreasonable request by suggesting an option based on the client's idea. It doesn't matter how little of the client's own idea you include in your response providing *something* is present. This might mean that your suggestion simply postpones the client's idea or that you respond with something like:

'I quite like the idea of your hair in that style but it would look *even* better if you had . . .'

This is far more positive than 'That would look *awful* on you'. You will need to explain the advantages and benefits of what you are suggesting to clients for them to be convinced that your idea is better. This can only be done if you have a sound knowledge to support what you are saying. You need to put into words how it will improve their appearance without sounding as though you are giving them 'a load of old flannel' or disbelieve what you are saying. If you have enthusiasm for what you are saying (because you have a positive belief in it) this will come across to the client and they will be more responsive to your ideas. Here are some examples of how the way in which you respond could affect a client's decisions.

Client: 'So you think it wouldn't look right if I had that style?'
Hairdresser: 'Well, you would look so much better with this one because it would make you look more youthful and it is very easy to manage.'
Client: 'But I really wanted a perm and you say my hair won't take another one.'
Hairdresser: 'I guarantee a perm at the moment would affect the condition of your hair but if you have a haircut and a treatment today, we will be able to tell whether it will be possible to do the perm by the end of the month. You'll get a much better result if you wait and we will be having a special offer on our perms then.'
Client: 'My husband will go mad if I go home with something as short as that!'
Hairdresser: 'How about leaving it a little longer at the back? – you can always have it shorter the next time you come in and by leaving it slightly longer today, it will give you and your husband time to get used to your new look.'

Client: 'But I want to be the same colour that I was when I was younger – and that colour was black.'

Hairdresser: 'I'm sure it looked nice then but as our hair colour changes so does the colour of our skin. Having such a dark colour would not complement your present skin colour, and would make you look a bit too pale. This colour is very popular with our clients because it is very flattering and tends to make the complexion glow – it will look very natural on you.'

Can you see from these examples that the hairdresser responds with his or her own ideas in a confident and positive way? Also, the advantages and benefits of the hairdresser's ideas are given to help convince the client why this is the better option.

(4) *Gaining the client's agreement on the course of action*

When all the options have been investigated and discussed with your client, you need to confirm and agree a course of action. This will include outlining the following details for the client:

- to do the agreed service now or to postpone it;
- the procedure of the service that has been agreed;
- the length of time the service will take;
- the cost of the service;
- any special information relating to aftercare the client will need to follow.

Questions

1. What three courses of action are open to you if a client resists your professional advice?
2. Make a list of positive points that you should use in persuasive communication.
3. What are the four steps involved in such communication?
4. How would you establish a relationship with the client?
5. What are the three categories of question that you should ask?
6. How can you offer the client alternatives that they might accept?
7. When you gain agreement on a course of action what kind of details should be explained to the client?

Dealing with clients' complaints

There will be times when clients will complain about the service they have received. Clients do not usually complain without cause, but you may come across the 'funny' client who will always find something to criticise.

Everybody working with the public needs to receive training in how to respond to dissatisfied customers or clients. This is true for those employed in shops, public houses, restaurants, hospitals, hairdressing salons, etc. If you deal with people, it is inevitable that you will be faced with this situation at some time. Usually, your employer will outline the procedure for dealing with complaints as soon as you start your job. After all, if there is a particular procedure to be followed, it is within your employer's interests to inform you of it. The procedure that you will be asked to follow will differ from other salons, because a lot depends on the size of the salon that employs you and the management structure. Salons that belong to large organisations usually have a corporate procedure for dealing with complaints. That means all the salon managers employed by the company have been trained to deal with complaints in a particular way. Unfortunately, such organisation is not usually evident in some of the smaller salons, where clear lines of seniority amongst the staff are less defined, often leaving new employees to sort out any problems.

Health and safety legislation

If you do not know the procedure for dealing with complaints in your salon, find this out *now*. You need to know who deals with the complaint and if they are not around, who replaces them. You will also need to find out the policy in your salon regarding re-doing the complainant's hair, whether or not you give refunds and how such complaints are recorded. Usually, it is the salon manager or supervisor that deals with complaints but as we have said, this may vary in different salons.

There are laws which are designed to protect the public from inadequate standards of health and safety, quality of service or purchase and also confidentiality. A few of the Acts pertaining to hairdressing salons, the employers, employees and clients are set out below.

The *Data Protection Act* protects the rights of individuals so that they have the right to know any information concerning them that is stored on computer. That means *any* organisation keeping records on clients, employees, patients, customers etc. on a computer system must declare that they are doing so to the Data Protection Registrar.

The Environmental Health Officer is charged with the responsibility of checking that health and safety standards of public premises meet with local authority requirements. If the officer finds that these standards are not being met, the owner of the premises may be fined and given a period of time to correct the offence. If this is not done within the specified time limit, the officer has the power to apply for a court injunction to close the premises and prevent it from operating. The *Health and Safety at Work Act 1974* protects almost everyone involved in working situations and sets out the responsibilities of the employer and the employee in terms of:

- the first aid arrangements and procedures for reporting accidents;
- general health and safety;
- the enforcement of the Act by Area Offices and the Inspectors.

For further information on the Health and Safety at Work Act 1974 please refer to *Hygiene – A Salon Handbook*.

The *Public Liability Act 1969* makes it compulsory for employers to have an insurance policy which protects themselves, employees and clients in terms of compensation for accidents. This policy must be displayed in the salon premises.

The *Fire Precautions Act 1971* is enforced by your local fire authority and requires premises to apply for a fire certificate if there are more than twenty people at one time on the premises, or ten people on one floor of the premises. The Act also requires all premises to have fire fighting equipment in good working order, readily available and suitable for the types of fire likely to occur. Doors, that would enable people to escape from a fire, must be unlocked when the premises is in use and must not be obstructed by the contents of the room, as these could prevent a quick exit in the event of a fire.

Complaints about services

A client dissatisfied with a hairdressing service can take a hairdresser to court, and the hairdresser will be sued if negligence is proved. It is usually quite difficult for clients to prove negligence, because it usually takes so long for cases to reach court that their hair will not look as bad as at the time the alleged negligence took place. However, solicitors will advise the person taking the court action to take photographs of their hair as soon as possible after the event as proof. The prosecuting and defending lawyers may call upon independent expert witnesses to give evidence. Sometimes such cases can go on for several years involving large sums of money. This is why so many complaints never reach the stage of going to court. It is often less troublesome and costly to make a settlement out of court.

Dealing with complaints

If a client feels they have reason for complaint, the hairdresser must deal with the situation in a polite, calm and understanding way. Getting irritated or emotionally involved will make the problem more difficult to resolve. If you are able to maintain self-discipline and control how you respond and what you say, it is more likely that the client will respond in a similar way. As most complaints will be referred to managers and supervisors, it is valuable to observe (unobtrusively) how the situation is dealt with and learn from what you witness.

Dealing with a complaint involves three steps as set out below:

Step 1 – Acknowledging the complaint.
This should be done politely and, if possible, the client should be taken to a quieter part of the salon to deal with the complaint. Audiences can make people behave irrationally and hysterically, so it is always better to be in a less busy area of the salon than the reception area. Also, it is not good for business for other customers to hear someone complaining.

Step 2 − Analysing and defining the complaint.
You will need to examine the hair and scalp to determine the nature and validity of the complaint. You will also need to question the client in detail with regard to how the hair has been treated and cared for since the date of the appointment.

Step 3 − Propose a solution to the problem.
The alternative solutions to the problem need to be taken into account and the best course of action needs to be chosen. This course of action is then proposed to the client.

Here are some examples of typical causes of complaint with the responses of the hairdresser. Please think about how the two different responses from the first and second hairdresser could affect the level of communication.

Client: 'I can't go out like this! My hair looks awful!'
Hairdresser (1): 'It looks all right to me.'
Hairdresser (2): 'Perhaps you'd like it more if I did this (making a change). What do you think of it now?'

Client: 'This isn't good enough. My perm has gone completely straight.'
Hairdresser (1): 'It's not meant to be curly.'
Hairdresser (2) : 'Let me have a look at it to see what the problem is.'

Client: 'I spent twenty pounds on this and I can't see any difference in the colour at all.'
Hairdresser (1): 'I can.'
Hairdresser (2): 'Let's go over to a better light so I can look at it properly for you.'

Questions
1. What is the procedure for dealing with client complaints in your salon?
2. Who usually deals with them?
3. What is the Data Protection Act?
4. Why is the Environmental Health Officer important to a salon?
5. Who does the Health and Safety at Work Act protect?
6. What is the Public Liability Act?
7. What are the main points of the Fire Precautions Act?
8. What are the three steps in dealing with a complaint?
9. Find out what kinds of complaints stylists in your salon have had to deal with in their careers and how they were handled.

Chapter Three
Treatments for the Hair and Scalp

Introduction to treatments

The one area of potential growth for attracting more clients into salons and which is wholly concerned with hair is treatments. Your clients enter the salon to have services such as a cut and blow-dry, yet there may be other things that you can offer, depending on the condition of the hair and scalp.

Just as fashions inevitably change, so does the way people treat their hair. Recent statistics prove that women shampoo their hair far more frequently today than in the past, a trend that men are also following. About 10 per cent shampoo their hair every day, while an incredible 65 per cent do so every two or three days. Of the 10 per cent that shampoo their hair every day, 44 per cent use a conditioner every time. Surveys definitely show that the public are concerned but ill-informed about their hair, and that is why *we*, the experts, should guide them. Those salons that provide a range of in-salon conditioners and treatments, backed up by a comprehensive retail range, will benefit financially from increased services and contented customers. If you think back to Chapter 2 you will remember that in your diagnosis of hair, conditioning may be necessary before you can attempt some chemical work safely.

If we were absolutely candid about the services that we can offer in a salon, most of us would realise that some treatments and special shampoos do little to improve the hair and scalp, no matter what the rep or salesman says about the new wonder product. We are rather like the doctor giving harmless sugar pills or coloured liquids to his patients, so that they will believe they are being treated and respond positively. Many of our hairdressing treatments make the hair look better and relax the clients, making them feel more positive about themselves. When you feel good, you look good. Clients should never be 'conned', told a product will permanently mend split ends or make their hair grow thicker or faster. If the product does not live up to its high expectations it will not be used again.

Conditioners

There are a wide range of conditioners available, marketed by the major manufacturers as ranges of hair care products, usually in distinctive packaging. You will find it far easier to persuade clients to use a 'name' product which is nicely packaged, and even easier still if that product has become familiar through advertising. If you take on a range, there are often demonstrations given on how to use them, retail display stands and advertising literature. If clients buy a conditioner which pleases them, they will be more likely to purchase shampoo and other items from the same range. An alternative to this is to have your own products made, bearing the salon name and motif. This is an excellent form of publicity for your salon, as it is something that usually only top salons do. Your salon can appear more successful than it really is! One major manufacturer supplies excellent products which are then repackaged by the salons.

What are the different types of conditioner and how does a conditioner affect the hair?

A conditioner is a special chemical which can be applied to the hair to help restore its strength, protect it against chemical damage and leave it shiny and manageable.

Today's conditioners are the sophisticated scientific expression of the earlier ones which were based mostly on vegetable oils and eggs. They may be formulated to be applied either before or after a hairdressing procedure (a pre- or post-treatment). To a great extent conditioners must be substantive to hair, that is, be attracted to it. Because keratin has more negative charges than positive ones, this is easily achieved by having a conditioner with positive charges. Unlike charges attract (rather like the opposite poles of a magnet) and the positive conditioner is attracted to the negative charges. The more damaged or porous a head of hair is, the more conditioner it can attract and hold. The first conditioners introduced in 1945 were based on cationic (positively charged) compounds. (A word of warning: because cationic compounds are positive they are incompatible with anionic (that is negative) ones, and their action will be neutralised or cancelled out. The majority of shampoos are anionic so you should avoid using a shampoo after a conditioner, because it is likely to be a pointless exercise!)

Conditioners can be grouped into three main categories: (1) oils, (2) acids and (3) substantive.

(1) Oils

Since antiquity oils have been used to provide the hair with lubrication and lustre. They have a high refractive index (the refractive index is the degree to which light is bent on passing from one substance to another; substances like diamond which have high refractive indexes reflect light more) and so give the hair lustre. A thin layer of oil will reduce friction when the hair is combed or brushed and help the hair to retain moisture. Oils must be used sparingly, however, to avoid excessive greasiness. A small amount should be spread over a large area of hair or, if more is applied, the excess should be rinsed out. The oil is usually in the form of a dilute oil-in-water emulsion and may contain lanolin (sheep sebum) or a synthetic product made to resemble sebum. Lanolin is used in a number of products because it is a natural compound similar to our own sebum. (A word of warning: a number of people are allergic to lanolin so if redness or itchiness of the scalp develops, discontinue use of the product.) Silicones have a good conditioning effect on the hair and leave behind a film of protective polymer after rinsing. They are now added to many products used to chemically process the hair which need built-in conditioners to prevent damage.

(2) Acids

Traditionally, weak acid rinses were used to remove soap scum which was produced in shampooing (see Chapter 4), neutralise any excess alkali left on the hair after a chemical processing treatment or to impart a sheen to the hair. Weak organic acids such as acetic acid (vinegar) and citric acid (lemon juice) were used to close the cuticle. Their main use today is after chemical processing (see later), because shampoos today are soapless and have no scum. The preferred acid today is ascorbic acid (actually vitamin C), because it is also an antioxidant, helping to stop the action of hydrogen peroxide after bleaching, perming and tinting. If it were not used unnecessary damage would occur. Rupture of peptide bonds by hydrogen peroxide or ammonium thioglycollate produces water-soluble products which would be lost on subsequent shampooing, thus weakening the hair fibres. Acids cause these soluble products to precipitate or solidify, thus preventing their loss. They also help to prevent such loss because they close the cuticle of the hair. This also makes the hair less likely to be damaged by brushing or combing as the cuticle scales are flattened.

(3) Substantive conditioners

This group includes cationic detergents and protein hydrolysates. There are other chemicals with conditioning properties, such as PVP (see Chapter 4) or non-ionic detergents (detergents without a charge) which are added to hairdressing products. Something which is *substantive* is attracted to hair.

The best-known cationic conditioner is cetrimide (chemically a quaternary ammonium compound), its positive charge being attracted to the negatively charged hair. It reduces static, softens the hair, and makes it easier to comb. The antistatic effect is due to the retention of moisture by the hair.

The so-called protein conditioners are actually mixtures of the breakdown products of proteins (polypeptide chains, peptides and amino acids), which have been prepared by hydrolysing protein. (Hydrolysis is the breakdown of something by its reaction with water.) The protein hydrolysates thus formed are attracted to the hair in much the same way as opposite charges. Some amino acids in the hair have free, unattached basic groups (positive), which are attracted to free acid groups (negative). This attraction forms what is known as a 'salt linkage' (see Chapter 8 for further details). As hair damaged by chemical processes contains more of these free groups, such hair will attract more protein than undamaged hair. There is no real need to have exotic sources of protein such as placenta, but it certainly sounds impressive! If a conditioner contains hydrolysed keratin it is usually from sources such as animal hoofs and horns, while if it is human keratin, from old hair cuttings! Again, salesmen will tell you that because it is like adding small fragments of hair it must be better. Recently cystine, one of the amino acids which make up keratin, has been put forward as the wonder ingredient of protein conditioners.

A number of experiments have been conducted with protein conditioners to prove that they do combine with the hair. These include the use of radioactive labels, amino acid analysis and staining. They have been shown to protect damaged hair during bleaching and perming. Little damage was caused to protein-treated hair while untreated damaged hair suffered extensive damage. It is recommended, therefore, that protein hydrolysates are used before chemical treatment. They have also been shown to help make split ends cling together by electrostatic attraction. You can tell clients that there is solid scientific evidence to support the use of conditioners.

Hair restructurants

As their name implies these are products which help to make good, temporarily some of the damage that the hair may have suffered. They are usually packaged individually because their ingredients can deteriorate after opening. They are applied to towel-dried hair which has been shampooed. Mix the ingredients as required and apply to the hair, before combing through. Hair restructurants normally contain a setting agent and are not rinsed out of the hair after application. The restructurant contains chemicals which help to establish new cross-links between the hair fibres. They usually contain an acid catalyst which forms a hair-strengthening resin within the hair fibres, making the hair virtually insoluble in water.

What are surface and penetrating conditioners?

Many hairdressers refer to the conditioners that work on the cuticle alone as 'surface conditioners'. These will remove tangles from the hair by smoothing down the cuticle and are usually very quick-acting, so do not need to be left on the hair too long. As the name implies, penetrating conditioners are intended to help repair the cortex and may take longer to work than surface conditioners. You should be able to classify conditioners into these two groups by what the manufacturers claim they can do, or if heat needs to be applied to aid penetration. In general, surface conditioners will be those that contain natural (lanolin) or synthetic (silicone) oils to coat and lubricate the cuticle or acids to close it. Penetrating conditioners may also be referred to as reconditioning creams and restructurants. They contain protein fragments, quarternary ammonium compounds and synthetic chemicals, often containing urea.

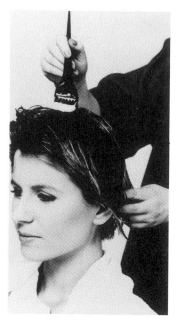

Figure 3.1 Applying conditioner with a tint brush. (Courtesy Trevor Sorbie.)

How are conditioners applied to hair?

This depends to some extent on the manufacturer and the purpose of the conditioner. Some are used to protect the hair before chemical processing (see later in this chapter) while others are used to repair damage, sometimes on a regular basis after shampooing the hair. In the latter case, towel-dry the hair after shampooing and before applying the conditioner, to remove excessive moisture, or the conditioner will be diluted. Conditioners can be applied with a tint brush, as shown in Figure 3.1, in much the same way as you would apply a tint.

Alternatively, they can be applied directly with the hands. Pour the conditioner into the palm of your hand and then distribute between your hands. Smooth your hands through the hair, distributing the conditioner as evenly as possible throughout the hair. Gently massage the product through the hair, ensuring that all the hair is treated with the conditioner. Use your fingers like a comb to disentangle the hair or alternatively use a wide-toothed comb to remove tangles. The application may look like that in Figure 3.2. More of the product will be taken up where the hair is most damaged. Leave the conditioner on the hair as long as is recommended by the manufacturer. Leaving it on longer will not make it work any better.

Why should the conditioner be rinsed from the hair?

The conditioner should be rinsed out of the hair, or otherwise it will become greasy, flop and be difficult to manage. Check that rinsing has been thorough by running a comb through the hair. If a foam appears on the comb, there is still conditioner present which needs to be rinsed off.

What type of heat can be used to assist the penetration of the conditioner?

Some conditioners will require heat to aid penetration into the cortex. This can be supplied by using hot towels (to form a turban as shown in Figure 3.3), steamers, accelerators (Climazon) or hood driers (place a plastic cap over the client's hair). Remember to switch on steamers and hairdryers before they are needed so that they have time to warm up. If you use hot towels they will have to be replaced as they cool down. A hot towel is made by soaking it in very hot water and squeezing it out; however, it should not be so hot as to scald the client or your hands as you prepare it!

Questions
1. Why are treatments likely to attract clients into salons?
2. Why should you not misinform a client about the benefits of a product?

Figure 3.2 Completed application of conditioner. (Courtesy L'Oréal.)

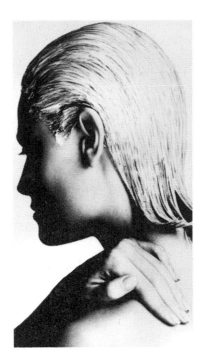

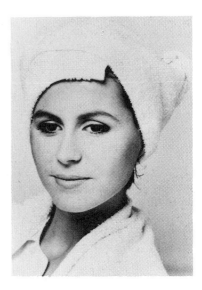

Figure 3.3 Hot towels applied in the form of a turban. (Courtesy Trevor Sorbie.)

3. Why might it be easier to sell products to clients which are made by major manufacturers?
4. What benefits does a salon get from having its own product range?
5. What does a conditioner do?
6. What were the early conditioners based on?
7. Explain the terms pre- and post-treatment.
8. Why are conditioners with positive charges attracted to hair?
9. What are cationic and anionic compounds?
10. What does the term 'incompatible' mean to you?
11. List the three categories conditioners can be grouped into.
12. Why do oils give the hair lustre?
13. What is lanolin?
14. Why might it not be suitable for some clients?
15. Why are silicones added to some products which are used to process the hair?
16. What were the three reasons acid rinses were used on the hair?
17. What three acids are commonly used in such rinses?
18. Why is ascorbic acid preferred?
19. How can the hair be weakened by hydrogen peroxide or ammonium thioglycollate?
20. What chemicals are classed as substantive?
21. What do cationic conditioners do for the hair?
22. What are protein conditioners made from?
23. How are protein conditioners attracted to the hair?
24. Why does damaged hair attract more protein conditioner to it than undamaged hair?

25. What proof have we that protein-treated hair is harmed less in chemical processing?
26. What is a hair restructurant?
27. How does a hair restructurant work?
28. What is the difference between surface and penetrating conditioners?
29. Give examples of each.
30. Why should hair be towel-dried before applying conditioner?
31. How can conditioners be applied?
32. How should tangles be removed from the hair?
33. Why should the conditioner be rinsed from the hair?
34. Describe the different ways of supplying heat in conditioning treatments.

Treating hair conditions

In this section we will be looking at the treatment of the following conditions: (1) fragilitis crinium (split ends), (2) damaged cuticle, (3) seborrhoea, (4) trichorrhexis nodosa.

(1) Fragilitis crinium

Fragilitis crinium, or as it is more commonly known, split ends, cannot be permanently repaired by the use of conditioners. The only treatment to get rid of the split ends is to cut them off. However, the client should be consulted about the way they treat their hair and the products that they use because something has caused the hair to split. If the reason for the damage can be identified, clients can be educated about how they should care for their hair to prevent future damage.

Clients will need to be given a conditioning treatment to nourish the middle lengths and ends of their hair, to make them less brittle and then have the split ends cut off. Sometimes, the hair will be split quite a long way up the hair shaft. If the affected hairs are not cut, the splitting can continue up the entire length of the hair. Cutting off split ends does not necessarily mean that clients must have their hair cut very short. The hairdresser can remove the affected parts of the hair without altering the overall appearance of the hairstyle. This is done by taking meshes of

Figure 3.4 Cutting off split ends from a twist of hair.

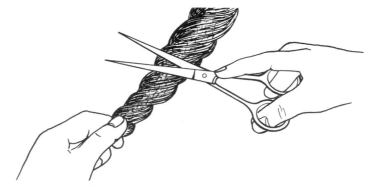

hair about 3 cms square and twisting the hair from the scalp to the points. By running the thumb and forefinger up the twist of hair towards the scalp, the split ends will stand out. Starting at the root end, you can begin cutting off the split ends with the points of your scissors, working towards the hair points. This is shown in Figure 3.4, and is carried out on any part of the head where the hair is split.

(2) *Damaged cuticle*

A damaged cuticle can be caused by either physical or chemical abuse. Instead of lying flat and closed, the cuticle scales are open, often leading to cuticle abrasion when scales will actually shear or break off. As the cuticle is responsible for protecting the internal structure of the hair and giving the hair shine, the hair will be susceptible to further damage and will appear to be dull as it diffuses, rather than reflects, light (see Chapter 10 for an explanation).

The application of a conditioner will coat the outside of the hair shaft, smoothing down the open scales and 'filling in' areas where the cuticle scales are missing. A conditioner will cover the hair with a coating of oil, wax or protein, and because the outside will now be made smooth, light will reflect off the smooth surface and the hair will shine. Remember that the effect of a conditioner on the outside of the hair is temporary and that normal brushing and combing will cause friction on the hair, wearing away the coating of conditioner. Also, shampooing will remove conditioner from the hair. Therefore, a conditioner will need to be applied each time the hair is shampooed. If any clients buy shampoos from you, tell them about the conditioner that goes with it and give them information about how long it should be left on, etc.

Hair that is porous (a term used to describe hair with a damaged cuticle) will tangle more easily than hair which has a cuticle that is lying flat. This is because the open scales make the individual hairs mat together. You may notice this after shampooing porous hair, because the physical handling of the hair during shampooing encourages the hair to mat together. As soon as a conditioner is applied to such hair, it will feel softer from the lubricating effect of the conditioner and will be easier to comb through.

(3) *Seborrhoea*

Seborrhoea is the condition of greasy hair caused by overactive sebaceous glands. This condition is seen particularly amongst teenagers because the hormone levels in the body change at puberty, causing the sebaceous glands to produce more oil than the hair or skin needs. This condition is not, however, confined to those experiencing puberty; people with high levels of male hormone or a particular sensitivity to it, and people with fine hair, may find the amount of sebum that is produced exceeds what is actually necessary to lubricate and protect the skin and hair. This results in greasy hair and an oily skin.

It is far more difficult to control overactivity of the sebaceous glands than it is to stimulate them into action. This is because the activity of the glands is under the control of the hormones in the body and actions such as massaging during a shampoo will stimulate the glands into working harder.

The treatments for dealing with seborrhoea act like blotting paper to soak up excess sebum and have an astringent effect on the glands which, with regular and continuous use, will gradually cause them to shrink and produce less sebum. These treatments are available in a shampoo base and are applied to the root area and left on for a while before they are rinsed from the hair. Other products include those which are applied to the roots and left on the hair, or they can be a combination of the two products; a special shampoo which is followed by the application of a lotion that is not rinsed from the hair.

When dealing with a client who has seborrhoea, try not to stimulate the scalp too much as this will increase the blood flow and activate the sebaceous glands. Therefore try to use minimum massage and tepid rather than hot water. Make the suggestion to the client that they purchase products from you that will enable them to continue the treatment at home between salon visits. The range of products available for clients to buy from chemist shops and supermarkets to treat this condition at home is very restricted. Those with seborrhoea are usually willing to spend quite a lot of money when they eventually find a product that does have a significant effect. Shampoos for greasy hair simply contain more detergent so are not treatments, they only clean the hair more thoroughly than a shampoo for normal hair would. Advise the client to avoid stimulating the scalp too much at home. They should avoid hot water, vigorous brushing, and use minimal massage in shampooing.

(4) Trichorrhexis nodosa

Trichorrhexis nodosa is a nodule on the hair shaft caused by the loss of cuticle scales and a resultant swelling of the cortex in the damaged area (see Chapter 2). Normal conditioners that coat the outside of the hair with a film of oil or wax will do nothing to restore the hair's internal strength. Although the damage cannot be permanently repaired, there is a type of treatment that can be applied which will help to strengthen the hair and make it less likely to break. These treatments, described earlier in this chapter, are called restructurants and usually come in the form of a lotion that is applied to the hair and either left on or rinsed out. Ordinary conditioner may then need to be applied to make the hair feel softer and easier to comb through. Check with the clients about their home haircare routine and advise them to avoid too much heat (curling tongs, heated rollers). Natural bristle brushes will also be kinder to the hair.

Questions

1. What is the only permanent cure for split ends?
2. Why is it important to question clients about the way they treat their hair?
3. Do you have to cut the client's hair short to treat split ends?
4. Describe how you would cut off split ends.
5. Why does hair with damaged cuticle look dull?
6. How do conditioners improve damaged cuticle on hair?
7. What causes seborrhoea?
8. How do treatments for seborrhoea work?
9. Are shampoos for greasy hair actually treatments to reduce it?
10. What haircare advice would you give a client with seborrhoea?
11. What is the treatment used for trichorrhexis nodosa?
12. What haircare advice would you give a client with trichorrhexis nodosa?

Treating dandruff

Pityriasis capitis, or as it is more commonly known, dandruff, is a scalp condition that can be treated in the salon. Dandruff is a non-infectious scalp condition that is caused by the cells of the epidermis rejuvenating and multiplying too quickly, with the result that they cannot be shed as fast as they are produced. The scalp will be covered all over or in patches, by silvery skin scales that come away easily from the scalp if it is lightly scratched. The client will sometimes experience slight scalp irritation and this will be accompanied by the scalp feeling tight. Clients will often say that they have a 'dry scalp' or 'scurf', as alternative names for the condition.

The treatment for dandruff is to apply a lotion that will lift the skin flakes off the scalp, leaving the scalp free of the scales. Treatments that will do this contain ingredients such as zinc pyrithione (this is the same as zinc omadine), selenium sulphide or coal tar and are normally available in a shampoo base or a lotion that is allowed to rest on the scalp before being rinsed from the hair. Selenium sulphide is claimed to slow down cell division in the epidermis but can increase sebum production so should only really be used on dry scalps. Some clients will also be allergic to sulphur and dermatitis will result. Zinc pyrithione is slightly antiseptic and helps to control the population of yeast found on the scalp when someone has dandruff. Regular and continuous treatment with such shampoos and lotions is usually necessary to arrest the problem and keep the multiplication of the epidermal cells under control. Do not tell the client that you can cure it as the condition may last some time. Advise the client to use the same products at home between salon visits: don't waste the opportunity to sell!

Questions
1. How might clients describe their scalp when they have dandruff?
2. What are the ingredients of the treatments used for dandruff?
3. What disadvantages have the ones containing selenium sulphide?
4. Can dandruff be cured quickly?

Conditioning hair before and after chemical treatment

There are special types of conditioners that can be applied to help protect the hair before it is given chemical treatment. These conditioners are special because they provide protection for the hair without forming a barrier that is impenetrable to the chemicals which will be applied to process the hair chemically. Ordinary conditioners should not be used before chemical processing because they will inhibit the performance of the chemicals which need to penetrate the cuticle in order to work effectively in the cortex.

Pre-perm treatments are lotions which are applied to the hair before the hair is permed. They are not rinsed out of the hair and help to equalise the porosity of the hair shaft. This has the effect that the speed at which the perm lotion penetrates the cuticle is controlled equally along the length of the hair rather than acting really fast in the heavily damaged areas.

Certain conditioners can also be applied before some colouring processes when the hair is prepared by shampooing and towel-drying, as in the case of using semi-permanents and toners after bleaching. Again, the application of these special conditioners helps to level out uneven porosity, with the aim of achieving more even colour results.

After chemical treatment, the hair will benefit from the application of conditioners that are acid (pH of about 4) because these help to restore the hair's natural pH. Conditioners which are reducing agents as well as acids are described as 'anti-oxidants' because they react with any remaining hydrogen peroxide in the cortex of the hair so that it cannot oxidise the hair further. They thus prevent damage rather than repair it. If conditioners claim to be 'pH balanced' they will have a pH of about 4.5 which is the same as the hair and skin. It is important to use an acidic product to close the cuticle of the hair so that it is easier to handle.

Questions
1. What is special about conditioners which are designed to be used before chemical treatments?
2. Why should normal conditioners not be used?
3. Why are pre-perm treatments used?
4. Why are conditioners used before colouring?
5. What types of conditioners are used after chemically processing the hair?

6. Why are some conditioners referred to as anti-oxidants?
7. What advantage would you say conditioners were to a client if you were asked after you had permed a client's hair and an extra charge were being made for the conditioner?
8. Why do we use acidic conditioners after alkaline treatments?

Additional information – other treatments which may be offered in salons

Scalp massage

Massage is best described as the physical manipulation of the soft outer tissues of the body. It is one of the most ancient ways to reduce pain and tension. People who can give a good massage are often referred to as having 'magic hands'.

What effects has a massage on the scalp?

There has been some controversy in the past about the real physiological value of massage. Basically it stimulates the scalp. The blood vessels dilate and the scalp becomes redder in colour (this redness of the skin is referred to as a hyperaemia), giving the benefit of an increased blood supply to the papillae of the hair follicles (this gives extra oxygen, glucose and amino acids for cell growth). The drainage of blood is also increased from the scalp, which helps remove waste respiratory gases such as carbon dioxide. The lymphatic system is also stimulated which helps with the removal of waste products. The mechanical stimulation of the nerve supply increases the secretion of sweat from the eccrine sweat glands, again increasing the removal of waste products. Stimulation of the arrector pili muscle attached to each hair follicle causes the hair to rise and increases the rupture of fat cells. This indirectly stimulates the constriction of the sebaceous glands which secrete more sebum (hence massage can be good for a dry scalp). Besides these physiological benefits, the massage can decrease tension and pain, making someone more relaxed.

Contra-indications to massage

If the client has an infectious condition such as impetigo or ringworm a massage should not be given. The scalp should be checked for head lice and if these are present you must not proceed. If a client has broken skin check for reasons such as infections; do not proceed if any are present or you might open up the breaks further. If the scalp is inflamed (red and tender-looking) do not proceed. Never massage if a client has just been on a sunbed or is sunburnt or they might pass out on you. Do not massage a client who has low blood pressure or any kind of heart or circulatory disorder; ask about this or you may cause your client to black-out. Massage should not be performed on a client with an above normal temperature, as might occur with flu or a fever.

How should you prepare yourself to give a massage?

Wash your hands and thoroughly dry them before beginning the massage. If your hands are very cold, your client will appreciate your doing this in hot water to warm them up! Stand behind the client with your weight evenly distributed on both feet. (A word of warning: your nails should not be too long or you could scratch your client's scalp.)

How should you prepare the client for a massage?

You should already have checked the client's scalp for infections, etc. It is essential that clients are completely relaxed before commencing the massage. If they are nervous about it, calm them down and tell them how much they will enjoy it. Seat the client in an upright but comfortable position. Loosen any constrictive clothing around the neck. The hair should be free from tangles. Since the threshold of discomfort and pain varies from person to person, you should question the client frequently about any uncomfortable sensations.

What are the techniques of hand massage?

There are five basic techniques of hand massage:
(1) effleurage, (2) petrissage, (3) tapotement, (4) friction, and (5) vibration.

(1) Effleurage

This is a stroking movement which should be used to begin and end a massage. With the fingers together, mould your hands to the head. Stroke the scalp from the frontal hairline right back to the base of the occipital bone (almost to the top of the shoulder blades) in one continuous movement. Be careful not to pull the hair. Try to build up an even, firm pressure with these stroking movements. Cover the left and right sides of the head, always stroking from the front hairline towards the nape. Many people will tell you that you should use both hands together, but it does not matter if you make alternate strokes with each hand. If it is your first massage, do it whichever way feels most natural to you. This type of massage should be continued for at least a couple of minutes and will soothe and relax your client. If you tell your clients that you can already feel the scalp loosening they will be very happy!

(2) Petrissage

This is described as a kneading movement, because the scalp is kneaded in almost the same way a baker kneads dough. The pads of the fingers are placed a little apart on the scalp, with one hand on each side of the head. While exerting light pressure, move the scalp with your finger tips in a circular direction. You should be moving the client's scalp and not your fingertips! If you move your fingers against the skin and hair you might damage the hair. Use your hands to support the client's head. Do not be shocked if clients fall asleep during their massage as they will be so relaxed – it is a compliment to your skill. If you look at Figure 3.5 you will see how the hairdresser is standing behind the client making these kneading movements. Keep this massage up for between 5 – 10 minutes. You will actually notice the scalp loosening with this movement, which breaks down the fat and increases the removal of waste products. If you do not proceed to the next movement, finish the client off with a few minutes of effleurage. Gradually decrease the pressure of your stroking movements as you massage again for a couple of minutes.

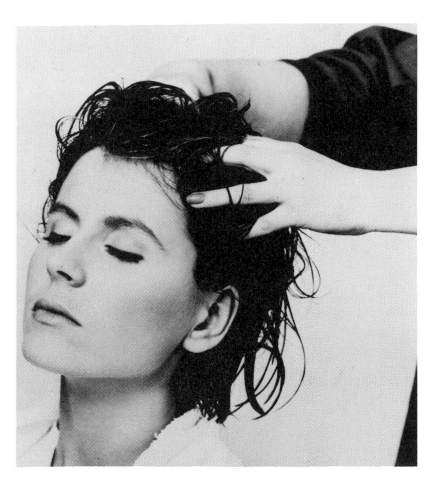

Figure 3.5 Petrissage is used to loosen the scalp. Notice that the hairdresser stands behind the client. (Courtesy Trevor Sorbie.)

(3) Tapotement

This means percussion or tapping. In hairdressing this is carried out with the tips of the fingers. The tapping should be as quick as possible and it quickly gets tiring! It is very difficult to achieve the proper intensity. This movement is not particularly effective on the scalp. On the body the same term is used to describe quick 'chopping' with the sides of the hands.

(4) Friction

This type of massage refers to a small deep movement with great pressure, performed in a circular direction with the thumb and fingertips (some people wrongly refer to it as a 'light rubbing' movement with the fingertips, the friction thus created producing heat). Surface rubbing of the skin is likely to produce irritation and possible inflammatory reactions as well as hair breakage. The skin should therefore be moved against the skull below.

(4) Vibration

This can be referred to as a shaking movement. The hands or fingertips are placed firmly against the skin and a fine trembling or shaking of the scalp is produced. Light vibrations are soothing while heavier shaking is stimulating. An electrical machine can be strapped to the back of the hand to make this type of massage easier. The machine, sold under the trade name of 'Stimulux' can be set to provide weak or strong vibrations. You simply place your fingertips onto the client's scalp. When first using the machine it may shake itself off your hand but you will soon learn to position it properly so that this does not happen. Be careful not to let the retaining bands, which are often wire, get caught up in the clients hair.

What is a vibro?

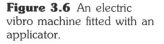
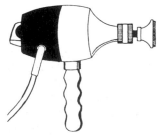

Figure 3.6 An electric vibro machine fitted with an applicator.

This is an electrically operated vibratory machine which on first sight resembles a hairdryer. It can produce vibratory movements similar to those of friction. One is illustrated in Figure 3.6, fitted with a spiked applicator that consists of rubber prongs on a base that is screwed into the machine. This is for use on the scalp and the surface of the prongs vibrates rapidly as it is held against the skin. The machine should be held lightly, but firmly, against the skin, lifting occasionally to prevent hair tangles. Use the vibro in small circular movements to cover the scalp, or in lines from frontal hairline to nape. Other applicators are available for use on the face which consist of soft rubber sponge. Remember to clean applicators after every client. Finish your massage with effleurage by hand.

After any massage, allow the client to rest for a few minutes before standing up or they may become dizzy and faint. Wash your own hands.

Questions

1. What is massage?
2. What benefits has massage?
3. What are the contra-indications to massage?
4. How would you prepare yourself to give massage?
5. How would you prepare the client?
6. What is effleurage?
7. When would you use it?
8. What is petrissage?
9. When would you use it?
10. What is tapotement?
11. What is friction?
12. What is vibration?
13. Besides using the hands what machine can be used to give vibration?
14. What is a vibro machine and when would you use it?
15. Why should the client rest for a while before standing up after a massage?

High frequency

This is something that is still taught in most colleges but has become a rare service in the majority of salons. The high frequency machine produces a high voltage with a low current, so is safe (when used properly); car batteries have a low voltage but a high current, so can give a nasty shock. The machine is usually seen as a small portable black box, like the one illustrated in Figure 3.7. It is plugged into the mains and the electrodes are fitted into an insulated holder.

Why give high frequency treatments?

High frequency treatments will stimulate the scalp and when used frequently will benefit hair loss conditions. It can produce hyperaemia, redness of skin due to increased blood flow, which increases the supply of nutrients to hair follicles. Do not tell your client that it will stop such loss as it will not, but it may help slow it down. The gas ozone is produced during high frequency which has a slight antiseptic action. This is a form of oxygen which contains three atoms of oxygen per

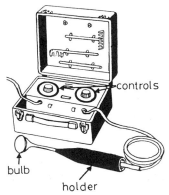

Figure 3.7 A high frequency machine complete with electrodes.

controls

bulb

holder

molecule rather than the normal two that we would breathe in. You will be able to smell the ozone, which might remind you of the seaside because this is another area where ozone is produced. This is why the sea air is said to be so 'bracing'. Like hand massage, high frequency is relaxing and can have a positive psychological effect if carried out correctly.

Are there any contra-indications to giving high frequency?

Yes. It should never be given to anyone who has an infectious skin condition such as ringworm or impetigo, head lice or inflamed skin. Also, ask your clients if they have any kind of heart trouble, including a pacemaker; if so, do not give treatment. Never give treatment to pregnant women or anyone on medication.

How do I prepare to give high frequency to my client?

Check the high frequency machine first before any treatment, checking for any damaged cables or cracks to the holder or glass electrodes. Any loose jewellery, such as bracelets or earrings should be removed from both your client and yourself. Otherwise there can be irritation caused by sparking of electricity when skin contact is made. The client should be placed away from water and metal objects. Sit clients comfortably in a chair and try to get them relaxed before starting a treatment. Electrodes should be cleaned if this was not done by the last person to use the machine. Remove tangles from the *dry* hair. Never give high frequency if a client has had any kind of alcohol lotion applied to the scalp, or the vapour could ignite.

How do I carry out high frequency?

High frequency can be carried out either (1) directly, or (2) indirectly.

The *direct method* is carried out by inserting the glass electrodes into the holder and drawing them through the hair. The electrodes should be inserted with the current turned off. They should fit snuggly into the holder. Never force them in or out of the holder or the glass could break. If you look at the lid of the high frequency box in Figure 3.7 you will see the electrodes held by clips. From top to bottom they are the glass bulb, rake and comb, below which is the metal saturator rod. Use the bulb on bald areas or areas with little hair and the rake and comb on the normal scalp hair. Grip the holder in one hand, turn the current on low to start with and place one finger of your free hand onto the top of the glass electrode you are using. This is illustrated in Figure 3.8 with a rake. Do not remove your finger until the electrode is in contact with the client. This prevents sudden sparking, which may be uncomfortable for the client, between the hair and skin. Do this every time the electrode is removed from scalp contact before reapplying. Use the bulb in a small circular movement for between 2–5 minutes. As the client gets used to

Figure 3.8 The tip of the index finger should be kept on the electrode until it is in contact with the head.

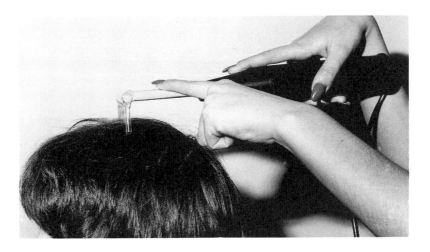

the treatment you will be able to increase the current by turning one of the dials on the machine. Do not be frightened by the violet light that is produced in the glass electrodes. When using the rake or comb be careful not to get them tangled in the hair. Starting at the front hairline, gradually work towards the nape by drawing the electrode through the hair. Be careful to avoid lifting the electrode clear of the scalp or hair − painful sparking may result. A treatment should last no longer than about ten minutes. The direct method of application may be combined with the indirect method to wind up a treatment.

The *indirect method* is carried out by inserting the metal saturating bar into the holder and asking the client to hold it, one hand on the metal bar and the other on the holder as shown in Figure 3.9. Emphasise to clients that they should not release their hands or they will get a sudden

Figure 3.9 Indirect high frequency treatment.

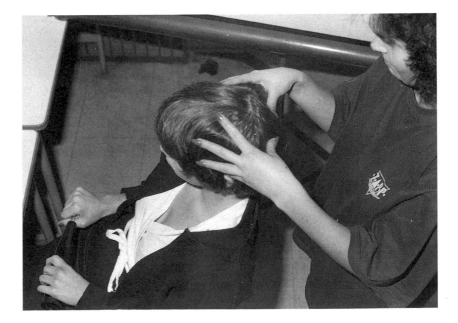

shock. Clients will not feel anything until you place your hands onto their scalp. As the fingers touch the skin the current flows from the bar through the client's body to the point of contact with the client—your fingers. Carry out a gentle massage. With practice you will be able to create a slight spark gap which will stimulate the scalp without causing the client discomfort.

After use clean all electrodes which have been used remembering that if you use some type of spirit (alcohol) it must be done some time before using on another client.

Questions
1. What are the benefits of high frequency?
2. What gas is produced during high frequency?
3. What are the contra-indications to high frequency being given?
4. How should you prepare the client for high frequency?
5. Describe how you would give high frequency directly.
6. Describe how you would give high frequency indirectly.

Chapter Four
Shampooing

Shampooing is carried out for a number of reasons in the salon and it will be discussed fully in this chapter. No shampooing could be carried out without water, so we will discuss the salon water supply first.

Water in the salon

Water, like electricity, is one of the most important things that we use each day in the salon. Just like electricity, we take it for granted, always expecting it to be there. Whoever runs a salon and pays the monthly bills, however, certainly does not take them for granted because they both cost money! How much they cost can depend largely on the staff who use them. Currently we pay for our supply of mains water by paying the water rates set by the local water board. This charge also takes sewerage into account. In the future there is a possibility that we may have meters fitted to our mains supply so that we will pay for the amount of water used, and not simply a fixed yearly amount.

The salon water supply

From the street outside the salon one pipe enters to supply water. This is the mains pipe which is under considerable pressure. Somewhere in your salon there should be at least one tap which is connected up directly to this mains pipe, providing a safe source of drinking water. If you look at the diagram of a typical salon water supply (Figure 4.1) you will see that a stopcock is fitted to this pipe so that water can be turned off in an emergency such as burst pipes, or if you simply want to have something done to the plumbing. You should know where this mains stopcock is just in case something ever goes wrong. The mains goes on from this point to supply a water tank, usually found in a loft space. This tank should then feed both the hot and cold water supplies of the rest of the salon. The higher the bottom of the tank is above the taps being used the greater the water pressure should be. It is the weight of the water in the tank pushing through the pipes when you turn a tap on that creates the pressure. As a rule, the wider the diameter of a pipe, the greater the pressure and the flow rate of water that can be provided. This is why the taps on a bath have larger pipes than, say, a sink. In your particular salon you may notice that the water pressure fluctuates if more than one tap is turned on. This is usually because all the pipes have the same diameter. To stop loss of pressure smaller pipes for each sink should come off a larger pipe. The reason this does not always happen

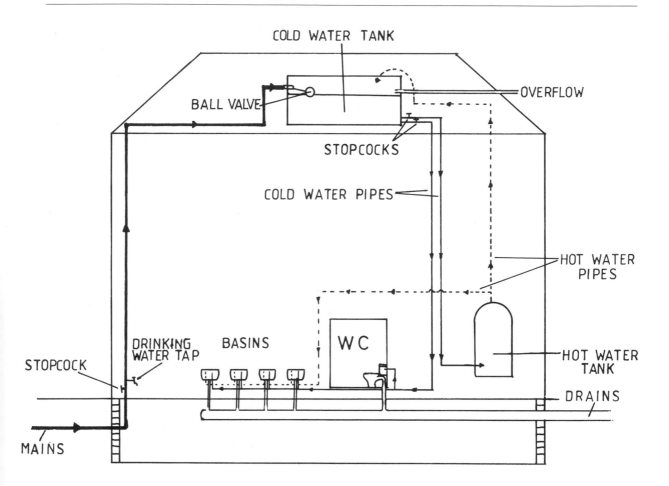

COLD WATER TANK

OVERFLOW

BALL VALVE

STOPCOCKS

COLD WATER PIPES

HOT WATER PIPES

BASINS

WC

HOT WATER TANK

DRINKING WATER TAP

DRAINS

STOPCOCK

MAINS

Figure 4.1 A salon water supply.

is purely financial, as the wider pipe is more expensive. You will notice stopcocks should also be on the pipes that emerge from the cold water storage tank, again so that water can be shut off if required.

What causes burst pipes?

As most things are heated up they expand and get bigger. When they cool down they contract and get smaller. Water, unfortunately for us, is different. Between 4°C and 0°C, as water is cooling, it expands by about one-tenth of its volume. This does not matter when water is not enclosed, but when it is enclosed in a pipe the expansion can rip the pipe apart. This will not be noticed until the frozen ice melts and suddenly water flows from the burst pipe. This water can seriously damage walls, bring ceilings down and be a hazard with electricity. Never switch on a light if the walls are wet or you could be electrocuted. Burst pipes usually occur in loft spaces where the pipes or water tank itself are not protected by insulation or lagging. Because there is no heating in the loft it should be the coldest place in the building if the loft space has been properly insulated from the rooms below. To protect the tank and pipes many people run the insulation from ceiling level up and over the tank. Insulation acts in the same way as a thermos flask with hot or cold drinks. Because it is a poor conductor of heat, water in an insulated pipe will take a long time to cool down.

Try the following simple experiment using a thermometer, paper cup, polystyrene cup, two lids, a large dish and some ice. Place the two cups in the dish and surround them with ice. Pour some hot water into both cups from a kettle or straight from the tap (but make sure that the water is the same temperature). Place a lid on each cup and leave for at least ten minutes. Remove the lids and record the temperature using your thermometer. The one which is warmest is the best insulator because it has not lost its heat so quickly to the ice. The polystyrene can be compared to the insulation around a cold water tank or pipe.

Types of water

Depending on where you live the water that comes out of your taps will be either hard or soft. These terms for water have been with us for a long time and often give people strange ideas about what they actually mean!

All water originally starts off as clouds of water vapour in the sky which eventually condenses and falls to the ground as rain. On its way down from the clouds each drop of rain will dissolve a small amount of carbon dioxide from the air. In doing so the rain becomes slightly acidic. The acid formed is called carbonic acid, and has nothing to do with the industrial pollution in the air that forms the much stronger acid rain. The drop of rain will soak into the ground and eventually it will end up in some kind of water supply. This could be natural lakes, rivers, wells or springs, or in a man-made reservoir.

If the ground through which the rain passed contained some types of rock, this water will dissolve tiny traces of chemicals and become 'hard'. If you live in an area where the main rock is limestone or chalk, the water will contain dissolved calcium and magnesium bicarbonates or sulphates. Some people refer to bicarbonate as 'hydrogen carbonate'. These dissolved salts give the water certain properties that make us refer to it as being hard − mainly forming scum with soap and depositing scale on heating. This will be explained a little further on in this section. If you live in an area without rocks containing calcium and magnesium salts your water will be soft. Even though it may contain other salts it will not form scum with soap or deposit scale on heating.

How can I tell if my water is hard or soft?

The simplest test is to look inside an electric kettle. In areas where the water is hard there is usually a pale-coloured layer of limescale. Basically, if the water contains calcium (or magnesium) bicarbonate and it is heated, it will change this salt into calcium carbonate which is deposited as limescale. Any water that deposits this scale is referred to as being temporary hard water, because it can be softened (i.e. have the calcium removed) by boiling. If the water contains calcium or magnesium sulphates it is referred to as being permanently hard, because it is not softened by boiling.

The scientific way to tell the difference between hard and soft water is fairly simple: add some soapflakes and stir! If after two minutes there is still a lather the water is soft, however, if the lather has collapsed, it is hard. What happens is that soap, which is chemically sodium stearate, reacts with the calcium (or magnesium) bicarbonate or sulphate to form scum. Chemically scum is calcium stearate, so all that has happened is that the calcium has replaced the sodium in the soap lather.

Back in the 1950s when shampoos were based on soap, if the salon had hard water the clients ended up with scum in their hair! This meant that special rinses had to be used to clean the hair of the scum. Modern shampoos are all based on soapless detergents that do not react with hard water so now we do not have this problem. This may explain to you why people today wash their hair more as there is far less hassle! The aspect of hard water that can really cause trouble in the salon is scale. This is most obvious when you look at the spray heads fitted at shampoo basins. After a while some of the holes in the spray head become blocked with scale or spray water to the sides instead of in the direction you want. Spray heads can easily be removed and the holes can be cleared with a fine pin or by pouring in some liquid descaler and leaving it until cleared. (It is best to use the liquid type sold for plastic jug kettles.) This scale will also block the nozzles in steamers if hard tap water is used in them. For this reason it is recommended that distilled or deionised water is used in steamers (both of these types of water are free from dissolved salts so are safe to use). If taps are left dripping, deposits of brown limescale will build up where the water drips. This can not only look unsightly but can also cause damage when you try to clean it off. Some of the most serious damage is not obvious as it takes place in the hot water system. The scale can be deposited throughout boilers, pipes and radiators as a layer of 'fur'. Special chemicals can be added to central heating systems either to stop this happening or to descale it once it has happened. If pipes are furred up the water pressure will gradually be reduced as it makes the diameter of the pipes shorter. Although hard water has its problems it has a nicer taste than soft water and also contains calcium, needed for teeth and bones.

You can check out these facts about hard and soft water by taking some distilled or deionised water and placing some in three beakers. Leave the first as it is and label it A. Into the second stir in some calcium bicarbonate and label it B. Into the third stir in some calcium sulphate and label it C. Stir some soap flakes into each beaker to produce a lather. The one with soft water will still have a lather after two minutes. Now heat the remaining two beakers until they boil. After they have cooled add some more soapflakes and stir. One of the beakers will still have a lather after two minutes. This is the beaker containing temporary hard water, while the remaining beaker must contain the permanently hard water because it was not softened by boiling. Now record which beaker contained each type of water.

Water softeners

Many salon owners have been persuaded by salesmen to install a water softening unit in their salons. These can be fitted to the single incoming mains pipe so that all the water in the salon is softened. They work by simply swapping sodium for the calcium or magnesium that makes the water hard. So instead of water containing calcium bicarbonate (it works in exactly the same way with calcium sulphate) it will end up with sodium bicarbonate instead. The sodium bicarbonate does not form scum with soap or deposit itself as scale when heated. Eventually the water softener runs out of sodium so this must be replaced at regular intervals. Many of you may have seen people adding sodium, in the form of salt, to their dishwashers to do this. If this were not done in an area of hard water, everything would be streaked with limescale.

There are also some chemicals which can be added to water to soften it. Calgon (sodium hexametaphosphate) is sometimes added to washing powder as a water softener while sodium carbonate is used as a water softener in bath salts. Many people say that the water feels slightly slimy against their skin once it is softened. These water softeners all work in the same way, sodium replacing the calcium of hard water.

Heating water

One of the most expensive aspects of the salon water supply is heating it up. When a client comes into your salon there must always be adequate hot water, no matter if it is first thing in the morning or last thing at night. If a salon has central heating there is usually a hot water tank as part of this. It may need to be a larger tank than the size that you would have at home, depending on the number of clients that you have at your busiest period of the week. Some salons have a water tank that is fitted with an electric immersion heater. This is rather like having a gigantic electric kettle, as the water is heated by a long electric element inside the tank. Unlike an electric kettle, this element can be fitted with a device that controls the final temperature the water reaches (called a thermostat). This means that you can have a tank of water kept at the right temperature and save money! Once the required temperature is reached, the electricity switches itself off until either someone uses the water, or it simply cools down.

Economy

The tank of water should be covered with some kind of insulation. Modern tanks come covered with a layer of hard yellow foam which does not allow much heat to escape from the tank. This means that the water will stay at the right temperature for long periods without having to be heated up again. Older tanks may have a covering of fibreglass in plastic (usually red). Although this covering will help retain heat it is not as efficient as the first type of covering mentioned, so more power must be used to keep the water hot. Having no form of insulation at all will mean paying much higher bills for water heating!

When you are using hot water in the salon the most important tip for economy is to turn off the taps whenever you can. Many hairdressers, who do not pay the bills themselves, leave the water running from the time they wet the clients hair until they are ready to rinse the second lot of shampoo off! Instead of using enough water to fill a couple of buckets they may have used enough to fill a bath tub!

Many salons now use instantaneous water heaters housed in small shower units. They are usually electric and although expensive to buy and install, they are extremely economical as you only pay to heat the water that you use. Some washrooms have them fitted above sinks for washing hands.

Shampoo basins

The typical shampoo basin in most salons is made of glazed white stoneware or porcelain. With salons reflecting fashion, some are having coloured basins fitted. Basins should be cleaned regularly with a non-abrasive cleaner so that they do not become scratched, as this would enable bacteria to breed in the scratches. If basins are cracked they should be replaced for the same reason. Basins are referred to as either front or backwashes, depending on whether clients put their heads forward or lie back to have their hair washed. Today, most new salons have backwashes fitted so that the hairdresser can get at the hair without having to stand over the client. The backwash is also safer to use when rinsing off chemicals as you are less likely to wash the chemical off the hair and into the eyes.

Because of the amount of hair that will end up in a salon basin many are fitted with a filter to stop the hair going down the sink waste and blocking it. This filter should be cleaned regularly so that water flows away freely down the waste pipe. If you look down a sink plug hole into the waste pipe you should see water. This water is held in a trap and forms a seal on the waste pipe. If it were not there unpleasant odours and air-borne bacteria could enter the salon from the drains. Because you use the basin regularly the water in the trap is being constantly replaced and so remains fresh. The water in a toilet pan works in exactly the same way to form a seal. The two types of trap found under most shampoo basins are shown in Figure 4.2. Both can be easily taken apart should they become blocked. Simply turn off the taps, place an empty bucket underneath and unscrew the seal nuts. Because bottle traps have only one seal nut to unscrew many hairdressers prefer them to S traps which have two. If ever you do this wear rubber gloves as it can be very mucky!

The taps fitted in most modern salons are referred to as 'mixer' taps, because they mix the hot and cold water before it enters the spray fitting. As long as the water pressure is constant (remember the diameter of pipes above) this means that the water temperature remains stable for the client. Each tap is fitted with a small rubber washer that enables you

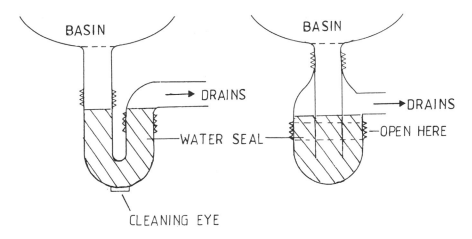

BASIN   BASIN

→ DRAINS   →DRAINS

WATER SEAL   OPEN HERE

CLEANING EYE

Figure 4.2 An S trap and a bottle trap.

to turn off the water totally. If a tap drips this means that the washer needs replacing. Never try to do this without turning off the stopcocks that supply the tap, so that you can drain the pipes down when you turn the tap on. Otherwise when you remove the top of the tap and the washer you will get very wet! There are taps available with ceramic discs instead of washers. Although much more expensive you will never have to replace a washer and the flow of water from the tap can be controlled in a quarter of a turn, rather than several full turns as with a conventional tap.

Questions
1. How does your salon pay for its water supply?
2. Find out how much it costs per year for this supply?
3. How does water get into your salon from the street outside?
4. How many drinking water taps are there in your salon?
5. Where is the stopcock on the mains pipe in your salon?
6. Why are water tanks usually found in loft spaces?
7. Why is the diameter of pipe used important to the supply of water?
8. Does water pressure in your salon drop if more than one set of taps is in use?
9. How is water different from other substances in the way that it reacts to cooling?
10. How much does water expand on cooling between 4°C and 0°C?
11. Why are burst pipes not always noticed immediately?
12. How does insulation help prevent burst pipes?
13. Explain how you can show that polystyrene is a good insulator.
14. What are the different types of water?
15. How does water become hard?
16. What are the two properties that would tell you that your water was hard?
17. What type of water do you have in your salon?
18. How does limescale form?
19. What is the difference between permanent and temporary hard water?

20. What is 'scum' chemically?
21. How is it formed?
22. Why was this a problem in the 1950s?
23. How can scale be a problem with salon basins?
24. How can the problem be overcome?
25. Why should distilled water be used in steamers?
26. Why should taps not be allowed to drip?
27. What 'unseen' damage can hard water cause?
28. How can this affect water pressure?
29. What benefits are there for health from hard water?
30. Describe an experiment to show how the different types of water can be identified.
31. How does a water softener work?
32. What is calgon?
33. What do chemicals which soften hard water have in common?
34. How is water for shampooing heated in your salon?
35. Why is it important to lag hot water tanks?
36. Why are instantaneous water heaters useful in salons?
37. How should basins be cleaned?
38. Why are backwash basins safer to use?
39. Why do some basins have hair filters fitted?
40. What is a trap?
41. Why are traps fitted to basins?
42. How do you unblock a basin?
43. What are mixer taps?

Shampooing

The word shampoo is derived from a Hindu word which means 'to clean'. How this is achieved is a little more complex, but shampooing hair is probably one of the first things most hairdressers learn when they start work in a salon. As a junior or trainee, you may be at the basins shampooing clients' hair for what seems like an eternity! So many services that a salon offers require the hair to be shampooed first before going any further. For this reason we will be concentrating on *why*, *when* and *how* you would shampoo for a range of salon services, and answer the technical questions about shampooing and handcare that you should know about.

Are today's shampoos soap or soapless?

Shampoos today contain soapless detergents that do not react with hard water like the older soap shampoos. A soap shampoo would react with the calcium in hard water to form insoluble soap scum so is of no real use in the modern salon (see earlier in this chapter). Soap shampoos were alkaline and made the cuticle of the hair swell, whereas soapless shampoos are naturally neutral or slightly alkaline, but can easily be made acidic by the addition of weak organic acids (citric acid, for example). Modern soapless detergents are very strong and can clean the hair too well (degreasing the scalp); they also have a greater tendency to produce dermatitis in the hairdresser's hands or on the client's scalp. These two drawbacks are fully accepted by the industry, but you may suffer from dermatitis in your early years so should know how to avoid it.

How do I avoid shampoo dermatitis?

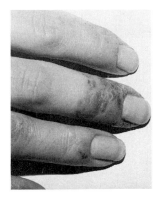

Figure 4.3 Shampoo dermatitis on a hairdresser's hands.

In an examination answer one candidate came up with the perfect answer, 'get the junior to do it'. This is not practical for all of us, however, so here are some tips which should help matters, but cannot always guarantee avoidance. Figure 4.3 shows dermatitis on a hairdresser's hands. The main cause is degreasing of the skin by detergent, so follow the following routine:

- Remove rings and bracelets which might get wet as these can cause irritation when your skin dries. Dermatitis is always worse around rings.
- Wash your hands thoroughly of all shampoo when you finish *each* client, even if you have another one within minutes.
- Dry your hands thoroughly, particularly at the base of the fingers where there are skin flexure points.
- Moisturise the skin with a hand cream. These contain chemicals called humectants which attract moisture into the skin from the atmosphere. This does not have to be expensive; try a few brands until you find the one that suits your skin. If you have sensitive skin avoid ones which have a fragrance or colour. Petroleum jelly is not suitable for your hands.
- Do not waste money on barrier creams as these are removed by the strong detergents found in shampoos.
- If you begin to get trouble with dermatitis you may have to buy special hand creams which contain steroids, so seek medical advice. If you have to use these creams for any length of time you will find that your epidermis becomes thinner, so use only when necessary. It takes the epidermis a year to recover fully from the effects of the steroids and get back to normal.
- Wear gloves when in doubt with any hairdressing chemicals. If you react to them it could make you sensitive to shampoo as well.

How do shampoos clean hair?

We say that shampoos contain detergents. The selected detergent must not be too alkaline as this will roughen the hair, nor must it damage the eyes or irritate the scalp too much. The shampoo must also produce a good lather as it is the lather that keeps the detergent in close contact with the skin and hair, enabling it to be clearly seen where the shampoo has been applied.

Actual detergency depends on the detergent molecule having both hydrophilic (water-loving) and hydrophobic (water-hating) groups of

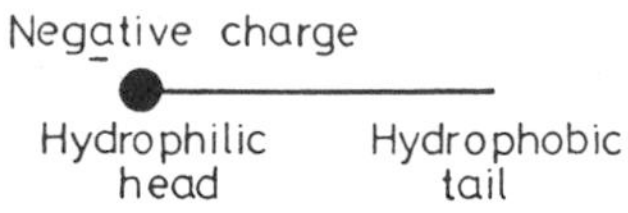

Figure 4.4 A molecule of detergent.

Negative charge

Hydrophilic head   Hydrophobic tail

atoms. These are usually arranged into a hydrophilic head (which may have a positive or negative charge, or no charge at all) and a hydrophobic tail (consisting of a chain of carbon and hydrogen atoms). Such a molecule of detergent is illustrated in Figure 4.4. If it is at an interface (the place where air and water meet, such as at the surface of some water in a glass) the hydrophilic head will be attracted to the water while the hydrophobic tail will stick out into the air. The detergent will form a single layer on the water surface. With grease and water, such as would be found on a dirty hair, the hydrophilic heads stick out into water while the hydrophobic tails are attracted by the grease. Although these two facts may not explain too much to you straight away, Figures 4.5 and 4.6 should do.

In Figure 4.5 a droplet of water has been dropped onto a hair. Because of surface tension, an inward pulling force that is exerted at the outer surface of liquids, it stays as a rounded globule (at the surface of a liquid the molecules are attracted to the ones next to each other and below – this is why you can overfill a beaker slightly without its overflowing). As soon as some detergent is added the hydrophilic heads break this surface tension (they get between the surface molecules and break the attraction) and the water droplet flattens out.

Figure 4.5 How a detergent improves the wetting of hair by reducing the surface tension of water.

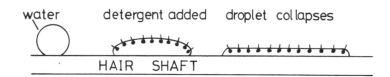

The detergent, being a surface active agent (often shortened to the word surfactant), has lowered the surface tension of water. This is important because it means that the detergent allows hair to be wetted better than by water alone. For this reason surfactants are also referred to as wetting agents.

In Figure 4.6, a globule of grease is present on the hair. As it is attracted to the hair it is flattened out onto the hair surface. Once detergent is applied to the hair the hydrophilic tails penetrate the surface of the grease and cause it to roll up into a globule. This gives the greaseless surface contact with the hair, until eventually it is suspended in the water to form an emulsion (oil droplets suspended in water), which can easily be removed as the hair is rinsed. Thus a detergent is also an emulsifying agent.

Figure 4.6 How a detergent removes grease from the hair during shampooing.

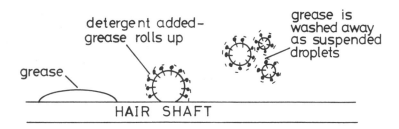

Emulsions are mixtures of oil and water. Normally oil would float on the surface of water and they would not mix for very long if shaken together. Because the detergent, as an emulsifying agent, is partially soluble in both oil and water, it forms a bridge between the two and stops them from separating out into two layers again.

Why is hair shampooed?

There are two main reasons for shampooing hair:

(a) to cleanse the hair and scalp by removing dirt, scales of keratin, stale perspiration, grease and other debris such as hairspray or oil-based styling products;
(b) to prepare the hair for subsequent hairdressing processes − shampooed hair absorbs more moisture than hair that is simply wetted with water. Also, the action of shampooing opens the cuticle scales.

Although we have given two reasons above, many of you might also want to include the fact that a shampoo helps to relax a client and serves as the psychological 'beginning' of the salon visit.

To expand on the two reasons given above, if the hair is not properly cleansed, a barrier could be left on the hair that interferes with the following service. Also, it is impossible to achieve body and bounce in hair which is greasy. A stylist would be none too pleased if her client had to be sent back to have another shampoo because the hair was not cleansed properly in the first place. We can remember seeing a trainee really struggling with a blow-dry and having great difficulty getting any root lift. Looking more closely, we could see 'smoke' coming off the hair which in fact was the grease evaporating from the heat of the hand dryer! Apart from the blow-dry being an absolute flop (literally!) the smell of heated sebum is not the most pleasant. Needless to say, the client's hair had to be shampooed again before a decent blow-dry was achieved. What a waste of time for the trainee and we don't think the client returned to the salon again either!

Because detergent lowers the surface tension of water, the application of shampoo is more efficient at wetting the hair than water on its own. If you have ever dampened a person's hair before a haircut as opposed to shampooing it, you will have found that the hair dried out a lot more quickly. Many hairdressers insist that the hair is kept wet during cutting and keep a water spray close at hand to dampen the hair regularly. If you are a person that prefers to cut very wet hair it is worth remembering that shampooing makes the hair absorb more moisture. For clients who have shampooed their hair on the day of the appointment, massage a little shampoo through the hair and then immediately rinse. You may find it amusing that there are many clients who shampoo their own hair before visiting the salon because they don't like the idea of going to the hairdresser's with dirty hair!

When should the hair be shampooed?

It would be easier to begin the answer to this question by stating when the hair should *not* be shampooed. The natural oil of the hair and skin (sebum) *lubricates and protects* – without it the skin and hair would become more susceptible to dryness and damage. It therefore makes sense that if you remove the sebum the scalp and hair has no means of protection against potentially harmful chemicals such as tint, bleach and relaxer cream. In fact we often *increase* the skin's own protection by applying barrier creams before these treatments. Apart from removing the protecting sebum, the action of massaging the scalp during the shampoo increases the blood flow to the skin's surface, making it more sensitive to chemicals. This means that the client would experience a burning sensation or irritation when the chemical product was applied. Therefore, it is recommended by manufacturers that the hair is *not* shampooed before a tint, bleach or relaxer application.

We expect that you are now thinking about a particular client who always comes into the salon for her regular tint application with her hair absolutely coated in oils and styling products and you are wondering whether this rule applies in her case? There are always exceptions that prove the rule, and there will be the few occasions when you have to shampoo the hair first. Also, the hair would have to be heavily oiled to impair the effectiveness of many chemical products. If the occasion should arise, follow these guidelines to help minimise scalp sensitivity:

- Remove any tangles with a brush or comb, but do not allow the tool to touch the scalp, as this could scratch the skin leaving an abrasion where the chemical could penetrate.
- Use tepid water (tepid means a temperature between cool and warm) to avoid stimulating the blood flow too much.
- Do not give a firm massage. Simply smooth the shampoo through the hair and leave it on for about a minute before rinsing.
- Apply the shampoo *once* only.
- Because you will need to dry the hair before applying the chemical product (tints, etc., are designed to be applied to dry hair) do so by using either a warm (not hot) hood or hand dryer and avoid rubbing or stimulating the scalp in any way.

Now that we have said when the hair should not be shampooed, you can presume that a shampoo can be safely carried out before all other salon treatments.

Shampooing the hair for a range of services/processes

(1) Before a perm

Hair is cleansed before perming to remove any possible barriers on the hair shaft that might prevent the lotion from penetrating the cuticle. The action of shampooing also swells the hair by opening up the cuticle scales, making it easier for the lotion to get into the hair structure. Because a chemical will be applied to the hair (perm lotion) it is important that the scalp is not stimulated too much or it will be very sensitive. Use tepid water, gentle massage and if possible, give only one shampoo. The type of shampoo to use before a perm is one which contains no additives. These shampoos are often referred to as 'plain' or 'pre-perm' shampoos. The reason for not using other shampoos is that they could contain substances that could leave a barrier on the hair shaft.

(2) Removing a tint

After a permanent tint has developed, the colorant will need to be removed from the hair by shampooing. When doing this, the aim of the operator should be for the client to leave the basin without any traces of tint remaining on the hair and scalp. There should be no need to use stain removers if a tint is shampooed off correctly.

The first thing to do is to add a little warm water to the hair and begin massaging to loosen the tint from the hair and skin. This is called *emulsifying*. Gradually, more water is added and the massage is continued until all the tint is loosened. Please note that not a drop of shampoo has been used yet. The hair is then thoroughly rinsed until the water runs clear and there should now be no tint left in the hair. The shampoo is now applied and the recommended shampoo for use after a tint is pH-balanced because this will not only reduce oxidation damage, caused by the tint, but will also help to restore the hair back to its natural pH of between 4.5 and 5.5. One application of shampoo should be sufficient because the tint contains a detergent and you will have emulsified the tint before adding the extra detergent.

(3) Shampooing for a semi-permanent colorant

Most semi-permanent colorants are applied to shampooed, towel-dried hair. As for perming, shampooing removes unwanted barriers on the hair shaft and helps to open the cuticle scales, enabling the colour molecules to penetrate more easily. Because this type of colorant contains detergent, one shampoo should be sufficient. After the semi-permanent colorant has been applied and developed according to the manufacturers' instructions, it is ready to be removed from the hair. Shampoo is *not* used for this. Instead, a little water is added and the operator emulsifies the colorant the same as would be done for a tint. When all the colorant has been loosened from the hair and scalp, the hair is thoroughly rinsed until the water runs clear. The hair is then ready for further treatment. Semi-permanent colours are designed to last for approximately four to eight shampoos (an average of six); if shampoo were used to remove the colorant, its life expectancy would be made shorter.

(4) Removing a bleach

After bleach has developed for the required time it is rinsed from the hair using tepid water. Remember that the client's scalp may be sensitive because of the bleach. Hot water and firm massage will cause the client discomfort. If a pastel toner is to be applied after the bleach application, this is even more important. The hair should be rinsed until all the bleach is out of the hair. Either a pH-balanced shampoo or a cream shampoo (one for dry hair) can then be applied. Remember that the massage should be gentle so that the scalp is not irritated and also because a rigorous rub makes bleached hair (which is more porous) tangle very easily.

(5) Shampooing after a relaxer

The shampoo that occurs after a relaxer application is very important because the special type of shampoo that is used has ingredients that neutralise the alkali left in the hair and return it to an acid state. The relaxer is first flushed out of the hair completely using the force of water from the basin water spray. Then, one to three shampoos are given with the manufacturer's acidic neutralising shampoo. Never intermix product ranges and always follow the manufacturer's instructions exactly.

(6) Shampooing for a hair/scalp treatment

Brands for treating hair and scalp disorders have become very sophisticated over the last few years and will often comprise a comprehensive range of shampoos, treatments and styling products. The product range stocked by a salon will determine whether the hair is shampooed or not before the treatment and also the products to be used. Many salons do not use such specialised products and rely upon offering re-conditioning treatments using a heavy conditioner such as henna wax (no relation to the type of henna colorant) and scalp treatments using oils such as olive, almond or jojoba. If this is the case, for re-conditioning treatments the hair should first be cleansed using a shampoo for dry hair.

If you are to give an oil treatment the hair is *not* shampooed before the oil is applied. The shampoo is omitted because the oil would simply lie on top of the water on the hair and scalp and would have little or no chance of making any difference. These treatments are described in Chapter 3. When the oil is ready to be removed from the hair after an oil treatment, shampoo is applied to the hair *without* wetting the hair with water first. The hair and scalp are massaged thoroughly before rinsing. A second shampoo is given in the normal manner and may be repeated as often as three times until the hair is 'squeaky clean', telling you that all the oil has been removed.

(7) Shampooing for all other services

Shampooing for services such as cutting, blow-drying and setting is probably carried out most often. It is the choice of the shampoo to be used for each particular client which is the most important factor. This involves consulting the client and recommending the shampoo which will be of most benefit to her hair. Too many hairdressers *ask* clients what shampoo they want – that is like the dentist asking you how many fillings you think you should have! Another commonly used expression, is to ask clients if they would like a shampoo other than the 'ordinary' one. The usual response to this is 'no' because the client presumes that anything which is not ordinary must be special for which they will be charged more. *You* are the professional and *you* should be able to diagnose the client's hair and select the appropriate shampoo.

How should the client be positioned during a shampoo?

Figure 4.7 Client's position at a backwash basin.

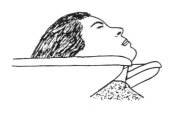

The best position for a client having a shampoo is reclined at a backwash basin, as illustrated in Figure 4.7. Because the client is leaning backwards the face remains dry and the risk of anything entering the eyes is reduced. Forward wash basins are becoming much less popular as even with a cloth held over the eyes the face can still get wet, possibly ruining make-up. The client should be comfortably seated when reclined and you may need to adjust the chair so that the client's neck rests in the central neck rest of the basin. Clients should be asked to lean back more if the head is too upright otherwise water could run down the face.

Depending on how the basins are fitted, you will be standing either at the side of the client or behind. You should always try and keep your back as straight as possible to help reduce fatigue and avoid backache. If you are standing alongside clients, try not to lean across too much and smother them with your body. Needless to say, you will be in very close contact with the client when standing at the side so your own personal hygiene needs careful consideration. Few people would appreciate another person's armpit under their nose that stank of body odour! The same advice is given to those hairdressers who smoke or who enjoy eating strong-smelling foods such as garlic and onions: when you are this close to clients you must make sure you are 'nice to know'. The gowning of a client for a shampoo is described in Chapter 1.

How is the water temperature tested and controlled?

The cold water should always be turned on first to prevent scalding and also to prolong the life of the hose, which is usually a rubber tube covered with a flexible metal covering. Gradually, hot water is added until a comfortable temperature is achieved. The temperature of the water should be tested on either the back of your hand or the inside of your wrist before it is put onto the client. Some mixer taps can control the water temperature better than others because much depends on the plumbing in individual salons. You may sometimes find that the water pressure or temperature changes when another basin is being used or even when someone flushes the toilet! If this is the case in your salon, you could hold the hose so that one of your fingers remains in the flow of the water all the time, keeping a continuous check on its temperature. Always check with your client if the water temperature is comfortable. If it needs readjusting, move the spray away from the client's head to do this, just in case you adjust the wrong tap!

How is the flow of water controlled during rinsing?

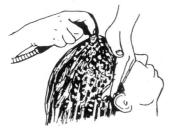

Figure 4.8 Shielding the client's face during the rinsing.

The client's face should be shielded from any splashes by placing your hand on the hairline as shown in Figure 4.8. The palm of your hand should always be facing the jet of water and it is moved to whichever part of the front hairline needs protection. Hold the water spray near to the client's head to avoid unnecessary splashing.

How should shampoo be applied to the hair?

Pour the shampoo into the palm of your hand. Spread it between your hands and smooth it through the hair to distribute it evenly. *Never* put the shampoo directly onto one area of the head, or it will not spread out evenly and will feel uncomfortably cold to the client. If shampoo is applied in one area like this it is concentrated and might cause dermatitis on the client's scalp. You are advised to apply too little shampoo rather than too much as it is easy to apply more but difficult to rinse out a copious amount of lather. You will also avoid wasting extra hot water.

How should the hair and scalp be massaged during a shampoo?

When you are applying the shampoo to the hair you are using a stroking movement to distribute the product: this stroking movement that begins at the front hairline and finishes at the nape is called the *effleurage* massage technique (see Chapter 3). Once the shampoo is evenly distributed through the hair, you would then begin a more stimulating massage technique called *rotary*. As the name infers, the hands move in a circular motion using the pads of the fingers on the scalp. The pressure of the fingers should be adjusted according to particular clients so that they find it comfortable. This varies from client to client but many prefer what is often called a 'hard rub'. Also, do remember that there are times when minimum massage is necessary because of scalp sensitivity before or after chemical treatment. Make sure that your massage covers the entire scalp – a common complaint from clients is that the nape area is missed.

When shampooing hair that tangles very easily (e.g. bleached) or delicate hair that could be damaged by harsh treatment, adjust your massage accordingly, perhaps using only the effleurage massage technique. Unfortunately, many clients (and some hairdressers!) believe that the hair will only be cleansed properly if the water is really hot, a great deal of shampoo is used and the client is subjected to a 'really good scrub'. This is not the case at all. Hair should be treated with the same respect that you would take if you were washing a silk blouse.

Why should hair be thoroughly rinsed?

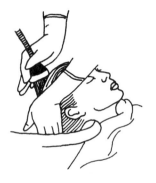

Figure 4.9 Lifting the hair with the fingers to ensure that the water can penetrate during rinsing.

Rinsing hair means allowing water to go onto the hair either to make it wet or to remove something from it, like shampoo. Shampoos are designed to be applied to wet hair — if they should be applied to dry hair, their concentration will be too strong because they are not adequately diluted. This can cause dermatitis on a person's scalp. After applying the shampoo to wet hair and performing the required massage, the shampoo will need to be rinsed out of the hair. If any shampoo is left in the hair it can cause scalp irritation and interfere with the performance of other products to be used. During rinsing, the hand which is not holding the spray should be used not only to shield the face from splashes but also to lift the hair to assist the water penetrating and flushing out the detergent (see Figure 4.9). Do look for the presence of lather when rinsing and continue to rinse until you are positive no shampoo remains.

Are all hair textures and lengths shampooed in the same way?

Greater care has to be taken when shampooing hair which is damaged or weak from chemical or physical abuse. This is because such hair has a tendency to tangle easily and break when subjected to undue tension and stress when it is rigorously rubbed or rinsed with hot water. Hot water opens the cuticle, while rubbing roughens the cuticle, causing the hairs to mat together. Very long hair can be a problem to shampoo because the plug hole can become blocked by the hair lying in the basin, making rinsing difficult. One manufacturer has even produced a basin to help cope with long hair! You will need to lift up the hair every so often to allow the water to flow away. The weight of the long hair may make it difficult for your fingers to penetrate the hair. As rigorous massage will make the hair tangle a lot anyway, try to use the stroking massage technique (effleurage) to assist the shampoo in its work.

What is the sequence and procedure for a shampoo?

The sequence and procedure for a shampoo will depend upon *why* you are doing it. For example, if it is to be carried out to remove a tint from the hair, you will only need to give one shampoo because the emulsifying will have loosened the tint from the hair and scalp. If the client had not shampooed her hair for four weeks, perhaps because of illness or injury to the head, it may be necessary to give more than two shampoos to clean the hair adequately. Below is a recommended procedure and sequence for shampooing, but this will vary according to the client you are dealing with and the service for which the client has booked.

1. Gown the client for a shampoo according to salon procedures. This might include the additional use of neck strips and a disposable plastic cape.
2. Disentangle the hair, making sure that the scalp is not scratched by the comb or brush.
3. Select the appropriate shampoo according to the condition of the hair and scalp or the service that follows shampooing. In the case of shampooing for a perm, a pre-perm shampoo is used which contains no barrier-forming additives and so is not chosen according to the client's hair or scalp condition.
4. Turn on the cold water tap first and gradually add the hot water until you have achieved a comfortable and suitable temperature. Test this on either the back of your hand or the inside of your wrist before rinsing the hair.
5. During rinsing, shield the client's face from any splashes. When the hair is thoroughly wet, turn off the water and apply the shampoo.
6. Pour the shampoo into the palm of your hand. Spread it between your hands and distribute it evenly through the hair. If the shampoo is runny like water, apply the shampoo by placing your hand on the client's head and pour it over the back of your hand. This method avoids the difficult task of trying to hold the shampoo in your hands and also that uncomfortable cold feeling of shampoo running over the client's scalp.
7. Massage the hair according to the client's requirements or the service that is to follow the shampoo. Remember that before a perm minimum massage should be given.
8. When you are sure that all the scalp has been adequately massaged, smooth off the excess lather from your hands; turn on the water and adjust to the correct temperature as before. Rinse the lather from your hands before rinsing the hair as this will help you to avoid dermatitis.
9. Rinse all the lather from the hair, paying particular attention to areas that can easily be missed such as the nape. Remember that your hand which is not holding the spray should be shielding the client's face from splashes. When you are not rinsing around the hairline, your free hand can be used to lift the hair slightly to assist the flow of water to flush out the shampoo.
10. You may need to repeat the shampoo and rinse as before. This will depend on the service that the client is having or when the client last shampooed her hair.
11. When the hair has been sufficiently cleansed and rinsed, the excess water in the hair is squeezed out by using your hands in a firm stroking movement from hairline to nape (see Figure 4.10).

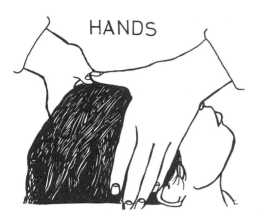 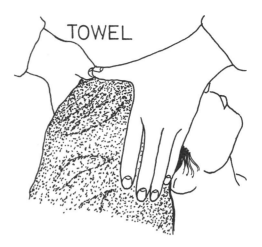

Figure 4.10 Squeezing out excess water after final rinsing.

12. A clean, dry towel is then placed over the client's wet hair to prevent drips while the client is gently raised to the upright position.

13. The client should then be seated at a styling unit and the hair gently towel-dried. Towel-drying the hair does not mean rubbing it so hard that it ends up a tangled mess. The towel should be pressed onto the hair using both hands in a stroking movement from front hairline to nape, so that the towel blots the hair of excess water.

14. Using a wide-toothed comb, the hair is disentangled and combed straight back from the face. The towel around the client's shoulders should be replaced if it has become wet, and if a plastic cape has been used which will no longer be needed, this can be removed.

Why is hair towel-dried for further processes after shampooing?

Most hairdressing processes require the hair to be towel-dried after it has been shampooed. Towel-drying means to dry the hair, with a towel, so no more water drips from it. Towel-drying is necessary because the majority of products applied to shampooed hair are designed to perform at their best on hair that is neither dripping wet nor too dry. An average head of hair can hold approximately 60 ml of water before it even drips. A setting lotion applied to hair holding that much water will obviously not work as effectively because it will be diluted. Conversely, if it were to be applied to dry hair it would be too strong and could be sticky. If the shampoo was given to remove bleach from the hair before the application of a pastel toner, it is also important that the hair is not too wet for the application. However, if a shampoo was given because the hair was coated in so much oil or styling products and the tint or relaxer would not have been able to penetrate this barrier, the hair should be dried before the hair is chemically processed as the products are designed to work on dry hair.

How is hair dried for further processes after a shampoo?

To towel-dry the hair a towel is held in both hands and the hair is pressed between the towel in a smoothing action that starts at the front hairline and ends at the nape on the points of the hair. The hair should never be harshly rubbed because this roughens the cuticle, making the hair tangle.

How is the hair disentangled after a shampoo?

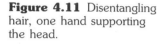

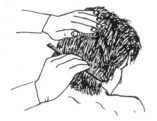

Figure 4.11 Disentangling hair, one hand supporting the head.

The hair is disentangled using a wide-toothed comb to avoid undue stress on the hair and discomfort to the client. Hair stretches more when it is wet than when it is dry so care should be taken not to over-stretch it, as it could break the hair. Brushes should not be used to remove tangles on wet hair: the hair will be stretched more because the number of filaments of a brush are far greater than the number of teeth in a comb. Disentangling should always begin at the nape region so that the hair is combed through section by section. The combing action begins at the points of the hair and gradually works up towards the roots (Figure 4.11). Hair should not be disentangled starting at the roots because the tangles will be pushed down to the points and when this happens, removing them is often damaging to the hair and uncomfortable for the client.

Different types of shampoo

Although we have said that soapless shampoos are the industry standard, the actual detergent and extra ingredients can vary in shampoos for different types of hair.

Shampoos for greasy hair

The actual percentage of soapless detergent in a shampoo for greasy hair varies from the usual 15−20 per cent to as high as 50 per cent of the shampoo. This means that the shampoo will remove the grease more quickly; but it does nothing to *prevent* greasy hair. Lemon shampoo is often mentioned as being the shampoo for greasy hair but lemon does nothing to prevent grease. A shampoo for greasy hair will contain few oily or fatty substances which would be found in shampoos for normal or dry hair.

Shampoos for dry hair

These shampoos are of two main types, those which degrease the hair less because of their reduced content of soapless detergent (about 10 per cent) or those with added oils. The added oils include coconut, olive and almond oils, residues of which are left on the hair. Lanolin (natural sheep's sebum) is also sometimes added but bear in mind that some people are allergic to lanolin. Other conditioners such as egg or beer are sometimes added and claimed to give the hair more body, but are, in truth, quickly rinsed from the hair when used as shampoo ingredients and are pretty ineffective. (One egg added to a 1,000 gallon vat of normal shampoo will still make it an egg shampoo!) Beware of herb shampoos as well; herb extracts do little for a shampoo except possibly scent it!

Anti-dandruff shampoos

These shampoos contain substances which claim to reduce the multiplication of the epidermal cells and thus reduce subsequent scaling. There are two main active ingredients found in such shampoos, but zinc pyrithione (also called zinc omadine) is by far the most popular of the two. It has a concentration of between 2−3 per cent in a soapless shampoo base and also has antiseptic properties. Those containing the other ingredient, selenium sulphide, are rare now because so many people are allergic to sulphur. This type of shampoo would contain between 2−5 per cent selenium sulphide and can be obtained through hairdressing manufacturers.

Shampoos for damaged hair

If the hair has a porous cuticle and structural damage such as split ends (fragilitis crinium) protein shampoos can be very beneficial. The shampoos contain broken down protein (often described in the ingredients as hydrolysed protein or keratin) in the form of short chains of amino acids. These are substantive to hair; that is, they cling to it, filling in some of the damaged areas and making split ends hold together. Any such repairs achieved are temporary, however, and there is no permanent change.

Psoriasis

If a client has psoriasis the use of a coal tar shampoo may be beneficial as it can reduce scaling. This type of shampoo often needs to be left on the hair and scalp for about five minutes to obtain maximum benefit.

Colour-treated hair

Shampoos which have a low pH (4.5−5.5) are most suitable for tinted or bleached hair because they help to reduce oxidation damage and close the cuticle. If the cuticle is closed, the degree of fade caused by colour molecules escaping through the cuticle is reduced.

Brightening shampoos

There are several types of shampoo that are designed to enhance and brighten the colour of the hair. These range from camomile, to gently lighten naturally blonde hair, henna for increasing the warmth (redness) of brown hair, to those containing varying amounts of temporary and semi-permanent colourants in shampoo bases. To lighten dark blonde hair, hydrogen peroxide (3 per cent or 10 volume strength) can be added to shampoo and is left on the hair for 5–10 minutes.

Itchy scalps

Clients with itchy scalps are likely to scratch them and this can cause subsequent infections. They should be encouraged to use a medicated shampoo which will be either cationic or have added antiseptics. Cationic shampoos have a positive charge which is attracted to the overall negative charge of hair. Most other shampoos are anionic, that is, they have a negative charge. The cationic detergent is usually cetrimide which coats the hair, leaving an antiseptic film behind. It does not lather very well and can cause damage to eyes (use a backwash basin as protection against this as cetrimide can cause the transparent cornea in front of the eye lens to become opaque) but can be a useful shampoo. Other shampoos contain anionic detergent together with an antiseptic such as hexachlorophene or resorcinol.

After alkaline treatments

The shampoo to be used should neutralise any excess alkalinity and close the cuticle, so has to be acid. The preferred acidity is similar to that of the skin and hair (a pH of 4.5–5.5, hence the term 'acid-balanced').

Pre-perm shampoos

The type of shampoo to be used to cleanse the hair before a perm should not contain additives that could form a film on the hair shaft and prevent the perm lotion from penetrating the cuticle. Sometimes, this type of shampoo is called 'plain' or 'regular'.

How do you choose a suitable shampoo for a client?

It is impossible to select the most suitable shampoo for a client without examining the hair and scalp and asking the client some questions. You need to do this to diagnose the client's hair type and recommend the shampoo which will be of most benefit to the hair and most suitable for the salon treatment the client is getting. *Never* ask the client which shampoo they want – this is highly unprofessional because as the person performing the shampoo, you should be able to recommend what type of shampoo the client should have. There are some important key questions that you should ask the client to help you in your consultation. For example:

'When did you last shampoo your hair?'

This helps you judge whether the client's hair has a tendency to being oily or dry. If you can feel a lot of sebum on the hair and they tell you that their was shampooed two days ago, you can be pretty sure that the client's hair has a tendency to being greasy.

'What shampoo and styling products do you use on your hair at home?'

This tells you whether the hair feels oily or dry because of the products they are using between salon visits. For example, one client who was asked this question said that she used a shampoo for treating dandruff. When asked if the dandruff was worrying her (as the hairdresser was about to recommend a treatment) she replied that she didn't have dandruff but liked the smell of the shampoo! In fact, the client was showing the first signs of dandruff due to using the shampoo.

'What treatment are you having today?'

This is an important question because certain services require the use of special shampoos, as in the case of a perm. Also, if the client has booked only for a cut and blow-dry and the hair would benefit from a conditioning treatment or other form of service, now is the time to suggest it to the client. Do remember, however, that if you recommend services or products to clients you must be able to tell them how it will benefit their hair and also how much it will cost.

How can wastage be controlled when shampooing?

There are a number of considerations to be taken to minimise wastage in the salon when shampooing. First, the water should always be turned off between rinses. Leaving the hot tap running can result in the salon running out of hot water! You should not require more than two towels per client for a shampoo. Unnecessary changing of towels increases the amount of laundry that the salon will need to do. Obviously, there is a limit to how much shampoo should be used for each application. Wastage is controlled by using pump dispensers as shown in Figure 4.12. This type of dispenser is pressed on top of the bottle and the pump is filled with sufficient shampoo for two applications. A great deal of wastage occurs by applying too much shampoo which results in a longer rinsing time and some of the product spilling down the plughole.

The last point to consider is how much time it takes you to carry out a shampoo. Time is money in a hairdressing salon and it is uneconomical for the salon if it takes you longer than necessary to complete a shampoo. Also, do remember that during the shampoo, you have the client's undivided attention and this golden opportunity is not to be wasted. Talk to your client about the latest products, special offers that your salon is running and tips on home hair care.

Figure 4.12 Shampoo bottle with pump dispenser. (Courtesy Goldwell Hair Cosmetics Ltd.)

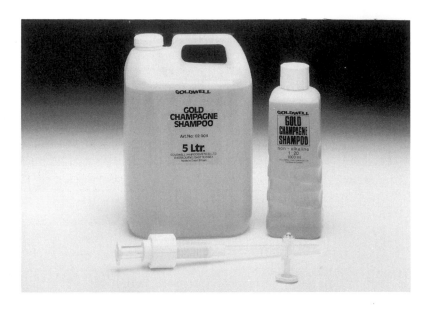

Questions
1. What does the word 'shampoo' mean?
2. Why are modern shampoos soapless?
3. What drawbacks do soapless shampoos have?
4. How would you look after your hands to prevent shampoo dermatitis?
5. Why is lather important?
6. What do the terms 'hydrophilic' and 'hydrophobic' mean?
7. Draw a diagram of a detergent molecule.
8. How does a detergent lower surface tension?
9. Why are detergents called 'wetting agents'?
10. Describe how a detergent removes grease from the hair.
11. What is an emulsion?
12. How does detergent act as an emulsifying agent?
13. What reasons are there for shampooing hair?
14. If you want to cut a head of hair wet, why is it better to shampoo it first?
15. When should hair not be shampooed?
16. How would you keep scalp sensitivity to a minimum?
17. Describe the shampooing procedure: (i) before perming, (ii) for removing a tint, (iii) before applying a semi-permanent, (iv) for removing bleach, (v) for removing a relaxer, (vi) for a hair or scalp treatment, (vii) for other services.
18. How should the client be positioned for a shampoo?
19. Describe how you should test and control the temperature of water for shampooing.
20. How should you protect the client from splashing during rinsing?
21. How should shampoo be applied to the hair?
22. Describe scalp massage during shampooing.
23. Why should more care be taken with bleached hair?

24. Why should hair be thoroughly rinsed?
25. How can long hair present difficulties when shampooing?
26. Describe the steps in the shampooing procedure.
27. Why do you towel-dry hair?
28. How should you disentangle hair after shampooing?
29. Make a table to show the various shampoo types and their uses from the information towards the end of the section on shampooing.
30. Make a similar table for the shampoos in use in your salon.
31. What kind of questions would you ask clients to determine the correct shampoo for their hair?
32. How can you minimise wastage when shampooing?

Chapter Five
Cutting

There is more to cutting hair than simply reducing its length. It takes technical skill, care and imagination to produce good results because every head presents its own problems. If you are following the Foundation Certificate in Hairdressing Syllabus there are a number of haircuts that you will be required to perform. We will be looking at cutting in its wider context so that you can apply the knowledge to the various styles. You will find some photographs of step-by-steps at the end of the chapter.

A good haircut is the basis of a manageable style and is usually a high priority when clients choose a stylist or a salon. A competent hairdresser is equipped with *all* the cutting skills necessary to carry out a client's requests and carefully selects the appropriate techniques to achieve the required effect.

Haircutting

The chapter is divided into sections which deal with different cutting methods. There are a number of skills and knowledge elements which will be dealt with first, because they are necessary for you to be able to understand how each of these is important to developing competence in cutting hair.

Why is the natural hair fall and movement important to the stylist when cutting hair?

Every head of hair is unique and will present you with a different set of problems to solve and decisions to make in order to achieve a satisfactory result. The stylist should always work *with* the natural fall and movement of the hair so that the finished style lies correctly and is not difficult for the client to maintain between salon visits.

The true lie of the hair can only be seen when the hair is wet because certain styling techniques can disguise the direction of how the hair falls naturally. When you are looking at a head of hair to observe the natural hair growth patterns, you will need to comb the hair and pay particular attention to the following hair growth characteristics: (1) the nape hairline, (2) the front hairline, (3) the crown, (4) amount of root lift, (5) natural partings, (6) degree and uniformity of curl formation (natural or chemical).

(1) The nape hairline

Situated at the back of the head, the nape hairline runs from ear to ear and is the perimeter of the hair growth on the neck. This line of hair growth will vary enormously between clients and men will usually have much lower hairlines at the nape. Some nape hairlines have particularly strong directions of growth and this can be limiting to what you can achieve with your scissors (or other cutting tools) so that the finished look lies properly. You will need to look for the direction and strength of the hair growth. Sometimes the direction of growth will be the same on both sides, being uniform and lying evenly. Other hairlines might have a tendency to grow towards one side while others may grow in opposite directions. A hairline which has both sides growing towards the centre is also common. The strength of the hair growth in this area will determine how you will cut the hair to achieve the best results. To see this properly you will need to comb the hair in this area in different directions (i.e. with and against the natural lie of the hair). If the hair is long and heavy, make sure that you are not deceived by the length of the hair weighing down the growth characteristics. Get all the unwanted hair out of the way so that you can clearly see which way the hair wants to lie on its own accord. You may find it easier to take very fine sections of hair, starting at the very bottom, and combing them to see the direction of growth and then gradually taking more hair until you have completed the observation.

(2) The front hairline

Front hairlines are situated at the front of the head; they are the outermost growth of hair that runs from ear to ear across the forehead. Like hairlines at the back of the head, these vary a great deal between people and, in the case of male pattern baldness, can gradually alter during a lifetime. It is not until you start looking at front hair lines that you begin to appreciate how they differ between people. Some front hairlines will be virtually straight across while others will recede at the temples or grow close to the eyebrows at the temples. Some of these growth characteristics are determined by our sex, age or ethnic group. For example, it is common for men to have receding hairlines and to have a lower growth of hair at the sides in front of the ears. Many females of Afro-Caribbean origin have a lower hairline growth in front of their ears than their European counterparts. As people get older, the amount of hair on the head decreases and may begin to recede at the temples. Apart from the characteristics already described, the two other growth patterns you will encounter on a front hairline are cowlicks and widow's peaks. A cowlick is a strong area of hair growth in the opposite or an unusual direction at the front hairline. The hair will 'kick' out and the cowlick will be clearly visible. A widow's peak is a strong growth of hair where the hair grows into a peak and is usually at or very near to the centre of the front hairline. The front hairline of Count Dracula is an exaggerated example of a widow's peak.

(3) The crown

The crown is situated at the top of the head but exact positions will vary. The crown determines the direction of hair growth on the top of the head and may be in the centre of the head, slightly to one side, high, low, or there might even be two of them! The term 'double crown' is used to describe a person that has two crowns. The hair at the crown might grow outwards from a visible point, sworling around in a strong circular pattern, while other crowns will be less distinct.

(4) Amount of root lift

The angle at which the follicle is set in the skin determines a hair's direction of growth and also how close it will naturally lie to the skin. This is the 'root lift'. If the follicle is set in the skin at an acute angle, the hair will lie closer to the skin's surface than a hair emerging from a follicle that is set in the skin at, say, seventy degrees. The quantity and position of a person's follicles is determined at birth and does not alter throughout a lifetime. Although hair may not grow from every follicle for ever, the follicle is still present, as in the case of alopecia. The amount of root lift will vary in different areas of the head and between clients. If a client requires lift at the roots there are cutting techniques that can be used to help do this but results will depend upon how heavy the hair is. Sometimes, perms are given to clients to help add lift and body at the roots.

(5) Natural partings

A natural parting is the position of where the hair falls naturally between the crown area and the front hairline to form a break (parting) in the lie of the hair. Some natural partings will be at the side, while others may be in the centre or off centre. The old myth about partings being worn on one side if you're male and on the other if you're female should be ignored. It is recommended that hairdressers style hair in accordance with a client's natural parting but we all know that this is not always possible because of the style the client wants. Therefore, you will often place partings elsewhere to achieve the desired look. Sometimes, working against the natural parting is useful for obtaining height in some styles, and the clever placing of a parting can make thin faces appear broader and wide faces appear narrower. A natural parting can only be found when the hair is wet. The hair is combed straight back from the face and using your free hand, the hair is gently nudged forward. The hair will then break to reveal the natural parting.

(6) Degree and uniformity of curl formation

There is an expression that says we always want what we haven't got.

Therefore people with straight hair often want it to be curly and vice versa. Ignoring natural curl and movement in the hair can often spoil a haircut, making it difficult for the client to manage and maintain. Working with any curl in the hair and using it to create the style is therefore recommended. If the curl in the client's hair is natural, it will probably be less curly when it is wet than when it has been wetted and allowed to dry naturally. However, if the curl was achieved chemically by perming, the hair has to be wet to see how much movement is present, because styling and drying methods can disguise the curl. The amount of movement in the hair might vary in different areas of the head. For example, the hair at the back may be less curly than the hair at the sides. If this is not spotted by you, it may result in the finished style not looking as it should.

Questions
1. Why is natural hair fall and movement important when cutting hair?
2. When can the true lie of the hair be seen?
3. Examine the nape hairline of some friends and describe the pattern of growth of each.
4. What is the front hairline?
5. How does it vary in different groups of people with ethnic origin and age?
6. What hair growth patterns might you find at the front hairline?
7. How can people's crowns vary?
8. What do you understand by the term 'root lift'?
9. How can extra root lift be obtained?
10. What is a natural parting?
11. How can partings be used in a hairstyle?
12. Why should you take curl into account when designing a style?

How can these hair growth characteristics be controlled when cutting?

We've already explained the importance of looking for the natural hair fall and movement, and when possible, working so that they are incorporated into the haircut. Below are some useful examples of how the natural hair fall and movement can be used and controlled.

Nape hair growth

Try not to cut above the natural hairline at the nape when possible. Sometimes this will be necessary, and scissors, clippers or a razor can be used for this. Reshaping the hairline, or in other words, cutting the hair so that it takes on a shape different from the way it has grown, is most often done when fashion cutting, or cutting Afro-Caribbean or men's hair. (A word of warning about reshaping men's hairlines: if a man is

Figure 5.1 Hairline shaping using a razor.

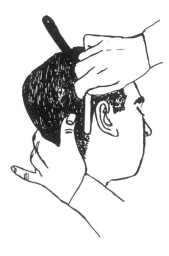

Figure 5.2 Hairline shaping using scissors.

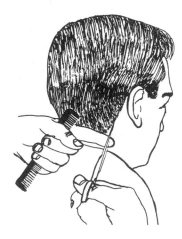

very hairy, the hair on his neck may join into the hair growing on his back and it is very easy to get carried away removing the unwanted hair. Before you realise it, you can have cut away some of the hair that would not have been seen anyway, because it would be covered by a shirt!)

Certain hairline shapes lend themselves better to particular hair growth patterns. Refer back to Chapter 2 which discusses this in more detail.

The hairline may be reshaped using either scissors, clippers or a razor. Examples are shown in Figures 5.1 and 5.2.

Front hairline

The growth characteristics you are most likely to encounter on the front hairline are cowlicks, widow's peaks and areas of recession. Cowlicks cause the hair to grow in a different direction to the rest of the hair on the hairline. It could cause the hair to move strongly to the left or right or perhaps push upwards. Try to use the direction of this movement in your cutting. If you attempt to cut a full fringe where a cowlick is present you will have difficulty because the fringe will kick out and appear uneven. If you use tension whilst cutting over a cowlick the result will be even more catastrophic. Tension will stretch the natural movement out of the hair and when the mesh of hair is released it will spring back and be surprisingly shorter than you anticipated. If the mesh is held with tension, and checked with the rest of the hair, it may appear to be technically correct and level, but as it is released, the ends will not be level.

Widow's peaks can also cause problems for the hairdresser. A widow's peak grows backwards from the face and trying to make the hair come forward onto the forehead should be avoided. That is to say, it is impossible to do this because it will very soon force itself back into its natural backward growing direction. Incidentally, did you know that the singer and actress Cher (of Sonny and Cher in the sixties) had electrolysis on her hairline to get rid of her widow's peak? This is proof in itself that there is nothing a hairdresser can do with their scissors to alter the way the hair grows naturally. Even if it is cut off down to the skin (as in the case of hairline re-shaping) the hair will still grow back in the same direction.

If the hair recedes on the front hairline of a female client, she will probably want this to be disguised. This can also be said for many male clients too, especially if they are sensitive about any hair loss caused by male pattern baldness. If the client is concerned about concealing areas of recession, try to leave the hair slightly longer and heavier in these areas so that the hair can be styled to cover the balding area.

Crown

If your client has a double crown, you must avoid cutting the hair too short in this area. Cutting hair short on a double crown will cause the hair to stick straight out because there is no weight to hold it down. Try to leave the hair longer over double crowns to provide sufficient weight to stop it from sticking out like a brush.

Amount of root lift

There are cutting techniques that will increase the amount of lift at the roots. All of these techniques involve cutting selected strands of hair shorter than the overall length of the style. Short hair is stronger than long hair and will push up and away from the scalp creating lift and volume by supporting the hair lying over it. Special scissors are available that make texturising faster because there is no need to weave out the selected strands to be cut shorter since these scissors are notched. Only the hair where there are no notches in the scissor blades will be cut leaving the remaining hair that is closed in the scissors untouched. If the hair appears too full because the amount of hair is so dense, excess bulk can be removed by thinning scissors which are very similar to the scissors used for texturising. If you are unsure of what texturising scissors look like, please refer to the back of this chapter where tools for cutting hair are described.

How does the degree and uniformity of curl formation affect your choice of cutting technique?

When cutting curly hair you must remember that it will spring back when the mesh is released, and thus appear shorter. The greater the tension put on the curl, the more it will stretch to being straight. As soon as the tension is taken off the hair, it will spring back to being curly. Depending on the tightness of the curl and the style to be achieved, it might be necessary to cut the hair 'free hand'. Free hand cutting is a technique used for cutting fringes (Fig. 5.3), over ears, on some hairlines and also natural Afro hair. It does not involve holding the hair between the fingers. Instead, the hair is first combed into the correct position to allow the hair to fall and lie naturally, then cut. Free hand cutting does not put any tension on the hair at all, so allows the hairdresser to reduce its length without being fooled by the effect that tension has on hair fall

Figure 5.3 Cutting a fringe free hand.

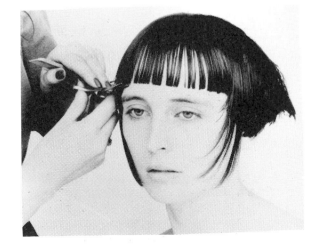

and movement. If the hair is very straight, as in the case of most Chinese hair, free hand cutting can also be used, allowing the hair to fall as gravity intends it to.

Questions

1. How can nape hair growth be disguised?
2. How can you disguise hair growth characteristics at the front hairline?
3. Why should hair be left longer at a double crown?
4. Why are some strands of hair cut short while others are left long to obtain root lift?
5. What is 'free hand' cutting?

Does cutting the hair wet or dry make any difference to the finished result or tools that can be used?

Today, the majority of haircuts are carried out on hair which has been shampooed. First, this enables the hairdresser to observe the natural fall and movement of the hair they are about to cut. Second, if the hairdresser is aware of the hair's growth characteristics, the hair can be cut with these in mind because they have an understanding of how the hair will respond and lie. Third, most haircuts are followed by some sort of finishing such as blow-drying, setting or moulding into shape with the use of styling products. Most hairdressers simply prefer to work with clean hair rather than hair which is greasy, coated in hairspray or smells, and will argue that a precision haircut is not possible to achieve on hair which is cut when it is dry. It is certainly a lot easier to control hair when it is wet and to make clean sections. It is also easier to follow a guideline because the moisture helps to bind the hair together and keep the hair in position. Often, the hair is repeatedly dampened with a water spray during the haircut to maintain the moisture content. Other hairdressers prefer not to use a water spray for they like to see how the cut is working as the hair gradually dries. Whether you re-damp with water or not could depend on who teaches you to cut in the first place or the type of hair you are working with.

The most important factor for the hairdresser to remember when cutting hair which is wet is that wet hair stretches more than dry hair. This means that if hair is cut wet, as it dries it will become shorter. You must make allowances for this when you are cutting wet hair. Unfortunately, many hairdressers learn this through the unfortunate experience of cutting a fringe whilst the hair is wet and getting a shock at how much shorter it is when it has been dried.

There are certain cutting techniques that should be carried out only on dry hair. We have already said that wet hair binds itself together and because moisture makes it do this, mistakes can be made if you try to texturise or thin hair which is soaking wet. You would be unable to predict precisely when you have removed sufficient bulk because the hair will not react in the same way as it does when it is dry. Also, because the hair will hold together when wet, too much hair can easily be removed by notched scissors. Electric clippers are also better used on hair which is dry.

Razors should only ever be used on wet hair. Trying to use a razor on hair which is dry will be extremely uncomfortable for the client. Ordinary hairdressing scissors can be used to equal effect on wet or dry hair. Thinning and texturising techniques using scissors and razors will be dealt with in more detail later on in this chapter.

Questions
1. Why do hairdressers like to cut hair when it is wet?
2. How is the hair kept wet during a cut?
3. Does everybody do this?
4. What must you allow for when cutting wet hair?
5. What cutting techniques should only be carried out on dry hair?
6. If you are using a razor, is it best to do so on dry or wet hair?

How do different cutting methods affect the shape of a style?

For you to understand the concept of hair shapes, you need to imagine hairstyles as being in silhouette. This means imagining a style so that you can only see the outside lines of the hair as if it were a shadow. The way in which the hair is cut and the angles at which the hair is held during cutting will make a significant difference to the overall shape (think silhouette!) of the finished result.

There are many cutting methods but variations in these and how they are combined can create an endless number of shapes. With simplicity in mind at this point, let us first consider these different cutting methods and how they form the final shape of the style.

One-length cutting (Bob)

A one-length haircut is done by cutting the hair to fall to the same outside length. The weight and fullness of the haircut is around the perimeter of the style while the inside hair has no shape. Due to this weight distribution, the overall shape is slightly triangular because all the weight falls to the same length on the perimeter. This is regardless of whether the hair is straight or curly, has a fringe or the position of a parting.

Basic layer cutting

There are different angles of holding the hair meshes for layer cutting but the basic layer cutting method requires all the hair meshes to be held at a 90 degree angle to the contours of the head. Basic layer cutting therefore produces a shape which is predominantly round because the weight and fullness of the hair has been evenly distributed.

Graduation

Graduation is a method of cutting that blends longer lengths of hair into shorter hair. This means that the meshes of hair are held at a position between 45 and 180 degrees, depending on the lengths of hair to be connected. There are two main types of graduation; one type of graduation leaves the inner hair length longer than the perimeter length, while the other leaves the reverse of this. A popular graduated hairstyle, which is cut so that the inner hair length is the longest part, is called the 'Wedge'. Cutting hair using this method causes the distribution of weight to move away from being just on the perimeter as in the example of a bob, or uniform as in a basic layer cut. Instead, the weight increases in a particular area to form an overall diamond shape.

Layering for long hair

Many clients with long hair want to retain its overall length but have layers to create fullness and a more interesting shape. This means cutting the hair so that the inner hair is shorter than the outside hair. This is a form of graduation because shorter lengths are connected to longer lengths (unlike basic layering when all meshes are held at the same angle). The overall shape leaves weight at the perimeter and reduces weight through the top where the shortest layers are.

Questions
1. How should you think of a hairstyle shape?
2. What is a one length haircut?
3. What will the overall shape be?
4. How do you hold the hair for a basic layer cut?
5. What shape is produced?
6. What is graduation?
7. How can the use of graduation vary?
8. What shape is produced?
9. How do you layer cut long hair to keep length?
10. How does this differ from basic layering?

Effects of other cutting techniques

In the examples above we have explained how the overall shape of a haircut depends on the distribution of weight and length. This is determined by the angle at which the hair is held when it is cut. Another way in which the shape is determined, is by the way the cutting tools are used on the hair. These techniques come under five headings:

(1) Texturising
(2) Thinning
(3) Taper cutting
(4) Club cutting
(5) Scissors over comb

(1) Texturising

This is a cutting technique which involves cutting selected strands of hair shorter than the overall style length with the intention of increasing root lift or softening a hard line. It can be done using specialised scissors or, as it is done more commonly, with conventional scissors. Unlike thinning, texturising is usually intended to show visible variations between hair lengths. Here are some examples of texturising techniques:

The weave cutting (Figure 5.4) technique works on the principle that the hairs which are cut shorter will push up and support the longer lengths — ideal for those hairstyles which need to be spiky or have a

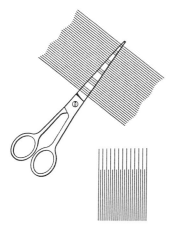

Figure 5.4 Weave cutting, using closed scissors to weave out selected strands. The result is on the right: shorter hairs are evenly dispersed amongst the longer ones.

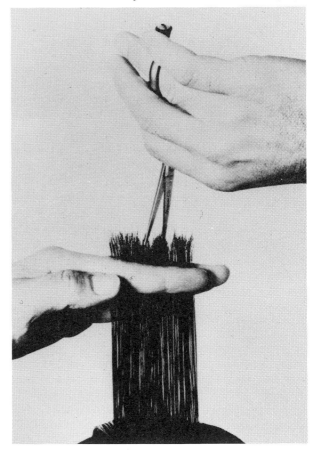

Figure 5.5 Vertical point cutting technique using conventional scissors. (Courtesy Rand Rocket Ltd.)

'strand' appearance. The width between the weaving should be evenly spaced. To achieve heavy texturising, the strands are woven out thickly and, for a more subtle look, the strands are finer. Weave cutting can be carried out over the whole head but is time-consuming because such narrow meshes (about 1 cm) are used. Therefore, weave cutting is usually restricted to specific areas.

Chipping and pointing reduce the weight from the points of the hair to create an uneven or jagged finish by cutting small 'V' shapes into the points. They can be used to soften or spike any area of a style, including fringes. Figure 5.5 shows how to hold sections vertically and point: this can be done all over the head, removing as much bulk as required.

Figure 5.6 The amount of hair cut with (a) double notch and (b) single notch thinning scissors.

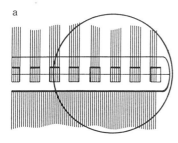
a

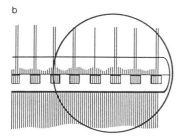
b

(2) Thinning

This is a term given to cutting techniques which remove bulk from the hair *without* affecting the overall length of the style. Conventional scissors or razors can be used although special thinning scissors are available with notched teeth instead of solid blades. Thinning scissors can also be referred to as aescalups and can have one or both blades notched. If both blades are notched, *less* hair will be removed than a pair with only one notched blade. This can be seen in Figure 5.6 which shows a magnified view of the two types of thinning scissors.

Thinning scissors should be used on dry hair and are held in the same way as conventional haircutting scissors (i.e. with the thumb and third finger). A mesh of hair is held between the fingers and the scissors are closed across the mesh at least 4 cms from the scalp. At this distance, you will prevent spiky hair sticking up through the top layers when the hair is combed flat. The scissors are closed once and then opened and moved down another 2−3 cms and another cut is made. If the hair is very long or dense, you will need to continue this movement down the length of the hair until the excess bulk is removed, but be careful not to remove too much hair! Use the finely spaced teeth of your comb to remove the cuttings from the mesh while thinning, as this will help you to estimate how many times the scissors will need to be closed. When using thinning scissors on men, they are usually used straight across the hair mesh as shown in Figure 5.7 while for ladies' hairdressing they are generally used at an angle or in a zig-zag pattern.

Avoid using thinning scissors in the following areas:

Figure 5.7 Using thinning scissors (aescalups).

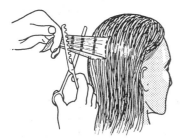

- closer than 4 cms to the scalp;
- on hairlines;
- at the crown;
- along partings.

Razors can also be used to thin out the hair but must only ever be used on wet hair because razor cutting dry hair would quickly blunt the razor and be painful for the client. To ensure that the overall length of the hair is not altered, minimum pressure is put on the razor as it is stroked over the mesh of hair towards you. The blade should be held flat to the hair when using a razor to remove excess bulk.

(3) Taper cutting

There are two cutting tools that can be used to taper cut hair: scissors or a razor. Taper cutting with scissors should be carried out on dry hair while a razor is used only on wet hair. Taper cutting removes length from the hair *and at the same time* removes bulk. The thinning effect of tapering creates shorter lengths of hair amongst each mesh. This results in each mesh being progressively finer towards the points, and this is responsible for increasing the hair's natural tendency to curl. The effect of taper cutting a mesh of hair can be seen in Figure 5.8.

Figure 5.8 Taper cut mesh of hair showing progressive reduction of bulk towards points.

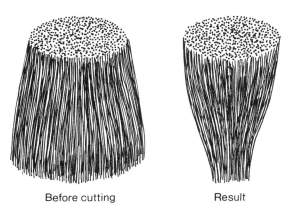

Before cutting   Result

Taper cutting with scissors is also referred to as slithering or feathering the hair. The scissors are used in a sliding action, backwards and forwards along the hair length. The heel of the scissors is used when tapering and the cutting occurs during the upward stroke of the blades, as they very slightly close on the hair. The method of holding a mesh of hair when taper cutting with scissors is shown in Figure 5.9.

When using a razor to taper cut, it is placed either underneath or above the mesh of hair to be cut. The hair is held and the razor blade is stroked down the hair in a scraping action from the middle lengths to the ends. Do be careful how much pressure you put on the blade; more pressure will remove a lot more hair! While razor cutting, both hands should move in unison. The hand holding the mesh moves away as the blade approaches – an important movement to remember to avoid cutting your fingers! The blade is *always* moved towards you, *never* towards the scalp and against the lie of the cuticle. This is shown in Figure 5.10.

Figure 5.9 Taper cutting with scissors.

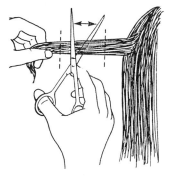

(4) Club cutting

Club cutting is also referred to as blunt cutting, and this cutting technique reduces the length of hair by making straight cuts with the scissor blades. The points of the hair are left the same length and blunt. Club cutting is

Figure 5.10 Using a razor to taper cut.

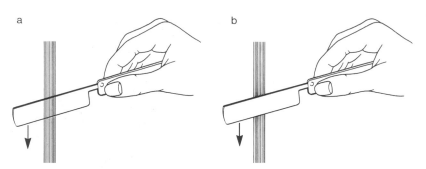

used today more than any other technique and is ideal for fine hair because it helps to make such hair feel and look heavier. Electric clippers can also be used to club cut the hair as shown in Figure 5.11 which shows hair being cut with the aid of a 'Flattopper'.

Figure 5.11 Club cutting with clippers. In this case a special comb called the Brian Drumm Flattopper is used to support and lift the hair so that it remains perfectly level for cutting. A spirit level in the handle lets the hairdresser know if it is being held straight. (Courtesy Brian Drumm.)

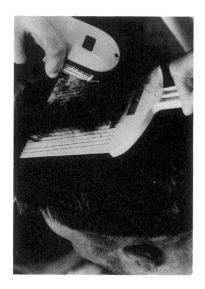

Figure 5.12 Scissors over comb technique.

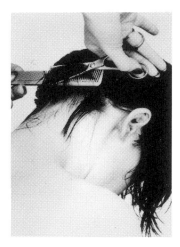

(5) Scissors over comb

This technique used to be called shingling when it was at the height of its popularity between the First and Second World Wars. Today, the term 'scissors over comb' describes hair being cut close to the contours of the head and is mostly used at the nape or sides of the head. A thin, flexible comb is needed so that the hair can be cut as close to the contours of the head as required. The comb is used in an upwards direction, lifting the hair as it moves through the hair. The scissors are held parallel with the comb all the time and your hands should move in unison with each other, in a flowing movement. As the hairs slip through the teeth of the comb they are cut off. This can be seen in Figure 5.12.

Electric clippers are often used instead of clippers to cut hair close to the head as shown in Figure 5.13. Clippers are generally used instead of scissors for this purpose when cutting Afro hair.

Figure 5.13 Clipper over comb technique.

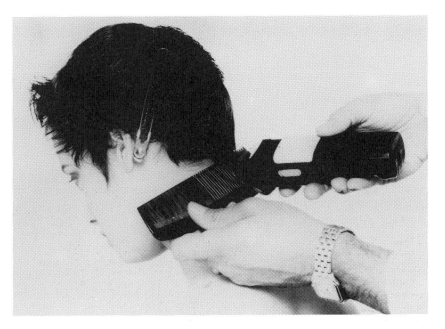

Questions
  1. What is 'texturising'?
  2. Distinguish between weave cutting and chipping/pointing.
  3. What is thinning?
  4. How do you use thinning scissors?
  5. When should you avoid using thinning scissors?
  6. How should you use a razor to thin hair?
  7. What is taper cutting?
  8. What other names are there for taper cutting?
  9. How do you use a razor to taper cut?
 10. What is club or blunt cutting?
 11. On what type of hair is it used?
 12. What is 'scissor over comb' cutting?
 13. When is it used?
 14. What can be used instead of scissors?

What effects can be achieved by different cutting angles and lines?

The angle at which the hair is cut to create different shapes and lines is limited only by your own imagination, technical skill and the particular head you are working on. Here are some examples of different cutting angles:

Nape outline shapes (Figure 5.14)

Figure 5.14 Nape outline shapes.

When deciding on the cutting angle which forms the shape at the nape, remember to look closely at the natural hair growth characteristics before beginning to cut.

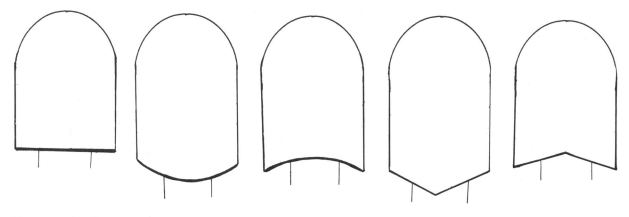

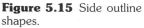

Figure 5.15 Side outline shapes.

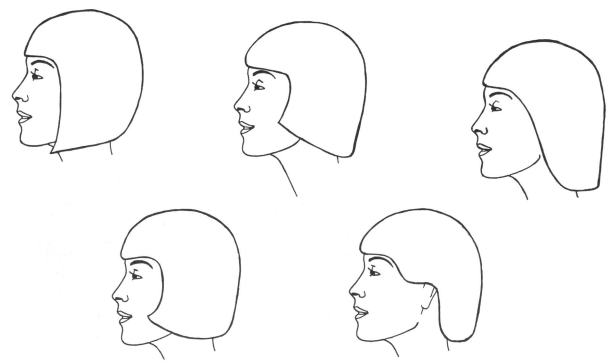

Side outline shapes (Figure 5.15)

It is helpful to 'plot' the angle of your cutting line using features of the face. For example, you can imagine a line which runs to the nose or corner of the eye from the chin, and use this imaginary line to help cut at the correct angle.

Fringe outline shapes (Figure 5.16)

If the hair is to be cut into a fringe, do check the hair growth pattern around the front hairline and the client's facial characteristics so that the most suitable shape is chosen.

Figure 5.16 Fringe outline shapes.

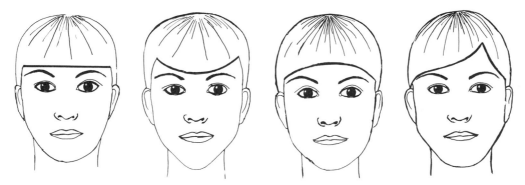

Geometric shapes (Figure 5.17)

Geometric styles are hair shapes which have been cut on lines to resemble angular shapes. They were made popular by Vidal Sassoon, in the 1960s, who created the 'five point' haircut for fashion designer Mary Quant (the lady who designed and introduced the mini skirt).

Figure 5.17 Geometric shapes.

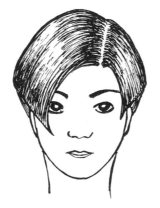
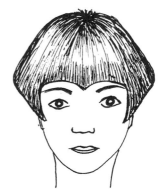

Figure 5.18 Asymmetric shapes.

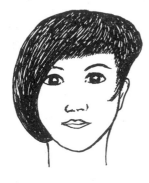

Asymmetric shapes (Figure 5.18)

The word asymmetric describes a shape that is unequal in line or size on both sides. (A shape which is equal in line or size on both sides is called symmetrical.)

Why is the balance and proportion of a haircut important?

There are two ways in which a haircut should be checked for balance and proportion. Firstly, the haircut should be *technically correct*. That means, the hair should be cut so that the hair lengths check into each other and do not show signs of disconnection or difference in length. Regardless of the shape of the haircut, or the method by which it was done, the style should always be checked during the haircut, when the cut is complete, and after the style is dried. If the haircut is not technically correct, the style will not be easy to manage for the client and could show the imperfections when it is finished. Secondly, the haircut should be correctly balanced and proportioned to the size and shape of the body and the facial characteristics. Too many hairdressers forget the importance of the total look. You will see clients standing up when their hairdresser has finished, and as they take off the gown, the style just doesn't look right. The haircut may be perfection in terms of technical skill but if it doesn't balance with, and therefore complement, the client's facial characteristics, you have not done justice to your client.

How is the balance of a haircut checked?

If you are cutting a one length style, such as a bob, you are going to be concentrating on checking that the lines are equally level on all sides. A one-length cut always shows any imperfections because the outside shape is so defined and strong. Do not be under the misapprehension that clients will not become aware of any mistakes. If they don't notice the imperfection whilst they are in the salon, you can guarantee that it will be noticed when they dry it themselves at home.

A one length shape can be checked by taking a small amount of hair in your hands from either side of the head at equal places and slowly sliding your fingers down the hair. If the hair is the same length on both sides, your hands will reach the points of the hair at the same time. It is not a good idea to try to check the balance by using the ears as a guide because they are very rarely equally positioned. To check the base line (outside edge) of a short bob, a hand mirror can be placed under the hairline to reflect any imperfections. You could also ask your client to stand up so that you have an eye level view for checking the cut.

When checking all other haircuts, you have a little more work to do because unlike a one length style, you have an outside and inside shape to check. It can be helpful to use the mirrors around the salon to check the shape of your cut from different angles and distances, because it is often easier to identify any discord or disproportion from a distance than it is close up. The client's chair or head can also be turned so that the haircut is seen more closely from different views. The inside shape of the cut is checked by picking up meshes of hair to see if the ends of the hair are level. If they are not, the stray strands are cut off. To check that the weight is evenly balanced, the fingers can be drawn through the hair in an outwards direction from roots to points. By looking in the mirror you will be able to see if any area has been left too long.

How is a back mirror handled to show clients their hair?

The hairdresser holds the mirror behind clients so that when they look in the mirror in front of them they can see the back of their hair reflected in the mirror being held by the stylist. (We have seen a trainee show the client her hair with a backmirror when there was no mirror in front of her to see it in!) Many trainees have a lot of difficulty in positioning the back mirror so that the client can see the back properly. They also tend to move it too quickly, making the client assume that this is done because something is wrong with the hair at the back. A back mirror should be held so that the hairdresser can see the reflection of the hair at the back of the client's head in the mirror in front of them. It should be moved slowly across so that the client has a full view of the back. If the client's hair is long and you want to show the entire length you will have to use a different method. Give the back mirror to the client and turn the chair 180 degrees so that he or she is facing away from the mirror. If clients hold the mirror at a slight angle and look into it, they will be able to see the back of their hair more easily. If their hair is very long, they might need to stand up and hold the mirror to see it all.

Questions
1. Why is the balance and proportion of a haircut important?
2. What happens if a style is not technically correct?
3. How is the balance checked?
4. Why is it easier to check a one length style?
5. What is a back mirror used for?
6. How do you use a backmirror to show a client (i) short hair, (ii) long hair?

How do cutting faults occur and how are they corrected?

You should be looking at the results of your cutting during the haircut as well as when it is complete. Using a vent brush to brush the hair in different directions during a haircut will allow you to see how well the hair is falling and responding to what you are doing. If something looks wrong, it can be corrected immediately. Problems occur when hairdressers do not spot the faults as they happen and continue the cut following a previously cut mesh of hair, which is the wrong length, or cut at the incorrect angle.

To avoid mistakes there are two very important things to remember:

- Always cut *exactly* on your guideline.
- Be aware of the angle at which you are cutting the hair.

If your hand is holding the mesh to be cut at the wrong angle for the desired result, the line of the cut will be lost. Your hand holding the mesh is as important as the hand holding the scissors and you should always be aware of where this hand is in relation to the contours of the head. For example, if you are cutting basic layers, the hair should be held at a 90 degree angle to the contours of the head for each mesh that is cut. If the hand holding the meshes is not controlling the angle correctly, the haircut will be unevenly balanced and shorter in some areas than others.

The most common mistake made by novice cutters on their first basic layer cut, is to cut the hair at the crown too short. This is usually because they fail to hold the meshes at 90 degrees *to the contours of the head*. Heads are not flat and square; heads are contoured. This means that the meshes must be held straight out at a 90 degrees angle with the curves and depressions of the head in mind.

A mistake that is often made when cutting a one-length style is to hold the meshes too far away from the skin. When this happens the ends of the hair become graduated, resulting in weight being removed from the outside shape.

If the hair is not cut to the guideline, steps may occur. Steps can also happen if even, flowing movements are not used when doing the scissor over comb technique. Steps are unsightly lines in the hair caused by meshes being cut shorter or left longer than the intended length in that area. If steps do occur, the only way to get rid of them is to find the shortest point in that area and cut the affected hair to that length. Depending on the seriousness of the error, the client could end up with very short hair! Do remember, that the checking of a haircut should require minimum scissor work if it was carried out competently in the first case.

Unfortunately, hair cannot be stuck back on once it has been cut off and an awful haircut will make a person's life a misery until it has grown again. Remember that a haircut is judged on the hair that you *leave* on the head and not the amount that is cut off. It takes no longer to cut off 10 cms of hair than it does to cut off 1 cm. It is the time you spend talking with your client before you start the haircut that is the most important and often time-consuming. If you do not *fully* understand the look the client wants to achieve before you begin cutting, it is a recipe for disaster. Conversely, if what you recommend to the client is very precise and the end result is not as you said, the client will be equally disappointed. You will be able to tell a lot about whether the client is liking what you are doing to her hair by looking at her face in the mirror. A displeased client will generally find it difficult to look at her reflection, and may frown, whereas a contented client will often smile as she talks and want to see the new cut from different angles while it is being cut. If you think your client is displeased, do not continue without offering reassurance or suggesting changes that will make it more satisfactory to the client.

Often, it is quite disconcerting to cut very long hair extremely short. The hairdresser is frightened that the client won't like it and is apprehensive about the client's wishes. In such cases, it is advisable to ask the client why they have made this decision. Is it something they have been meaning to do for a long time or is it a snap decision? In our experience, women that have asked for extreme amounts of hair to be cut off are usually trying to confirm that a big change has happened in their life, such as a new job, the end of a relationship, etc. It is helpful to show the client in the mirror how much hair you intend cutting off before you start. You will be surprised at the differences in people's concepts of how much they consider 1 cm to be!

Questions
1. How can faults be avoided during cutting?
2. What common faults do trainees make on basic layer cutting and one-length styles?
3. What are steps?
4. How do you get rid of steps?
5. How can you tell if clients like their haircut by watching them during the cut?
6. Why is it important to be certain that you understand what the client wants?

Why is the position of the client's head important during cutting?

We discussed earlier how cutting faults can be prevented and corrected, but did not mention how the client's head position during cutting can affect your judgement by distorting your perception of how the hair is falling. Perhaps the best example to give is that of trying to cut a one length bob for a client who is leaning on one arm of the chair. When a client does not sit straight in the chair, the head is inevitably slightly tilted towards one side. When the haircut is checked for balance, (perhaps by the client standing up) the hairdresser will be alarmed to discover that one side will be longer than the other, despite regular checks for balance during the cut. The fault has to be corrected and valuable time is lost. By frequently glancing in the mirror you can check whether the client's head is straight.

When asking a client to stand while the hair is cut or checked, make sure the client is standing with both legs straight. If the client leans towards one side, putting more weight on one leg than the other, their head will also be slightly over to one side. If you prefer to cut particular styles at eye level and frequently ask clients to stand, consider buying yourself a cutting stool. A cutting stool is set on wheels for easy manoeuvrability and has an adjustable seat.

How should the client's head be positioned during cutting?

When you are doing a haircut, you should either position the client's head so that your work is not hampered, or move yourself into a position that allows you to work effectively.

It can be very irritating for clients to have the hairdresser perpetually pushing their head in different directions. If you want a client to move the head into a particular position, tell her what you want her to do: e.g. 'Would you put your head down for me, please?' while at the same time holding the client's head between both hands and gently moving the head slowly into position. Often during cutting, the hair is cut as it lies flat against the skin's surface. By adjusting the client's head position, the amount that you will need to bend or stretch is reduced. When you are cutting against the skin at the neck, you will discover that it is more difficult to cut the hair that is situated on the skin at the outside of the neck (furthest away from the spine) because the neck is rounded and not as flat in this area as it is in the centre. If you gently turn the client's head to one side you will notice that the main muscle in the neck (the trapezius) will move, supplying a flatter and firmer surface on which to cut.

If your salon has revolving chairs, you will be able to turn clients so that they match your mobility. This is especially useful if the styling positions are closely arranged, as it avoids knocking the stylist or client next to you. If the chair is hydraulic, it means that the height of the seat can be altered to match the operator's stance. Continual bending at the waist will result in backache, fatigue and bad posture.

How is hair combed or brushed into position for cutting?

It is unusual to use a brush during a haircut except for checking how the hair is falling and laying in shape. Therefore, when it comes to controlling the hair for cutting, we will be concentrating on using a comb.

The angle at which the hair is held for cutting determines how much hair will be removed, and consequently, how it will lie. In order to get the hair in the correct position for cutting, the hair must be combed, and when necessary held in that position for cutting. The hair should obviously be tangle-free and should be combed until the hair passes freely between the teeth of the comb.

When combing hair for cutting a one length bob, it is important that the hair is combed so that it lies in the natural direction of the way it falls. If it is not combed into position in this way, the outline shape of the cut will not be level when the hair falls naturally.

To cut hair against the skin, the hair should be combed flat to the skin, making sure that every hair in the mesh has been thoroughly combed from roots to points. It is no good using the widely spaced teeth of your comb if you are aiming at precision. Using the finer teeth for positioning the hair ensures that every hair is completely under your control.

We have already mentioned free hand cutting and when it is used, but we now need to look at how hair is combed and positioned for cutting when it falls over the ear. If tension has been used to hold the hair falling over the ear, as the tension is released the hair will rise as the ear protrudes again. This is why the hair should be cut using free hand cutting. Again it is *very* important that the hair is thoroughly combed from roots to points and that the hair is allowed to fall naturally.

When using the scissor over comb technique, the hair is combed in an upwards movement and the hair that projects through the teeth of the comb is cut off. The closer the comb is positioned to the contours of the head, the shorter the result. The comb and scissors should move in an even, flowing movement or steps can occur.

When layering or graduating, the hair must be cleanly combed into position and then held exactly still to be cut. The angle that each mesh is held is the angle between the scalp and the mesh of hair you are holding.

When cutting natural Afro hair (not chemically relaxed or permed) the hair is usually cut free hand using scissors or electric clippers. Before the hair is cut it is thoroughly combed to remove tangles and to release the natural curl using an Afro comb. Sometimes, Afro hair is held in position during the cut using either an Afro comb or wide-toothed comb and the clippers or scissors are used to cut off the hair protruding through the teeth of the comb.

Questions
1. How can the way the client sits interfere with your cutting?
2. What should you beware of when checking a cut with the client standing?
3. How should you adjust the client's head during a cut?
4. What problems might you encounter when cutting in the neck area?
5. What benefits have revolving and hydraulic chairs?
6. When do you use a brush during cutting?
7. How is hair combed during cutting?
8. Why should you use the finer teeth of the comb when cutting?
9. Why is free-hand cutting used near the ears?
10. When using scissor over comb, what is the importance of the closeness of the comb to the head?
11. How is Afro hair cut?

How should different hair curl strengths be handled?

It is sometimes difficult to control curly hair during cutting because it takes greater effort to keep the hair in position for cutting. Also, it requires more tension to comb it, especially if the curl formation is tight. If you have difficulty, try using the wide spaced teeth of your comb as this will reduce tension on the hair and give you control without hurting the client. Even if the hair is wavy rather than curly you will need to remember that it will spring up more when it is dry than straight hair would. Bear this in mind when you cut your initial guideline. When hair is curly, it can be difficult to cut because it will have a tendency to wrap itself around your fingers.

Cutting straight hair can also present problems because it tends to show cutting faults much more than curly hair — so beware!

How should different hair lengths be controlled?

If the client arrives in the salon with very long hair and has decided to have it all cut short, the best thing to do is to remove the bulk of the unwanted hair before you begin work on the actual haircut. This always looks rather drastic, but it is much easier to control and it will save time in the long run. It is a good idea to offer the hair you initially cut off to the client, as they sometimes think hairdressers make a fortune out of selling hair to wigmakers!

If the client's hair is already quite short, you should be able to control it while you cut, so that you are able to follow a planned procedure and method even though sectioning clips just slip out of it because it is so short. If this is the case, keeping the hair wet and combing the other hair well out of the way should help.

Questions
1. When cutting curly hair, why are the wider teeth of the comb used?
2. What problems do curly or wavy hair give during cutting?
3. What is the first cut if you are dramatically reducing length?
4. How can you control very short hair during cutting?

Tools and equipment used when cutting hair

Scissors

Scissors can be the most expensive non-electrical tools that you possess. Prices range from a few pounds to hundreds. As you will be using them for much of your working life you must have a pair that you use effortlessly, as if they were an extension of your hands. Scissors vary in design and intended use, and the following text, illustrations and photographs will take you through the different types. Because of hygiene, you should have two pairs of normal cutting scissors so that you have one to work with while the other is being sterilised.

To work at their peak, all scissors should be sharp; just how sharp can be seen in Figure 5.19. If cutting tools are not sharp, they can damage the hair. This can clearly be seen from Figure 5.20.

Good quality scissors will be made of well-tempered stainless or cobalt steel and have free-moving, sharp-edged blades. They are available in different sizes ranging between 10 cms and 18 cms in length from the

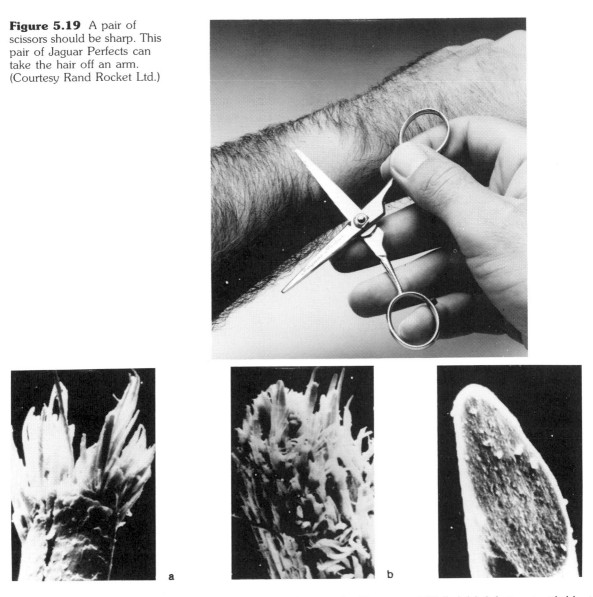

Figure 5.19 A pair of scissors should be sharp. This pair of Jaguar Perfects can take the hair off an arm. (Courtesy Rand Rocket Ltd.)

Figure 5.20 Effects of cutting hair using blunt and sharp tools. (Courtesy of Wella.) (a) A hair cut with blunt scissors; (b) A hair cut with a blunt razor; (c) A hair cut with a sharp razor.

tip of the blades to the handles. The size a stylist chooses to work with depends on whichever type feels most comfortable and easy to control for the particular job being done. It is usual for stylists to have more than one pair of scissors so that they can alternate which pair is used according to the work being done, and also when the other pair is being sterilised. The various parts of a pair of scissors are shown in Figure 5.21.

Figure 5.21 The parts of a pair of scissors.

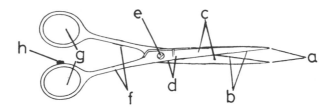

Caring for your scissors

- *Never* cut anything other than hair with them or they will become blunt very quickly.
- *Never* drop your scissors as this can upset their balance.
- *Always* carry them in their original protective case to prevent damage.
- *Do not* lend your scissors to others – they may not care for them as well as you.
- *Always* wipe the blades after cutting to remove moisture and clippings. This can be done with a piece of cotton wool soaked in surgical spirit which will also disinfect the blades.
- *Always* have your scissors maintained and sharpened by professionals – the trade magazines will carry advertisements for this.
- *Oil* between the blades at the base of the handles if you notice that the blades do not move easily.

Figure 5.22 (a) How to hold a pair of scissors correctly. (b) Holding a scissors and comb at the same time.

a

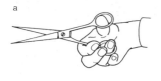

b

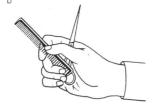

How are scissors held?

All haircutting scissors are held with the thumb and third finger as shown in Figure 5.22(a). This method of holding enables the user to have maximum control over the scissors. When the scissors are not actually cutting, the thumb should be slipped out of the handle so that they are cradled in the palm of the hand while still being supported by the third finger through the handle. By releasing the thumb from the handle, the user has the manoeuvrability to hold a comb in the same hand, while ensuring that the scissor blades are not open – this is shown in Figure 5.22(b). Only the thumb moves when using scissors. Time should be spent handling scissors before you attempt a haircut. As an exercise, open and close them using only your thumb, making sure the other blade remains stationary. Also, practise releasing and replacing your thumb through the handle and holding a comb in the same hand as your scissors.

Figure 5.23 Thinning scissors.

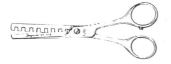

Thinning scissors

Thinning scissors remove bulk from the hair without affecting its length. They are available with either one or both blades notched as shown in Figure 5.23. Thinning scissors may also be called aescalups, texturising or serrated scissors.

Figure 5.24 Thinning scissors with different spaces between the teeth.

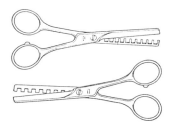

Several new types of thinning scissors have been developed which have wider and narrower spaces between the teeth to remove varying quantities of hair. Figure 5.24 shows two pairs of such thinning scissors.

Scissors with interchangeable blades are also available. Three different types are shown in Figure 5.25, while Figure 5.26 shows the result when used on the hair. These can achieve accurate cutting results in one snip of the scissors.

Scissors may be sterilised by autoclaving, boiling or using disinfectant solutions. They must always be disinfected if a client is cut.

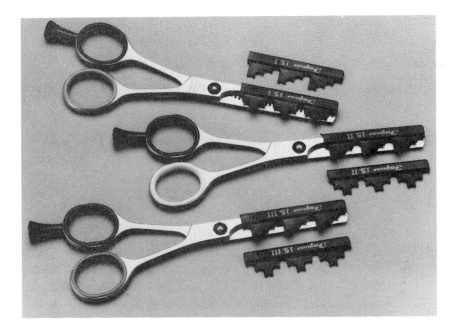

Figure 5.25 Scissors with interchangeable blades can be used to create a variety of effects when cutting hair. These are the Jaguar Detour Stylers, showing J. S. I, II and III attachments. The scissors have a removable finger rest. (Courtesy Rand Rocket Ltd.)

Figure 5.26 Removing bulk from the points of the hair in a single snip by using the Jaguar Detour J. S. II. (Courtesy Rand Rocket Ltd.)

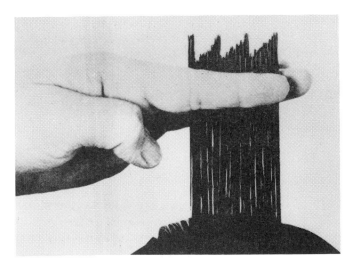

Electric clippers

Electric clippers work on the principle of one blade remaining fixed while the other blade moves across it. The action of the moving blade, operated by the motor, is similar to several pairs of scissors being used at the same time; as many as 14,400 cutting strokes can be made per minute with some types of clippers. A pair of electric clippers is shown in Figure 5.27. Some clippers have detachable blades so that the closeness of the cut can be altered. Such blades are numbered with 0000 for the closest and 3 for the longest.

Figure 5.27 A pair of electric clippers. (Courtesy Wahl Ltd.)

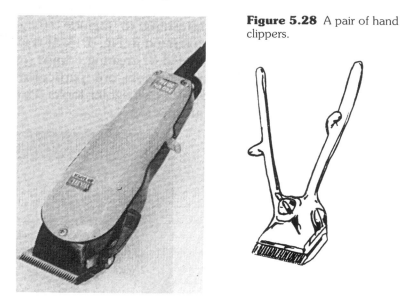

Figure 5.28 A pair of hand clippers.

It is important to keep the clipper blades well oiled (using an oil specifically designed for this purpose) and aligned. The blades should be aligned following the manufacturer's instructions. Clippers are available which run directly from the mains electricity or from rechargeable units. The latter can be used without leads trailing. Spray sterilising solutions are available for clippers, otherwise they have to be dismantled to sterilise them.

Hand clippers

Hand clippers are not frequently used in salons because of the greater popularity and extra safety of electric clippers. Their portability is also no longer unique with the development of rechargeable clippers. Hand clippers are operated by squeezing the handles together, making the movable upper blade move across the fixed blade underneath. A pair of hand clippers is illustrated in Figure 5.28.

Razors

Razors either have a fixed blade which will require regular sharpening or a replaceable blade. Open, or cut-throat, razors can be either hollow-ground or solid-ground. Solid-ground razors are commonly referred to as French razors. A cut-throat razor is illustrated in Figure 5.29.

Figure 5.29 (a) The parts of a cut-throat razor. (b) Cross-section of a hollow-ground blade. (c) Cross-section of a solid-ground blade.

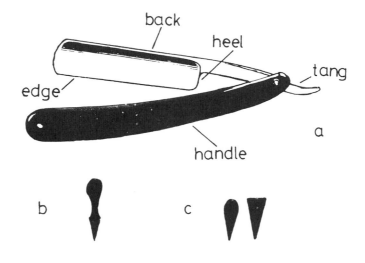

Open razors with disposable blades are now available like the one illustrated in Figure 5.30. They have the advantage of being extremely hygienic and you will also always have a sharp blade. This modern

Figure 5.30 A Wilkinson Sword disposable razor alongside a cassette of ten spare blades.

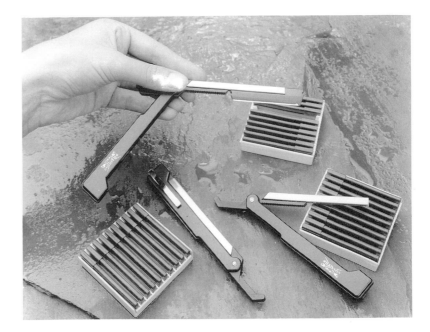

version is extremely safe because there is no risk of cutting yourself when loading from the cassette the blades are kept in. If ever you throw anything sharp away, try to place it in a small box or wrap it well. Sharps boxes are available for depositing all sharp objects.

Another type of razor is the hair shaper or safety razor. These are very similar to the cut-throat types except that they have disposable blades and have a metal guard over the cutting edge of the blade. An example of a hair shaper is shown in Figure 5.31.

Figure 5.31 A hair shaper is similar to an open razor but uses a disposable blade which has a guard over it.

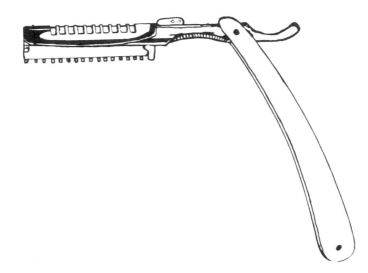

How is a razor held?

Razors should be held with the thumb on the underside of the shank and the little finger resting on top of the tang. The other fingers should rest on top of the shank, as shown in Figure 5.32. You should be able to hold the razor firmly with this particular grip, so that it can move freely in all directions.

Figure 5.32 Method of holding a razor.

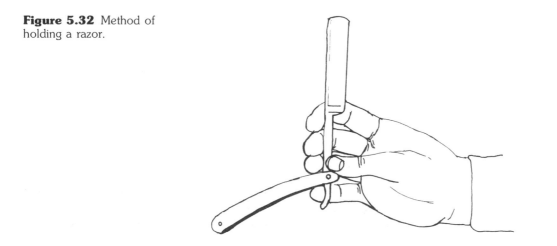

Figure 5.33 A straight comb.

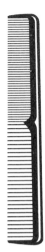

Caring for razors

Razors with fixed blades require regular maintenance to keep them sharp. If blunt razors are used they will damage the hair (or skin if used for shaving). This maintenance involves 'setting' and has nothing to do with wrapping hair on rollers! Setting a razor is the process of honing and stropping and is explained in *Cutting and Styling – A Salon Handbook*.

Cutting combs

Combs used when cutting are straight and usually have two sizes of teeth. Sizes of straight combs vary and the stylist should choose the type most suitable for the cutting technique to be used and the texture of hair to be cut. For example, when using the scissors over comb cutting technique, a comb which is flexible and thin allows it to bend to the contours of the head, permitting a close cut if required. When cutting very curly hair, it is sometimes better to use a comb with widely spaced teeth to avoid unnecessary pulling on the hair and for natural Afro hair an Afro comb might be used. A straight comb is shown in Figure 5.33.

Figure 5.34 A neck brush.

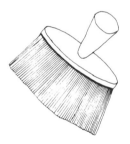

Neck brush

A neck brush is used to clean hair clippings away from the client's face and neck. The bristles should be long and soft so that they do not cause discomfort on sensitive skin. A neck brush should be used frequently during a cut to ensure client comfort. By putting a little talcum powder on the bristles, the clippings are removed easily from the skin. Alternatively, a powder puffer can be used.

Powder puffers

Powder puffers contain talcum powder which can be easily applied to the client's skin to help remove hair clippings. They are used by gently squeezing in quick repetition to make a fine dusting of powder emerge at the top. If they are squeezed too hard, the talcum powder will not come out as a fine dusting but like a jet.

Figure 5.35 A powder puff.

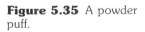
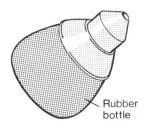
Rubber bottle

Water sprays

Water sprays are used to wet the hair without the need to take the client to the basin. When doing a wet cut, the hair can be remoistened easily and quickly if it should become too dry. The bottle should be filled with fresh water each day as seeing green algae caused by leaving the bottle in sunlight can be very off-putting! The amount of water that comes out

Figure 5.36 A water spray.

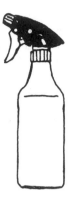

of the spray when the trigger is pulled can be adjusted by turning the nozzle. Try to remember to check that the spray is fine enough before using on a client by testing it on your hand first. Nobody will appreciate a jet of cold water being sprayed on the head! If you are wetting hair near the face, always use your free hand to shield the face. If for any reason a water spray contains something other than water, it should be clearly labelled to that effect.

Sectioning clips

There are a variety of clips used in hairdressing to hold the hair in place. During cutting, clips are used to secure hair out of the way while another part of the head is being cut. Clips used when cutting allow for large quantities of hair to be held in place and are made either of metal or plastic. Two types of clip suitable for use when cutting are shown in Figure 5.37.

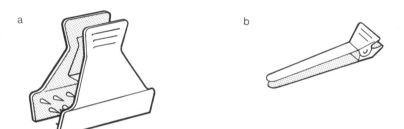

a   b

Figure 5.37 Sectioning clips which are used for securing the hair in place during cutting: (a) Plastic hair clamp or 'butterfly clip'; (b) metal sectioning clip.

Brushes

We said earlier that hairdressers will often use a brush during a haircut to check how the hair is lying. Usually the brush that will be used for this is a vent brush (Figure 5.38) because it has open filaments which allow the hair to pass freely through when it is drawn through the hair.

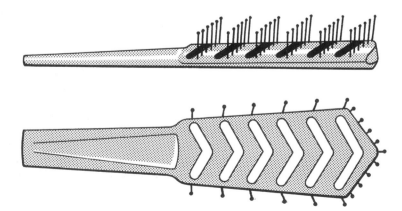

Figure 5.38 A vent brush.

Mirrors

When cutting hair you should be constantly checking the line and balance of your work in the mirror in front of the client. Also, you will need a hand mirror to show the client different views of the head. We explained earlier how a hand mirror can also be used to check the accuracy of a bob haircut. All mirrors should be kept spotlessly clean and this may mean polishing them several times during the day. Proprietary window and glass cleaners can be used to do this although many salons will swear by using methylated spirit to dissolve hairspray on mirrors. One salon we know uses wet newspaper to clean mirrors with excellent results!

Record cards

It is a necessary part of the hairdresser's work to record processes that clients have. For services such as perming, colouring and hair or scalp treatments up to date records are very important. It is a matter of opinion whether records should be kept on haircutting and this will rely on individual salon policy.

Questions
1. Why should you have two pairs of scissors?
2. Why must scissors be kept sharp?
3. What are the different parts of a pair of scissors called?
4. How should you look after your scissors?
5. How should you hold your scissors?
6. How can the blades of thinning scissors vary?
7. What other names are there for thinning scissors?
8. What different effects can they give on hair?
9. How should you look after clippers?
10. What advantage did hand clippers have in the past?
11. What types of fixed blade razor are available?
12. What advantage have disposable blades?
13. What is a hair shaper?
14. How should you hold a razor?
15. How do you chose the right comb for cutting?
16. What is a neck brush used for?
17. What is a powder puffer used for?
18. How should you use a water spray?
19. What are sectioning clips used for?
20. How can you keep mirrors clean?
21. Does your salon enter information about cutting on record cards?

Step by step cutting

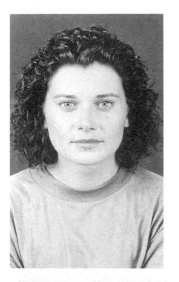

(A) Layer cut

1. Freshly permed hair ready for cutting.
2. Beginning at the nape, the guideline is cut with the hair held next to the skin.
3. The guideline is cut so that it curves up towards the ears. Narrow, horizontal sections are taken, and all the back hair is cut to the same guideline.
4. Using horizontal sections, the hair at the sides is blended with the guideline at the back. The hair is cut at an angle so that the longest point is level with the chin.
5. When both sides have been cut, the outside shape in the temporal area is blended with the longest point at the chin.
6. The hair on the front hairline, across the forehead, is cut by making 'V' shaped snips with the points of the scissors to achieve a textured finish.

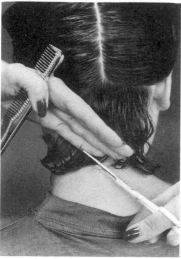
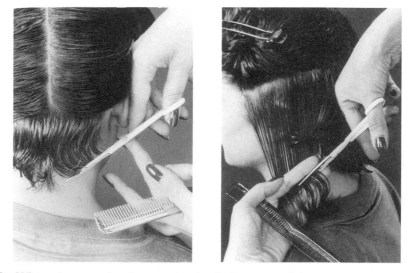

7. When the outside shape is finished, the internal layering is carried out. Taking a vertical section in the centre back of the head, the mesh is held straight out from the head. The guide for cutting the layers is taken from the shortest point seen in the hairdresser's fingers. i.e. the hair nearest to the client's nape.
8. Once cut, this mesh of hair will act as the guideline for all the internal layering. The sections are held at a 90 degrees angle for

this cutting technique. Remember that the angle at which the hair is cut is achieved by holding the meshes at right angles to the contours of the head.

9. The final shape is an easy to manage style that can be scrunch-dried using a hair dryer with a diffuser attachment.

10. In this photograph, the hair has been dried with the fingers and then tonged to create the deep waves.

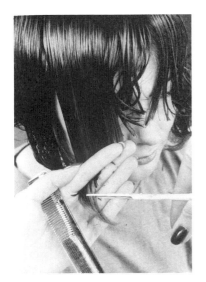
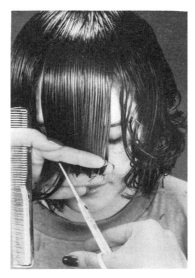
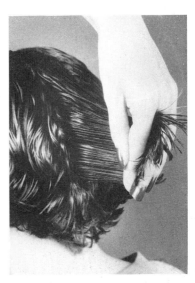
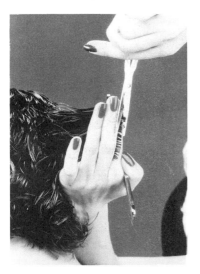
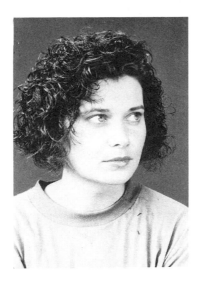
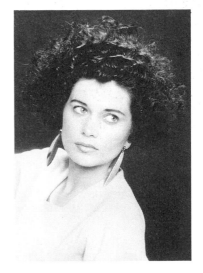

(B) Graduation

1. A freshly coloured head of hair is ready for cutting.
2. This haircut begins at the side of the head where the main bulk of the hair will fall, i.e. *not* the side of the head where the parting is positioned. All the hair from the parting is brought down and held closely to the head. In this example, the hair is held so that the angle of cutting is equivalent to the width of the hairdresser's middle finger.
3. This cutting line is continued to just behind the ear.
4. The cutting line can be clearly seen, showing the underneath hair which will be removed using the scissors over comb technique.
5. The underneath hair is cut by positioning the comb close to the contours of the head. The hair which protrudes through the teeth of the comb is cut off. The cutting line which is creating an area of weight is continued from behind the ears through the occipital region.

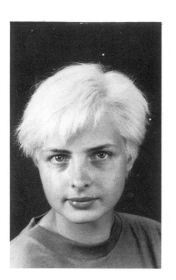

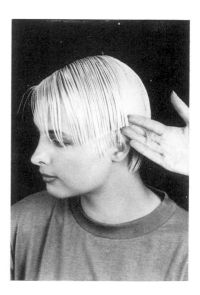

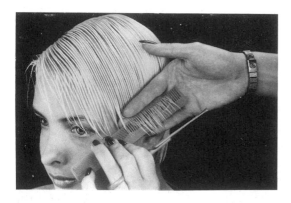

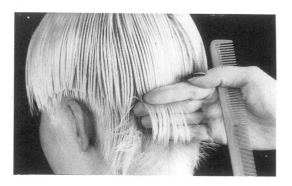

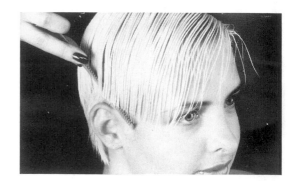

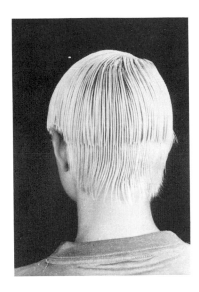 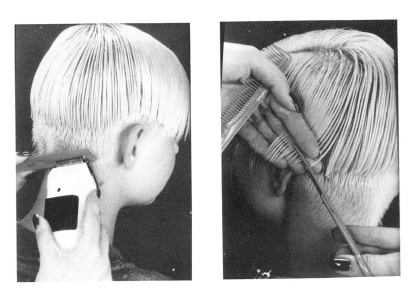

6. This photograph shows the completed cutting line at the back of the head.
7. The hair below the weight line is removed by using electric clippers. The comb is used to lift and hold the hair for cutting in the same way as for scissors over comb.
8. The side of the head where the parting is placed can now be cut. Notice that the cutting line is sloped up towards the eye.
9. The front hair is cut to blend the shortest hair at the parting, to the longest point over the other eye.
10. To add interest in the crown area, the hair is cut shorter to prevent it from being too flat.
11. This shorter area is blended into the rest of the hair by angling the fingers so that minimum length is removed from the weight line.

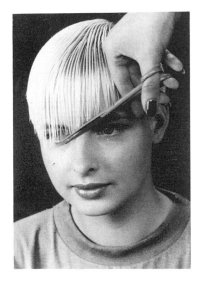 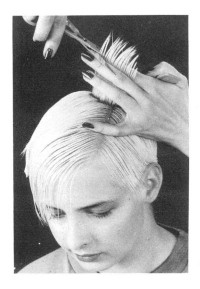 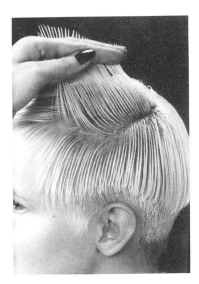

12. Point cutting through the crown area will reduce the bulk, giving the hair a more textured appearance.

13. Side view of the completed cut before it is dried.

14. The hair has been blow-dried to create a sleek finish.

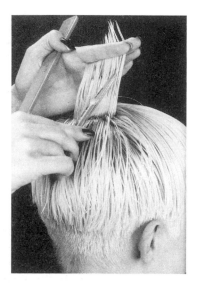
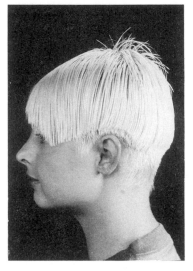
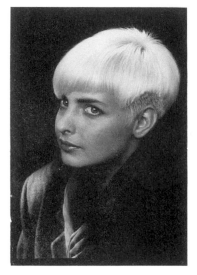

(Photographs in Step by Step Cutting are reproduced courtesy of Goldwell Hair Cosmetics Ltd.)

Chapter Six
Blow-drying

What is blow-drying?

Blow-drying is a method of drying and styling the hair using a hand-held dryer and brushes, combs, or the hands to create a variety of different effects. Blow-drying works on the principle of evaporating the moisture from the hair (with the dryer) and it is the way in which the hair is positioned during drying that will determine the final effect.

What effects can be achieved by blow-drying?

If the hair is wrapped around a circular brush and dried, the effect produced will be a curl. A mesh of hair dried while it is held straight will be straight. Hair that is 'scrunch-dried' will have movement and texture. Hair that is directed in a particular way and held with a comb during drying will result in a wave. Lift and volume can be achieved by over-directing a mesh of hair and directing the airflow at the roots. Conversely, styles that lie close to the head, requiring little or no volume, can be achieved. Blow-drying can also temporarily straighten hair. Smooth, sleek styles can be produced or spiky and 'rough' looks. The finished look can either be casual or sophisticated but there is one fact that is paramount in the success of a blow-dry; hair that is cut well and in good condition will always produce the best results.

Blow-drying techniques are set out in Figure 6.1 to describe their effects.

Figure 6.1 Effects of drying techniques.

Drying technique	Effect
Scrunch-drying	Produces a rough finish with curl and movement.
Finger-drying	Produces a natural, casual look.
Using a circular brush	Creates curl and movement in the hair – the smaller the brush, the tighter the curl.
Using a flat brush	Used to dry sleek styles but can also add bounce (e.g. bob).
Using a vent brush	Creates a natural finish to the hair with a soft, 'broken' effect.
Blow-waving	Creates waves in the hair to look like finger waves.
Natural dry using infra red	Achieves an effect that is totally natural because the hair is allowed to dry with minimum disturbance.
Finger-pressing	Creates a sleek finish to smooth straight one length styles.

How is the most suitable drying technique selected?

The skill of blow-drying is knowing when to use the various drying techniques on different hair types to produce the desired effect. The

Figure 6.2 Suitability of drying methods.

Drying technique	Suitability
Scrunch-drying	Not suitable if hair has no wave or curl. Also unsuitable for hair which is very short or long hair that is not layered.
Finger-drying	Suitable for straight, curly or wavy hair if the hair's curl formation is to remain virtually unchanged. This technique is best for fashion looks that require a casual finish.
Circular brush	Suitable for most hair lengths except very long hair which is not layered. Circular brushes can easily tangle in the hair if the hair is fine and long. The diameter of the brush determines the degree and tightness of the curl. Circular brushes are also good for adding bounce and curl to the points of one-length styles.
Flat brush	Curl cannot be achieved with a flat brush although the slight curve of the brush where the filaments are embedded can produce bounce. This brush can also be used to smooth out movement from the hair during drying. Suitable for most hair lengths, especially long hair. This is probably the most frequently used brush in salons today.
Vent brush	The filaments of a vent brush are arranged in pairs and the hair is brushed; the shorter filaments break up the hair so that it lies as if fingers have been drawn through it. Ideal for using on most hair lengths except very long hair which is fine because the filaments can get caught in the hair.
Blow-waving	Suitable for short hair if it is not too curly. Mostly used on male clients although it is equally good for female clients. Blow-waving is difficult to do on hair that is sparse and should be in the direction of the natural growth patterns on the front hairline.
Natural dry	Suitable for clients who want their hair to look natural and casual. Ideal for permed hair and naturally curly hair. Not suitable for clients that like a 'set' look or require a lot of root lift.
Finger-pressing	This technique is only used for styles that are straight. It is used to smooth the surface of the hair so that it is ultra-sleek and shiny.

finished result should also complement the client's facial characteristics.

Certain hair textures are better for achieving particular looks and effects than others, and selecting an unsuitable drying technique can result in the hairdresser struggling with the hair. In Figure 6.2 we have set out the various drying techniques to help you to select the most suitable method of blow drying.

A few clients are apprehensive about having a blow-dry, instead of their usual shampoo and set. If you are blow-drying an elderly client's hair, try to create soft lines around the face to prevent the style from looking severe. If the client is used to height and curl, blow-dry the hair to produce this effect. The style can always be finished with tongs or a hot brush after it has been dried. Do remember, that there are too many hairdressers who suggest styles which are typical 'granny' looks because of the person's age. It is the facial characteristics which should be the main consideration, not the client's age. Just because a client is seventy should not mean she should have a shapeless shampoo and set. A new style which is blow-dried can be more suitable if it is thoughtfully planned to complement the client.

Please refer to Chapter 7 for a discussion about the different styling aids which are available.

How are these drying techniques carried out?

Blow-drying a one-length shape

When drying a one-length shape, such as a bob, you will be aiming to produce a sleek look with some bend on the points of the hair. A flat brush is the ideal tool for drying this type of style and the curve of the brush is what you will be using to produce the bend on the hair points.

Figure 6.3 Sections which are as wide as the diameter of the brush you are using are taken.

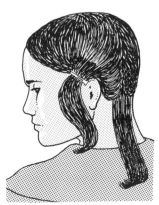

Method using a flat brush

1. Prepare hair with styling aid if desired and make any partings that are required.
2. Divide the hair into four sections (forehead to nape and across the top of the head from ear to ear) and secure each division with sectioning clips.
3. Take a section, equivalent to the diameter of the brush you are using, ready for drying. This is shown in Figure 6.3.
4. Working with the hand dryer in one hand and the brush in the other hand, place the brush underneath the mesh of hair at the roots. Keeping the tension on the mesh so that it is kept taut (without undue stress), direct the air flow in a downwards movement onto the hair following the downwards movement of the brush. Concentrate on drying the root area first, repeatedly introducing the brush to the roots once it has moved down the length of the hair. Repeat this movement until the hair is dry. Once the roots are dry, use the dryer

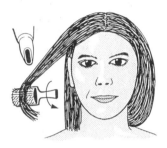

Figure 6.4 The final side of the style being blow-dried. The brush is turned in the hand once it reaches the points of the hair.

to style the middle lengths and ends, using the curve of the brush to achieve the bend on the hair points.

5. Once the whole of the mesh is dry, take another section of hair (the same depth as the diameter of the brush) above the section you have dried. Dry this section of hair in the same manner as the previous one, ensuring that the root area is dried first. Continue in this manner until all of the back hair is dried.

6. When you have completed the hair at the back, begin at the sides by taking horizontal meshes of hair on the underneath, gradually working upwards towards the parting or top hair. Figure 6.4 shows the final side being dried. Note how the brush is turned in the hand once it reaches the points of the hair, to utilise the curve of the brush, to create the bend on the points. The dryer is held so that the airflow is directed downwards, keeping the hair smooth and sleek.

7. To complete the blow-dry the hair can be 'finger-pressed' to achieve optimum smoothness. This is done by taking meshes of the top, overlaying hair between the first two fingers and sliding them down the hair, followed by the airflow. This helps to flatten and smooth the cuticle even more, thereby achieving the maximum degree of shine on the hair.

8. Once the blow-dry is completed, you should always check that the hair is completely dry by feeling it with your hands. When the freshly dried hair is brushed, it should fall into the desired shape. If the ends do not turn under properly and tend to stick out when brushed, check they are thoroughly dry; this will not occur if the hair is completely dry.

Method using a circular brush

There are many different sizes of circular brushes, varying from about 1 cm in diameter to as much as 5 cms. The smaller the diameter of brush that is used, the greater the amount of movement and curl that will be achieved. It is important to remember that the smaller circular brushes should be carefully used as longer hair has a tendency to tangle with such brushes, especially if the hair is fine.

Large circular brushes can be used to shape one-length hair shapes instead of flat brushes, but the smaller ones are mostly used on shorter lengths when curl is required.

1. Prepare hair with styling aid if desired and comb the hair into its intended direction (that is, make any required parting and comb the hair according to the finished result).

2. If the hair at the nape is long, it is recommended that the drying commences in this area. Otherwise, the drying could begin wherever the stylist prefers. The important thing is that the blow-dry is carried out in a systematic way, using clean partings, correct size meshes, and that each mesh of hair is thoroughly dried before moving onto the next one.

3. It is always important to dry the roots before the middle lengths and ends. Failing to do this will result in the stylist being unable to create any volume at the roots.

4. Dry each mesh of hair and avoid disturbing the movement or curl until it has completely cooled as this will pull out the newly formed shape. When working with a circular brush, make sure that the hair points are cleanly wrapped around the bristles or you could end up with frizzy, distorted ends (that is, fish hooks).

5. On completion of the blow-dry, check that the hair is fully dry and look for any areas that require further styling. Also, check that the style is well balanced in volume and that the hair is falling as intended. You may find it necessary to use tongs or a hot brush to achieve the desired degree of curl or movement, which is an acceptable practice. You should not rely on the tongs or hot brush to produce the style as your blow-drying should have formed the hair into shape.

Blow-drying using a vent brush

If you look at a vent brush, you will notice that the back of the brush has open spaces which allows the airflow from the drier to pass through. Also, the nylon bristles are of two different lengths. It is the venting on the back of the brush and these different length bristles that give the hair a casual, broken appearance when brushed. Therefore, blow-drying with a vent brush is recommended when a textured, casual result is required. Vent brushes can also be used to simply brush through the hair after drying with a flat or circular brush, to break up the hair and create a softer, casual look.

Blow-drying using the fingers

Sometimes there is no substitute for the fingers to dry the hair into shape. The fingers are used to lift and direct the hair into the intended style, giving a softer and more casual appearance than using a brush. To create lots of volume and texture, as would be seen in spiky styles, place the palm of your hand flat onto the scalp and rotate it in a circular movement, directing the airflow onto this area. The hair will become matted, causing the hair to stand up. Sometimes, stylists ask clients to bend their heads forward so that the airflow can be directed underneath the hair at the nape. This helps to increase the body at the roots, making the hair stand out on the supporting hair underneath.

Scrunch drying

Scrunch drying is a method of blow-drying using the hands. It helps to increase curl and texture in hair which already has some natural movement. The root area should be dried first, and the client perhaps asked to bend her head over to achieve maximum volume first. Then the middle lengths and ends are clasped tightly in the hands while directing heat onto them from the dryer. Sections are not normally necessary when drying hair using this technique and quite large quantities of hair can be scrunched as opposed to small meshes. Do not be tempted to brush or comb the hair after scrunch-drying. All your hard work will be lost as brushing would pull out the texture and movement you have created. Many stylists prefer to work with different diffuser attachments when drying hair using the scrunching technique.

Natural drying

There are certain looks that do not require shaping by a brush and hand dryer. Instead, they are combed or brushed into position and then allowed to dry naturally, perhaps occasionally lifting the hair with the fingers or an Afro comb. Such styles might be those which are permed and require no stretching by blow-drying. Because it would be unreasonable to expect clients to sit in the salon waiting for their hair to dry as they would if they were at home, we use an additional source of heat to accelerate the process.

Perhaps the most popular means of drying hair naturally is by using heat provided from infra red lamps in the form of some sort of accelerator, such as the Wella climazon, or an octopus lamp. The heat is dry and there is no airflow to disturb the lie of the hair. Care must be taken that the radiation is not directed into the client's face.

If you use a diffuser attachment on a hand hairdryer it will disperse the airflow and will give little disturbance to the lie of the hair. Never allow the client to leave the salon with wet hair as it is possible to catch cold easily as the moisture evaporates.

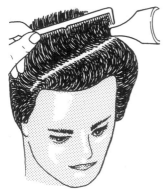

Figure 6.5 The airflow from the hairdryer is directed along the wave crest against the direction of the movement.

Blow-waving

The art of blow-waving was developed as a technique during the 1930s using a comb and hand dryer to produce waves in the hair, similar to those produced by finger-waving. A comb, traditionally made from vulcanite to withstand heat, as many plastics are softened (though some modern plastic combs are heat-resistant), was used. Blow-waving should start at the front hairline, following the natural hair growth movement and direction. The wide teeth of the comb are used to hold the hair in the wave direction and the airflow is directed onto the hair. Use a low power setting so that the hair does not blow out of position. An important rule of blow-waving is that the airflow is directed along the wave crest against the direction of the movement as shown in Figure 6.5. Use a nozzle attachment to concentrate the airflow of the hairdryer.

Relaxing over-curly hair

Blow-drying using a brush can be done after the hair has been set on rollers to loosen the hair if it is too curly. The hair is not dampened, as it is the heat from the dryer and the tension that you put on the hair that will relax the movement. When doing this, be careful to observe how the hair responds as it is very easy to over-relax the set, making it limp and lifeless. This technique is most frequently used after doing a wrap round to smooth out the hair.

Principles for blow-drying

- A style will always lie better and last longer if it follows the natural hair fall and movement.
- The hair should be directed to the movement of the intended style, taking its direction from the roots. This can only be achieved if the root area is dried before the middle lengths and ends. Lift at the roots cannot be successfully achieved if the roots are not dried first. To increase the volume at the roots, over-direct the mesh of hair and direct the airflow in at the roots.
- The dryer should always be kept moving to prevent damage to the hair or scalp.
- The depth of meshes to be dried should be no deeper than the diameter of the brush being used.
- Wherever you begin drying the hair, it is essential that the mesh is completely dry before going onto another mesh. If you fail to dry a particular area thoroughly, the remaining moisture will evaporate, causing the style to collapse.
- When blow-drying, the airflow should be directed so that it follows the lie of the cuticle (i.e. roots to points) because if the cuticle is kept smooth, the hair will shine.
- You will need to position yourself and the client so that you can get at the hair easily. Sometimes, you may need the client to lean right forward so that you can dry the hair at the nape. This is often done when scrunch-drying to achieve maximum volume and support in the underneath hair.
- During the blow-dry you will need to check the balance and shape of the style by looking in the mirror. You may also find it useful to bend down so that you are at eye level to the client's head when looking in the mirror. This will help you to notice any discord in the shape or balance much more easily.
- Only products intended for blow-drying should be applied. Ordinary setting lotion can dry to be sticky and makes the hair difficult to manage and control. Mousse, gel and other styling aids should be applied to the hair evenly (see Chapter 7). They should be applied to towel-dried hair and thoroughly combed to distribute them evenly throughout the hair. Too much styling product in one area will normally mean there will not be sufficient in another.
- When the blow-dry is finished, check that the hair is completely dry. Comb or brush the hair if necessary, to ensure that the style is blended and looks polished. This is also the opportunity to check that partings are clean and straight.

- The application of hair spray or fixative will help hold the blow style in place, and protect it from atmospheric moisture. If the style you have created is sleek, apply the fixing spray in downward movements to avoid disturbance. Any fine, stray hairs, can be gently smoothed down with the hands at this stage, to get the style looking really sleek. Remember that fixing sprays should be applied at a distance of approximately 30 cms and that the client's eyes should be protected during the application. You might also wish to apply finishing products such as gloss sprays, gels or waxes to complete the look. (Remember that this is the ideal time and opportunity for recommending retail products to your client.)
- Always show the client the back of the hair when it is finished by using a back mirror. It should be held so that you are able to see the reflection in the mirror which is in front of the client. Try not to move the mirror too quickly or the client may presume something is wrong with the hair at the back!

How can wastage be minimised?

Blow-drying can be tedious and time-consuming. Time can be saved if excess moisture is removed before styling begins. This can easily be done by towel-drying or rough-drying the hair a little using the dryer. Alternatively, the dryer can be directed at the roots while the hair is brushed. This will remove excess moisture and at the same time give lift and body to the roots. Only apply as much styling product as the manufacturers recommend. Careful application will prevent any product from ending up on the floor or simply making the towel around the client's shoulders wet. Finally, never waste the opportunity of having your client's undivided attention during a blow-dry, to offer them hair care advice and to recommend further services and retail products.

Questions

1. What is blow-drying?
2. What effects can be achieved?
3. Construct a table to show the effects of drying techniques.
4. Construct a table to show the suitability of various drying methods.
5. What kind of effects should you try to produce for clients who normally like their hair to be set?
6. How should you blow-dry a one-length shape?
7. Blow-dry a style on a model using a flat brush.
8. Blow-dry a style on a model using a circular brush.
9. Why should you blow-dry the roots before the middle lengths and ends?
10. What are 'fish hooks'?
11. Blow-dry a style on a model using a vent brush.
12. What type of style can be created using a vent brush?
13. Blow-dry a style on a model using your fingers.

14. What type of style can be created using the fingers?
15. What type of style can be created using scrunch-drying?
16. What is natural drying?
17. How can it be achieved in the salon?
18. What is blow-waving?
19. How should the airflow be directed when blow-waving?
20. How would you relax over-curly hair?
21. Make a list of the main principles of blow-drying.
22. Why should hair be towel-dried before you blow-dry it?

Tools and equipment

Hand-held dryers (blow-dryers)

A typical professional dryer is shown in Figure 6.6. It is lightweight, well-balanced and has variable controls for the heat and speed of the airflow. The back of this dryer has a filter which prevents dust particles from getting into the motor. This filter requires regular cleaning because a build-up of dust reduces the amount of air that the dryer can suck in. If this happens, the dryer will overheat and could cut out, this being a safety mechanism to prevent the hairdryer from damage and possibly from catching fire. Some of the latest hairdryers available cut out if they

Figure 6.6 A professional hairdryer complete with nozzle. Controls for variable airflow speed and temperature are incorporated into the handle. (Courtesy Babyliss Ltd.)

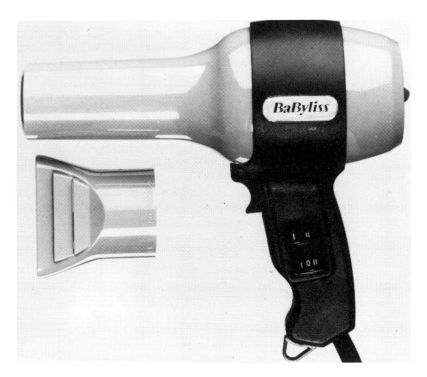

are held too close to the client's skin, thus preventing it from being burnt. If the filter does need cleaning, *always* disconnect the dryer. It is not safe to work with a dryer without its filter in place because hair could otherwise be sucked into the fan which would normally be guarded by the filter.

Safe working guide – hairdryers

- Always work with a clean filter in place.
- Never use a hairdryer if the plug is cracked or the flex is damaged.
- Never use a dryer with wet hands or close to a water supply (e.g. next to the basins).
- Never leave cables (the dryer flexes) where people could trip over them.
- Never hold a hairdryer too close to a client's hair or scalp. The hot air can burn the skin and scorch the hair. For the same reason, do not play a stream of hot air on one area for too long, especially if there are metal clips in the hair that will quickly heat up.
- Never cover the back of the dryer where the air is sucked in. If no air (or a reduced intake of air) gets to the motor, the dryer will overheat.
- Always switch off a dryer before putting it down on a surface. The vibration of the motor could cause it to move and fall onto the floor.

Blow-dryer attachments

Figure 6.7 The varying airflows: (a) without a nozzle, (b) with a nozzle, (c) with a diffuser.

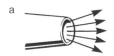

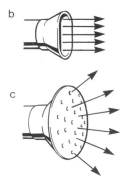

Hairdryers can be used with or without the nozzle, as all this does is change the concentration of the airflow. When a nozzle is used, the airflow if forced through the narrow slit of the nozzle, making the flow of air more forceful (see Figure 6.7). Without a nozzle, the airflow leaves the dryer at a much wider angle. Special attachments, called diffusers, can be used to disperse the airflow so that it is less forceful. Diffusers are particularly useful for drying styles that require minimal disturbance from the airflow.

Infra red dryers

Infra red dryers are used to dry hair when minimum disturbance to the style is required. Infra red dryers are available as either hand-held, pedestal or wall-mounted models. Hand-held infra red dryers can either be a single infra red bulb which is similar to the appearance of a hairdryer, or have the added function of a gentle airflow that can be switched on and used simultaneously with the heat given off by the bulb. Wall-mounted or pedestal models will have several infra red bulbs which are set onto adjustable 'arms' that are arranged so that the whole head can be dried, dispensing with the need for a stylist to hold the appliance. The models with multiple bulbs are commonly called by the name of an 'octopus' simply because of their appearance.

Safe working guide — infra red dryers

- Care should be taken not to direct the infra red rays into the client's eyes. Remember that although you cannot see infra red, it behaves in the same way as light. It can reflect off mirrors if an accelerator is placed next to one. Like any source of heat it can burn. Check that infra red equipment has been approved for use in this country. Some wavelengths of infra red can cause cataracts in the eyes.
- The bulbs can get very hot so be careful that you do not touch them.
- Do not have the bulbs too close to the hair or skin because the heat could burn.
- Infra red bulbs are expensive to replace so they should be handled with care.

Tongs

Tongs, otherwise known as curling irons, are a direct descendant of the curling irons which were used as long ago as Roman times. Of course in those days they did not have electricity so the irons were heated over a fire.

The tongs shown in Figure 6.8 have a built-in stand which can be used for resting the tongs when not in use. The black tip at the end of the metal rod is a safety tip which enables the stylist to hold the tongs for extra control. The flex has a swivel action to prevent the cord from getting twisted, allowing easier manipulation. When the lever is depressed, the tongs open.

Figure 6.8 Tongs shown resting on their own stand. (Courtesy Babyliss Ltd.)

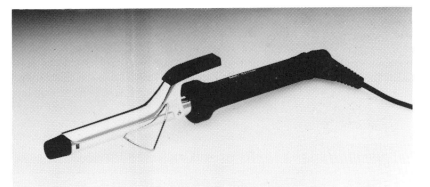

Tongs have a built-in thermostat to control the temperature and to prevent the appliance from overheating. Some models may also have variable heat controls which are adjusted according to the hair type and texture you are working on. Remember that excessive heat is very harmful to hair and that such damage is irreversible.

The points of the hair should be cleanly wrapped around the rod of the tongs to prevent distorted and buckled ends. The tongs are then wound up the length of hair and held in position until the heat has penetrated through the mesh of hair. If you intend to curl right up to the

Figure 6.9 Protecting the scalp while using curling tongs. A heat-resistant comb is placed between the scalp and the tongs.

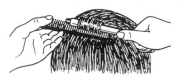

roots, place a vulcanite comb between the tongs and the scalp to act as a barrier against the heat, as shown in Figure 6.9. Once the hair is released from the tongs, it should be allowed to cool before it is combed or brushed.

Spiral tongs

Spiral tongs are curling irons which have a spiral groove running along the heated rod. The type shown in Figure 6.10 have the same features as the tongs previously described: built-in rest, protective safety tip, swivel flex. The lever is depressed and is closed on the hair points. As the tongs are turned, the mesh will automatically position itself in the spiral groove. When the mesh is released, the hair will be formed into a ringlet.

Figure 6.10 Spiral tongs shown resting on their stand. (Courtesy Babyliss Ltd.)

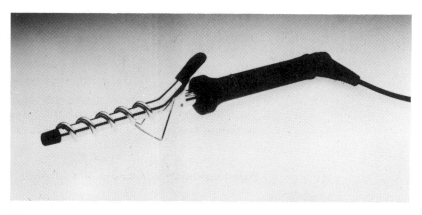

Safe working guide – tongs

- *Only use tongs on hair which is dry.*
- Do not leave tongs switched on for longer than is necessary as this shortens the life of the appliance and increases the chance of accidents.
- Use the built-in stand for resting the tongs to prevent scorching work surfaces. Alternatively, your salon may have special holes cut out of work surfaces specially for storing tongs.
- Clean the appliance regularly using cotton wool soaked in methylated spirit to remove grime on the rod. *Always* disconnect the appliance from the mains before doing this and *never* immerse the appliance in water.
- Use less heat on hair which already shows signs of damage. Once the hair has been scorched, the damage is irreversible.
- Never put hot tongs into a bag. Allow them to cool first.

Hot brushes

Hot brushes are preferred by some hairdressers because the teeth along the heated rod tend to help keep the hair in place while the hot brush is

Figure 6.11 A selection of different sized hot brushes. (Courtesy Babyliss Ltd.)

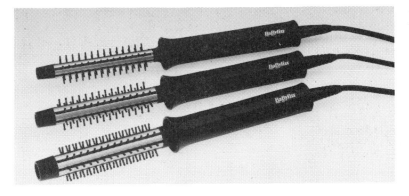

being turned. Hot brushes are available in different sizes to create tighter or looser curls. A selection of hot brushes is shown in Figure 6.11.

Hot brushes are used in the same way as tongs but care needs to be taken because messy sectioning can result in the hot brush getting tangled in the hair.

There are tongs and hot brushes available which are cordless and described as 'independent'. They use butane cartridges or batteries to provide the energy to produce the heat. They are popular to take on holidays and for hairdressers who are involved in photographic location work when a source of electricity is not always available.

Safe working guidelines – hot brushes

* *Only use a hot brush on hair which is dry.*
* Do not leave hot brushes switched on longer than necessary as this will ultimately affect the lifespan of the appliance and increase the chance of accidents.
* Clean hot brushes regularly in the same way as you would for tongs. *Always* disconnect them from the power supply first. *Never* immerse them in water.
* Take clean sections so that the appliance does not get tangled in the hair.
* Make allowances when using a hot brush on damaged hair by ensuring that the hair is not subjected to excessive and unnecessary heat.
* Wait until the appliance is cool before putting it away into a bag or cupboard.

Crimping irons

Crimpers are an electrical appliance which produce straight line crimps in the hair in a uniform pattern. Crimpers, such as those shown in Figure 6.12 can be used on partial areas only or the whole head to create a variety of interesting looks.

Figure 6.12 A pair of
crimpers. (Courtesy Babyliss
Ltd.)

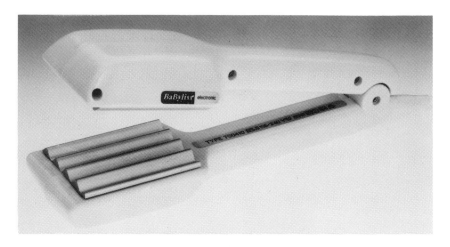

To use crimpers, neat sections are taken which are approximately
2 cms deep and no wider than the metal plates of the crimpers. The
mesh of hair to be crimped is held at an angle of between 45 and 90
degrees to the contours of the head and the crimpers are carefully
positioned so that the plates are on both sides of the mesh. The crimpers
are closed and held in position for 2–5 seconds before they are released.
Excessive pressure on the crimpers is not necessary – it is the heat
which is doing the work for you. This procedure is then continued down
the hair's length.

For safety guidelines see those for tongs and hot brushes, and for
more information on electrical styling appliances, see *Cutting and
Styling – A Salon Handbook*.

Brushes

An extensive range of quality brushes is available to hairdressers. Basically,
all brushes are made of filaments, which can be natural hog bristle,
nylon or wire, set into a wooden, plastic or rubber moulded handle.
Natural bristles are the most expensive and cause the least amount of
friction on the hair because they are composed of keratin, like hair.

The hairbrush you choose to use when blow-drying hair will determine
the final effect of the style and there are three types of brush which you
might use:

Figure 6.13 A flat brush.

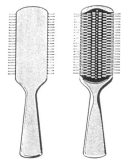

- flat brush,
- vent brush,
- circular brush.

Flat Brush

This type of brush is probably the most commonly used brush in salons
today for general use (see Figure 6.13). However, it is ideal for blow-

drying one length-shapes like bobs. The slight curve of the brush where the filaments are set helps create curve in the hair and encourages the hair to turn under.

Vent brush

The nylon tufts of this brush (see Figure 5.38) are set into the base in pairs with one tuft longer than the other. As the brush is drawn through the hair, the short and long filaments give the hair a broken, casual look. The back of the brush has spaces which allow the dryer airflow to pass through and encourage hair with natural movement to curl. Ideal for most hair lengths when blow-drying hair into casual looks.

Circular brushes

Circular brushes are available in different sizes varying from 1–6 cms. The diameter of the brush will determine the tightness of the curl

Figure 6.14 Types of circular brushes. (Courtesy Denman Ltd.)

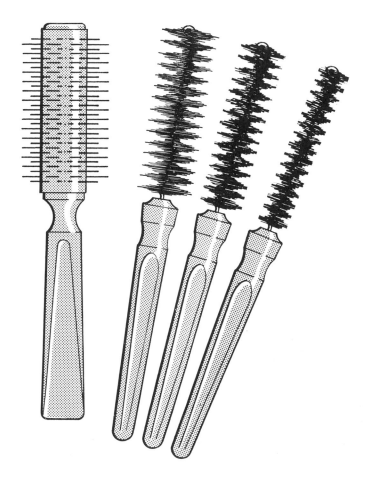

produced − just like a small roller will produce a tighter curl than a large roller. The size of the mesh that is taken when using a circular brush should be no deeper than the diameter of the brush being used. If meshes are too deep, the hair can tangle on the brush, especially if the hair is long.

Combs

Good quality combs are an indispensable tool for any hairdresser. They are available in a variety of shapes, colours and materials. Some combs are used for specific purposes only (like tail combs for sectioning hair into neat meshes for setting and perming) while others have a more general use. Quality combs are made from durable materials that have smooth, slightly rounded teeth that will not damage the hair or scratch the scalp. Cheap combs are often too flexible and the teeth are rough which snag the hair, causing it to tear. They can also be very sharp and consequently scratch the client's scalp.

If you are blow-waving, you will be using a comb instead of a brush. The best type to use for this is a vulcanite comb because it is heat-resistant. Vulcanite is a material which is made of rubber that has been treated with sulphur to make it more resistant to heat. Any plastic combs that you buy in future are likely one day to end up being sterilised in an autoclave, so make sure that they are heat-resistant beforehand.

Questions
1. Why should you clean the filter regularly in a blow dryer?
2. How do the latest dryers protect the skin from being burnt?
3. How can you be safe when cleaning electrical equipment?
4. Make a list of safe working rules when using dryers.
5. What effect does a nozzle have on the airflow of a dryer?
6. What effect does a diffuser have on a dryer's airflow?
7. When are infra red dryers used?
8. Make a list of safe working guidelines for infra red dryers.
9. Describe the safety points of a modern pair of electric tongs.
10. How do you use tongs on hair?
11. What are spiral tongs?
12. Make a list of safe working guidelines for using tongs.
13. When do some hairdressers like to use hot brushes?
14. What is an 'independent' hot brush?
15. Make a list of safe working guidelines for using hot brushes.
16. What are crimpers?
17. How do you use them?
18. Why are natural bristle brushes kinder to the hair?
19. What are the differences between flat, vent and circular brushes?
20. What is the difference between cheap and expensive combs?
21. What is vulcanite and when would it be required?
22. Why is it best to buy heat-resistant combs?

Chapter Seven
Setting

How setting and blow-drying work

Both setting and blow-drying involve a temporary change in the structure of the hair. Wet hair is stretched around rollers or with a brush and dried in its stretched state. The degree of curl introduced into the hair is always slightly tighter than actually desired, so that it can be brushed out into the planned style. The hair remains in this stretched position until it is wet again. Because no chemical reaction has taken place the change is physical; it only involves a change in the shape of the keratin, and can easily be reversed. This form of temporary set is known as a 'cohesive set'. Because it is a physical change the hair can be set as frequently as desired. This is the basis of finger-waving, pin curling, roller curling and all wet setting methods. The stylist should know whether each of these methods should be carried out individually on a head, or used in combination to produce the desired effect.

The cohesive set

As the setting of hair relies on its ability to stretch, it can only be carried out really successfully on hair that is in good condition. The stretching of dry hair is controlled to a great extent by the weak, but numerous, hydrogen bonds which are described in Chapter 8. Because there are millions of these bonds, they allow the hair to stretch slightly, while the stronger but less numerous disulphide bonds resist the movement. To obtain greater extension, the stretching is carried out on wet hair, by either winding tightly on rollers or by brushing when blow-drying. Figure 7.1(a) shows dry hair in its unstretched state, with a hydrogen bond between the hydrogen and oxygen atoms. When wet hair is stretched (Figure 7.1(b)) water molecules enter the hydrogen bonds allowing the hair to stretch further – this is known as 'bound water'. During drying, the bound water is evaporated off. In Figure 7.1(c) you can see that because the water is evaporated off while the hair is still in its stretched state, the bonds have reformed in different positions. When the rollers, or brush, are removed, the hair remains in its stretched state. It will not return to its normal state until the hair is wet, but because hair is hygroscopic (it absorbs moisture from the atmosphere – generally about 10 per cent of the cortex can be water) the cohesive set will be lost quickly unless it is protected from moisture. We protect it with various setting agents such as setting and blow-dry lotions, hairsprays, etc. If it were not protected the sequence shown in Figure 7.1 would be reversed and the set would be lost.

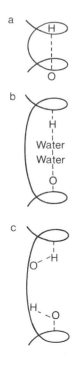

Figure 7.1 (a) Hair in its unstretched state. (b) Bound water enters the hair as it stretches. (c) During drying water is evaporated off and the hair is held in its stretched state when bonds are formed in different positions.

What are the two types of keratin involved in a cohesive set?

You may have heard people talking about two types of keratin as if they were totally different things. These are the magical alpha- and beta-keratins. Put simply, alpha-keratin is keratin in its unstretched state, while beta-keratin is keratin in its stretched state. It is rather like alpha-keratin being an unstretched spring, while beta-keratin is the stretched spring. Remember that it is the spring-like structure of the cortex that gives hair its elasticity. Set hair is hair which has been dried in a stretched state, so it is beta-keratin. If it is wetted it returns to being alpha-keratin. Remember that there are still powerful disulphide bonds intact in the cortex which will help pull the hair back to its original shape once the new hydrogen bonds are broken by absorbed water. The two types of keratin are summarised below:

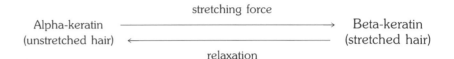

Alpha-keratin (unstretched hair) — stretching force → Beta-keratin (stretched hair), ← relaxation

Is there a difference between the cohesive set and the heat-setting carried out on dry hair with heated tongs?

The simple answer to this question is yes. The use of heated waving irons, tongs, crimpers, rollers, etc. is often thought by hairdressers to work in exactly the same way. Hair is both heated and stretched at the same time and then held under tension until it is cool. The hydrogen bonds between the polypeptide chains of keratin are broken by both the heat and the tension placed on the hair. The greater the heat applied, the more bonds will be broken. The hair takes up the shape of the tool used. As the hair cools under tension, the hydrogen and oxygen atoms of the original bonds are too far apart to reform, so they form new bonds with atoms close by which keep the hair in its new shape. Cold water has little effect on a heat set; hot water must be used to break the new bonds so that the hair can relax its structure and reform the original bonds. Remember that too much heat-setting will damage the cuticle of the hair.

Questions
1. What is a physical change?
2. Why must the hair be in good condition to take a set well?
3. Why is setting carried out on wet hair?
4. Describe what happens to the bonds in a cohesive set?
5. How is the set lost?
6. What are the two types of keratin?
7. What type of keratin is set hair?
8. What is the difference between heat and cohesive setting?

9. How can a heat-set be broken?

10. Which damages the hair least, heat or cohesive setting?

Setting

When hairdressers talk about setting, they are describing how hair is moulded into a shape while it is wet and then dried in that position. Once it is completely dry, the operator will dress the hair and the style is complete.

Hair can be set using rollers, pincurls, finger-waves and many of the alternative types of setting tools like spiral curlers, Molton Browners, chopsticks and even rags. Whichever setting tools are chosen the principle of setting remains the same – the hair takes on the shape of the mould it is stretched around and this is called cohesive setting. It stands to reason, then, that if you wrapped a mesh of wet hair around a match box and dried in that position the hair would take on the shape of the box. Setting is only a temporary method of changing the appearance of the hair and can achieve an array of different looks. We have said it is a physical rather than a chemical change (unlike perming) so is easily reversed. Hair can be set to make the hair straighter, more curly, fuller, flatter, sleeker or more wavy. All these effects can be achieved simply by the setting methods which the operator chooses to use and the imaginative way the rollers or whatever are positioned.

It is very disheartening to go into a salon and see a row of women sitting under the hood dryers with their hair set in exactly the same way. They don't all go out of the salon looking the same – or do they? Too often, hairdressers put in rollers in a mundane pattern with little or no thought given to the finished look or how the client will manage it at home. Do these hairdressers realise that they are in fact making their task more difficult? If you place rollers in a different position to the way you intend to dress it, of course you are going to meet problems. We have seen stylists frantically backcombing trying to dress the hair so that it takes on a decent shape. If only these hairdressers realised how much better the quality of their work would be if they practised the basic skill of setting hair. Such hairdressers do not become champion hairdressers nor fashion innovators. They are quite satisfied with their standard of work because they usually do not know any better. What is disturbing, though, is that these people will often be responsible for training others! With the competition of other salons and hairdressers operating in your area you cannot afford *not* to be able to set hair well. If you can't do something a client requests, or you do it badly, there is always a hairdresser who can do it well and will take that client from you.

What setting and finishing aids are available and how do they affect the hair?

Setting aids come in a variety of forms such as gels, mousses, sprays and lotions.

Setting lotions

The most commonly used form of setting aid is a setting lotion, which is generally supplied in individual application bottles. Setting lotions are available in different formulae designed to give gentle hold or maximum hold. Also, setting lotions may contain colour to add temporary colour to a person's hair. The lotions which contain colour are often referred to as 'rinses' or simply 'coloured lotions'.

Setting lotions prevent the hair from drying out too quickly during setting and also help to prolong the life of the set by excluding atmospheric moisture from the hair shaft. There are historically two types of setting lotion, those older ones based on gums and the more modern plastic setting lotions.

The gums were obtained when trees were damaged, as an exudation from the wounded bark. The two best-known ones are gum tragacanth (Turkish) and gum karaya (Indian). When added to a solution of water and alcohol the gums form a sticky solution called a mucilage. Their use is now obsolete because they yielded dull, brittle films, which crumbled into dust and became sticky in humid air because they were hygroscopic.

The modern setting lotions that you use in the salons contain plastic resins and polymers dissolved in a mixture of alcohol and water. The plastic resin is left as a flexible covering film on the hair when the water and alcohol have evaporated. They may contain resins or polymers such as polyvinyl pyrrolidone (PVP), polyvinyl acetate (PVA) or dimethyl-hydantoin formaldehyde resin (DMHF). Because PVP by itself is too hygroscopic, a copolymer of PVP and PVA is used in a ratio of 6:4; it is known as PVP-VA. To counteract any hardness of the plastic film, plasticisers are added. These are usually polyethyleneglycols and silicones. They make the film more flexible and water-resistant.

Setting lotions may also contain ingredients which are added to give the hair body and increased manageability. Plastic setting lotions intended for blow-drying often contain silicone oils; these lessen friction when brushing, by smoothing the cuticle of the hair, and reduce heat damage as they are heat-resistant. Conditioners, such as protein hydrolysates, are often added. Some setting lotions are available as temporary colours, containing acid dyes.

Hairsprays

Most salons use hairsprays which are supplied in aerosol cans. The actual spray is fine and makes an even application easier. They must be quick-drying and impart sufficient rigidity to the set to control it, without detracting from the natural sheen of the hair. They reached their height of popularity around 1970, but have fallen away since the advent of the mousse revolution of the 1980s. The resins could be shampooed off with ease yet not become powdery on brushing. The early ones contained shellac in alcohol. In 1948 this became available as an aerosol. Today it is the copolymers of PVP-VA which are most used. Other resins are also used, however, and about five new ones have been patented each year since the 1960s.

An aerosol is shown in Figure 7.2(a). It is one developed by Goldwell which dispenses from the large can into a small, hand-held spray. The one that you are most familiar with is shown in Figure 7.2(b). Once the spray button is depressed the hairspray is forced out of the can by the pressure of the propellant inside the can. Some propellants (chloro-fluorocarbons) were banned in the United States in 1979 because of their damaging effect on the ozone layer above the earth. The ozone layer acts as a shield against ultra violet radiation. If it were to deteriorate much further there would be increased skin cancer caused by more ultra violet (UVC) radiation reaching the earth. This ecological danger has led to the use of other propellants and hand pumps which are not as good as the original propellants for dispensing a fine spray. Within the next few years the use of chlorofluorocarbons will undoubtedly be banned worldwide.

Figure 7.2 (a) A can of Goldwell hairspray together with its small refillable spray which is filled by pressing down on to the large container. (b) A conventional aerosol can of hairspray. The nozzle of the button may become clogged from time to time.

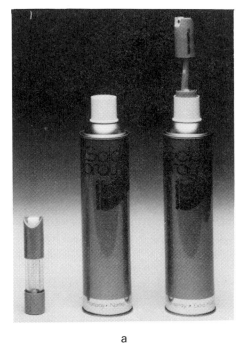

a

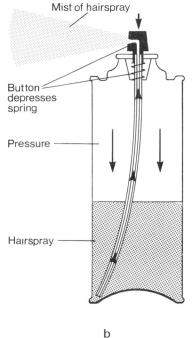

b

Because the propellant is volatile it forms a vapour at room temperature, which fills the space above the product in the can, the pressure of which drives out the hairspray (again, see Figure 7.2(b)). Never place aerosols near a source of heat or in direct sunlight on a hot day. The can could explode even after the contents have been used. Never dispose of empty cans in fires.

Mousses

Mousses are certainly the most popular styling aids of the 1980s. They

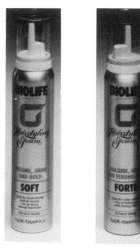

Figure 7.3 Mousse is available in different strengths to give varying degrees of hold and support. (Courtesy Goldwell Hair Cosmetics Ltd.)

are similar to setting lotions and hairsprays as far as ingredients are concerned, containing a solution of resins (polymers) and conditioning agents (silicone oils) in a mixture of water and alcohol in a pressurised container. The contents are dispensed in the form of a foam. Like hairsprays, the containers can explode if they become too hot, and the contents are flammable. Care should be taken near infra red dryers or even when smoking because of this.

Mousse is available in different strengths (see Figure 7.3) to give increased holding power and the addition of azo dyes has made it available in different temporary colours. It is usually applied to damp hair, although it may be applied to dry hair to increase curl and texture for scrunched looks.

Mousse can be revitalised the following day after application by running wet fingers or a wet brush against the direction of the finished look before final arrangement. Try different brands to see which one you like best. Some may be more greasy than others, depending on their exact formulations.

Gels

The popularity of hair gels has diminished with the advent of a broader range of mousses, which are firmer holding. Originally, gels were preferred by many stylists because of their holding power. In hairdressing terms, the two main types of gel available are: those which cannot be seen on the hair once it is dried, and those which create a wet look, just right for sleeked back styles. They can have added ingredients which make them fluoresce or glow in the dark — ideal to be seen on a bike at night! Modern gels contain water-soluble plastic resins with a plasticiser to allow flexibility, although some preparations are deliberately made to make the hair stiff and unnatural-looking (punk styles, for example). Some clear gels are oil-in-water emulsions where tiny microscopic particles of oil are dispersed in water, to give a less greasy feel than ordinary oil-in-water emulsions. They are sometimes called micro-gels.

Questions
1. What do hairdressers mean by setting?
2. How can hair be set?
3. What does the term 'mould' refer to?
4. What effects can be achieved by setting?
5. What ingredients did older setting lotions contain?
6. What benefits do the newer lotions offer?
7. Why are plasticisers added to modern setting lotions?
8. What other ingredients may be found in setting lotions?
9. Why should aerosols be kept away from heat?
10. What connection have aerosols with the ozone layer?
11. What are the main ingredients of hairsprays?

12. What are the main ingredients of mousses?

13. What kind of dye is sometimes added to a mousse?

14. How can mousses be revitalised?

15. Why do some people prefer gels to other styling products?

How are setting aids applied to the hair?

Whatever setting aid is being used there are three rules to observe about application techniques:

1. If the hair is supposed to be towel-dried before the product is applied make sure this is done.

The water in dripping wet hair will dilute the product and reduce its holding power. Alternatively, if the hair is too dry (perhaps the client has been waiting for a while with damp hair and the moisture has evaporated) the setting aid might become sticky and the hair will be difficult to manage.

2. Always ensure that the product is evenly distributed throughout the hair.

It's not much good if there are areas which have been missed due to a poor application.

Lotions should be carefully and evenly sprinkled through the hair, making sure that your free hand is used to protect the face and neck from drips. Too often, setting lotion is only liberally applied to the front and top areas leaving the back hair unaffected. If you find the lotion comes out of the bottle too quickly, use your index finger to cover the hole partially so that you have better control.

The hands are used to apply gel to the hair. Whether the gel is supplied in a tube, tub or pump dispenser the operator should place the required amount in the palm of one hand and then rub both hands together to spread it out before it is smoothed through the hair.

Mousses are applied in the same way as gels although some hair-dressers prefer to comb the mousse onto the hair. This is done by having the mousse in the palm of one hand and scooping it up with a comb and applying it in that way.

Setting aids which are in the form of sprays should also be evenly applied making very sure that the eyes and face are protected from the spray. The product instructions will always tell you the distance you should hold the container away from the head during the application.

3. Always make sure you know your product instructions before using it.

The instructions will tell you how much product you should expect to use, its formula and any special notes on health and safety. If you apply too much, the results can sometimes be worse than applying too little. A client with very dense hair will obviously require more than a client with very little hair. It's wasteful to use the whole bottle of setting lotion if the excess ends up on the towel around the client's shoulders because the hair has become saturated.

How is hair spray applied to the hair?

Again, you will find instructions on the product container telling you the distance at which the product should be applied to the hair. Usually, this distance is about 30 cms (about a foot away) and depending on the type of product and style you are creating, you may need to direct the spray at the roots of the hair or in slight sweeping movements so that all the hair is sprayed. If you spray it too close to the head the hair will become wet and will separate into strands. Alternatively, holding the spray too far away will result in most of the spray ending up on the floor! The client's eyes and skin must always be protected from the spray by the hairdresser's free hand. Some salons use special plastic shields that clients hold over their faces while their hair is being sprayed. Hairspray can play havoc with contact lenses because it can irritate the eyes and soft lenses will actually absorb particles of the spray. Also, as a hairdresser in the atmosphere of the salon, avoid inhaling hairspray and try to use it in a well-ventilated area. This warning is very important for people suffering from asthma. Also remember that a jet of hairspray could turn into a flame-thrower if it came into contact with a flame!

Sheen and gloss sprays should be applied sparingly as too much can make the hair greasy and lank. A light spray is usually sufficient. Gloss creams are also available and these are applied in the same way as gel although they can be applied to certain areas in the same way as you would for applying hair wax or dressing cream to add definition to a style.

How can wastage be minimised?

Most wastage that occurs in salons is due to careless product application and lack of product knowledge. We have said above how important it is to follow the manufacturers' instructions and to apply products in a careful and proper manner. The other waste that could be prevented is missing the opportunity to talk to your clients about retail products and future services while you are attending to them.

Questions
1. Why should the hair be dried before applying some setting aids?
2. How can you ensure even application of product?
3. Why should you read product instructions carefully?
4. How do you apply hairspray to the hair?
5. How should the client be protected?
6. What safety points should be remembered when applying hairspray?

Finger waving

Finger waving is the art of shaping hair into waves using a comb and the fingers. It is best carried out on wet hair which has had a setting aid applied because the hair can be controlled a lot more easily. Hair which has been taper cut (see Chapter 5) is much easier to finger wave than club (blunt) cut hair. Before rollers were introduced to Britain from the United States, all sets were done using a combination of finger waves and pincurls. It was around this time that long metal clips were also introduced to help form and hold finger waves. These looked very similar to the 'butterfly' clips in use today for sectioning but the metal ones were longer. Although these clips do not produce such a beautiful result as when the hair is waved with the fingers, we know of a few hairdressers who have been bequeathed these clips from grandmothers and think they should be relaunched!

If you watch the old movies on television you will notice the finger waves of the stars like Jean Harlow. However, this skill is fundamental to many styles and you will see waved hair in the top fashion magazines. The variations of the styles may change but the method of creating them still requires great skill.

Looking at a diagram of a wave (Figure 7.4) you will see that it is made up of crests and troughs. The crest is the raised part of the wave and the trough is the dip or hollow between two crests. Technically speaking to be called a wave, there must be two crests and one trough. The distance between two crests should ideally be about the diameter of a ten pence coin (30 mm) and this space is called the width of the wave. The height of the crest and the depth of the wave is determined by the way in which the hair is directed during combing. The S-shaped movements created by finger waving can look stunning. For those training in hairdressing it teaches the skills of controlling and directing hair. It also demands discipline and manipulative skills to become practised. The hair is moulded and shaped into waves to the form of the head and in the direction of the natural hair growth patterns. The waves encircle the head and can be formed with a parting (side or centre) or straight back from the face without a parting.

The best type of comb to use for waving is a straight comb with wide- and narrow-spaced teeth. The way the comb is held is important because it will help you to have maximum control over the hair. The comb should be held with the thumb and little finger on one side, with three fingers on the other. This may seem strange to you at first if you are not used to holding a comb in this way, but with practice it will seem like an extention of your hand. The method of holding of a comb for finger waving is shown in Figure 7.5.

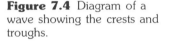

Figure 7.4 Diagram of a wave showing the crests and troughs.

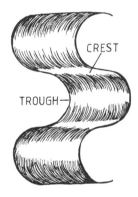

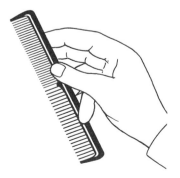

Figure 7.5 Method of holding a comb for finger-waving.

Guidelines for finger waving

- Keep your forearm up level with your hand when waving to give you maximum control.
- Always stand immediately behind the portion of the head you are waving.
- Hold the comb as shown in Figure 7.5.
- Keep the hair wet.
- Apply a setting aid to the hair.

- The hair should be combed away from the face before waving to look for the natural hair growth patterns.
- Use only the index finger and second finger during waving.

Finger waving practice

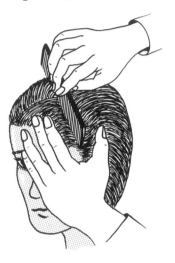

Figure 7.6 Directing the hair in preparation for a finger wave.

Like many hairdressing skills it is often best to practise on a tuition head (otherwise known as a block or 'dummy' head) before progressing to a live model. Before you attempt to wave a whole head we suggest the following exercise is practised:

1. If using a hair weft, secure this to a malleable block using postiche pins. If using a tuition head, make a parting across the back of the head from ear to ear just below the crown area and secure the front hair out of the way. Thoroughly comb the hair, wet it and apply a setting aid such as gel.
2. Begin by combing the hair in a semicircular movement which will direct the hair to the right. Remember that you should be standing immediately behind the portion of the head you are waving and keep your forearm up level with your hand. Place your index finger (of the hand not holding the comb) firmly against the head about 3 cms below the top of the weft or parting that you have made, to hold the curve you have just made in position as in Figure 7.6. Keep your finger firmly in position so that you are able to comb the rest of the hair without the curve being disturbed.

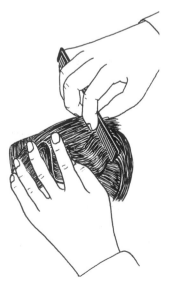

Figure 7.7 Holding the first crest in position while making the second crest to form a complete wave movement.

3. To form the crest (raised part) of the wave insert your comb about 2 cms below your index finger, and holding the comb flat against the head, push the comb up towards your finger in a movement directed to the left. Do not remove your comb from the hair at this stage. Move your hand position so that your second finger is resting on the teeth of your comb. Carefully slip out your comb so that you are able to hold the crest between your two fingers by pressure either side of the crest. Try not to pinch the crest too much or it will be distorted. While your fingers hold the crest in position, you can continue this sequence of movements down the rest of the hair.
4. The second crest can now be following the same series of movements but this time the hair is directed in the opposite direction. This is shown in Figure 7.7.
5. This series of movements continues all the way down the head and, to finish, the hair is pincurled using flat barrel curls. The pincurls are formed so that they continue the wave movement and are wound up to sit just below the final wave crest.

Finger waving a whole head

1. After the hair has been shampooed find the natural direction and fall of the hair so that you can see where the first wave should be placed. Apply a setting aid to the hair.

2. Combing the hair in its natural direction is the start of your first wave. Place your index finger below the crest you have just formed and your second finger above it. You can increase the height of this crest if you wish by inserting your comb at the root area and slightly lifting it upwards.

3. You should be able now to release your hold on the crest and it will remain in position. Following the same movement that you have just done, you are ready to wave the hair to the side of your first wave. Only allow your two fingers to touch the head so that you do not disturb your first crest.

4. Continue your waving around the head in the same direction so that you finish on the other side of the head at the hairline. You can then start to form your next crest right round the head. At the crown area the crest of the wave should be slightly faded to make it look more natural. This is called 'losing a wave' and is done by slightly flattening the crest.

5. It is important that you check the waves are equally balanced on both sides of the head if you decide to wave both sides of the head first and then join them up at the back.

6. When you have finished the waving the points of the hair at the nape and sides can be pincurled to the last crest. Try to avoid using clips to hold the waves in place for drying as these will leave marks on the hair. Instead, use tape positioned in the trough part of the waves.

7. When dry, the hair is combed through by retracing the movements of the waves and the pincurls dressed into curls or waves. Smoothing a little dressing cream through the hair before dressing the waves will give you better control if the hair is flyaway and make the hair shine. The result is shown in Figure 7.8.

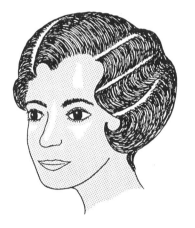

Figure 7.8 A finger-waved head.

Questions
1. What is finger-waving?
2. Why did finger-waving lose popularity in this country?
3. Describe the terms 'crest' and 'trough'.
4. What is the best type of comb to use when finger-waving?
5. How should it be held?
6. List the guidelines for finger-waving.
7. Undertake the finger-waving practice.
8. Finger-wave a whole head.

Pincurling

Pincurling is the sculpting of wet hair into a series of wound coils to form a curl. Once the curl is formed, it is secured in place with fine pins or clips. There are many types of pincurl, each producing a different effect, but they do fall into two main categories: flat pincurls and stand-up pincurls.

Figure 7.9 Securing flat
pincurls with a clip or fine
pins.

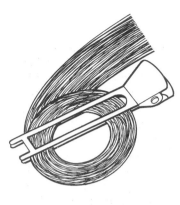

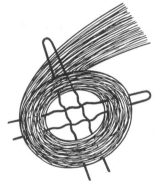

Figure 7.9 Securing flat
pincurls with a clip or fine
pins.

Flat pincurls

As the name implies, this type of pincurl is formed and then positioned so that it lies flat to the head. It does not therefore produce volume at the roots. Flat pincurls are secured either by fine pins or clips as shown in Figure 7.9. Fine pins will not mark the hair or distort the body of the pincurl and are recommended for securing hair that will mark easily as in the case of bleached hair and when setting good quality wigs. You will notice that two pins are needed and that they cross each other in the centre.

All pincurls take their direction from the roots and the stem of the pincurl so they are placed in the direction of the finished style. Just like when you put in a roller, your pincurls should be formed and positioned in the way you want the hair to lie in the final dressing. That means directing flat pincurls to the left or the right and stand-up pincurls under or over. The roots of pincurls should always be thoroughly combed so that they are not distorted. Pins or clips must be carefully placed so that the body of the pincurl is not disturbed. The points of the hair must be cleanly enclosed in the pincurl to prevent buckled and distorted ends. If you look at Figure 7.10 you will be able to see the labelled part of a flat, open pincurl. Can you say which direction the hair will lie when it is dressed?

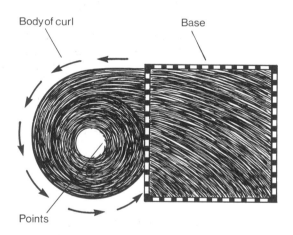

Body of curl   Base

Points

Figure 7.10 The parts of a
flat, even pincurl.

There are different types of flat pincurls and the hairdresser needs to choose the appropriate technique according to the result that is required. The four different types of flat pincurl are:

(a) open (barrelspring) pincurls;
(b) closed (clockspring) pincurls;
(c) reverse pincurls;
(d) long stem pincurls.

We will look at each of these in the order they are listed above. All you need to have clear in your mind at this stage is that all of them are flat pincurls, so they are positioned close to the head, thus creating little or no volume at the roots.

(a) Open (barrelspring) pincurls

These have an open centre and are sometimes referred to as barrelspring or barrel pincurls because they resemble the shape of the spring used in hand hair clippers. This type of pincurl is formed so that as each coil is made it is the same size as the previous one. The points of the hair are neatly enclosed with the coiled hair and should not stick out as this will cause them to be straight or distorted when the hair is dressed.

Because each coil of hair is of uniform size, the result is an even curl formation which can be seen in Figure 7.11. The smaller the loops are made the tighter the end result will be. On short hair, when it might only be possible to make one loop, the result will be a gentle curve in the direction the pincurl was made at the roots, i.e. clockwise (to the left) or anti-clockwise (to the right).

Really good results can be achieved when long hair is set using flat, open pincurls because it produces a similar effect to that of rollers but without the volume at the roots.

(b) Closed (clockspring) pincurls

These are called clockspring pincurls because they resemble the shape of the spring found in watches and clocks. You can see from Figure 7.12 that the centre of the pincurl is closed. They produce a more springy curl which is tightest at the points of the hair because each coil is formed around the previous one, which is smaller. Because forming this type of pincurl can only begin at the points of the hair, care must be taken that ends are not distorted and buckled. Closed pincurls are better to use than the open type on hair that drops easily and for tight curls at the nape.

(c) Reverse pincurls

Reverse pincurls are open, flat pincurls arranged so that they produce an S-shaped wave movement when they are dressed. The pincurls are formed so that they are in rows, and directed clockwise and anticlockwise in each alternate row. It is this change of stem direction that produces the wave movement. If you think back to the section on finger waving you will remember that the hair is directed first one way and then the other to form a wave. In reverse pincurling it is the arrangement of the pincurls that create the S-movement. The placement of reverse pincurls is shown in Figure 7.13 along with the dressed result.

Reverse pincurls are dressed in the same way as finger-waves. Closed pincurls are not suitable for creating waves because the movement they produce is not uniform and the hair points are too tight to dress into waves successfully.

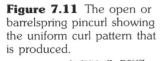

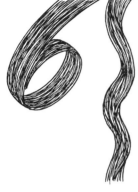

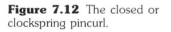

Figure 7.11 The open or barrelspring pincurl showing the uniform curl pattern that is produced.

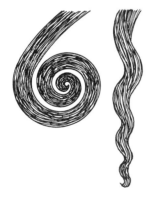

Figure 7.12 The closed or clockspring pincurl.

Figure 7.13 Reverse pincurls showing how rows of flat, open pincurls can be used to produce a wave pattern.

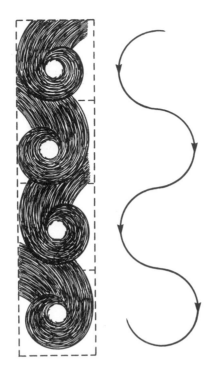

Figure 7.14 A long stem pincurl.

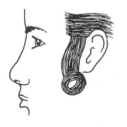

Figure 7.15 A stand-up pincurl.

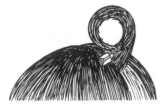

(d) Long stem pincurls

You have already seen a labelled diagram of a pincurl so you should have some idea of what a long stem pincurl is, based purely on its name. Long stem pincurls have a long stem which results in straight or slightly curved roots with curl on the ends (see Figure 7.14). Obviously, the stem of the pincurl creates no volume at all so is often used on fringes and hairline when soft movement is required. Remember that all pincurls take their direction from their stem. This means that long stem pincurls can be formed to create a movement which is slightly curved at the roots to come onto the face or away from it. Alternatively, if you use them on a fringe, you may want the stems to be straight so that the body of the pincurl is responsible for any movement that is produced.

Stand-up pincurls

Stand-up pincurls are always open in the centre and unlike the flat pincurls, create lift and volume at the roots. This volume is produced because a stand-up pincurl actually sits up on the head like a roller. This can be seen in Figure 7.15. Just as the diameter of a roller determines the amount of curl that is put into the hair, the diameter of the open centre of a stand-up pincurl also does the same. Stand-up pincurls can be successfully used to create the same results as rollers because they will create volume at the roots. Like all other pincurls, they take their

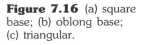

Figure 7.16 (a) square base; (b) oblong base; (c) triangular.

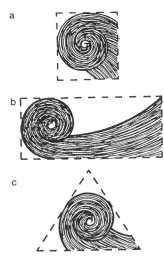

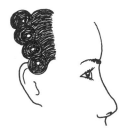

Figure 7.17 Oblong bases used with open, long stem pincurls at the side of the head.

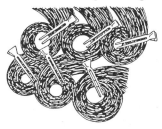

Figure 7.18 Square bases used for reverse pincurling.

direction from the stem. The body of the curl may often need support to stop it from distorting or collapsing. Small pieces of cotton wool or crepe hair are slipped through the open centre which will keep the body of the curl from becoming misshapen. To secure a stand-up pincurl, only a clip can be used rather than a choice of fine pins or clips. This is because the clip is slipped through the centre of the curl and holds it in place at the base. They are secured at the base so that the body of the curl is not marked or distorted by the clip. Stand-up pincurls can be formed to produce either a curl movement that turns under or one which flicks upwards just as you can with rollers.

Methods of pincurling

Now that you are aware of the different types of pincurls and the effects that each produces, you need to know how a pincurl is actually formed and the rules governing the shape and size of bases that are used.

Pincurl bases

The base is the foundation of a pincurl. It is the area of the head from which the hair mesh has been taken to form the pincurl and in most cases, where the pincurl will be secured. We will be describing three different types of bases for pincurls as these are the most commonly used and they are shown in Figure 7.16.

Square base: This shape of base is probably the one that is used most. This is not because it is the best of the four that we will describe. Many hairdressers are unaware that other shapes of base can be used that would, in fact, improve their pincurl results.

Oblong base: This base is used along the front sides of the hairline and allows for the placement of long stem pincurls that are directed away from the face.

Triangular base: Triangular bases are ideal for using on the hairline because they help to stop obvious breaks in the finished dressing. This is because the shape of the base allows part of the body of each pincurl slightly to overlap the curl next to it.

Let's look at how these pincurl bases are used in conjunction with the different types of pincurls.

If you wanted to create a movement at the side of the head which went away from the face and was flat, what type of base and pincurl do you think would be needed? Take a look at Figure 7.17 and you will be able to see that the pincurl bases are oblong allowing the long stem pincurls to sit correctly.

Square bases are best for reverse pincurls because pincurls do not usually have a long stem that needs accommodating as in the example above.

Triangular bases are best for the top front hairline because they help to prevent splits in the final dressing.

Figure 7.19 Winding the strand of hair around the index finger.

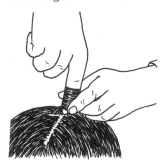

Figure 7.20 Sliding the curl off the finger.

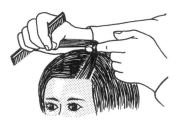

Figure 7.21 Forming the curl.

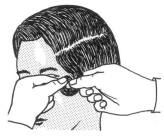

Figure 7.22 Angle for holding a mesh of hair for a stand-up pincurl.

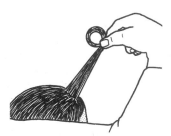

Forming a pincurl

There are two basic techniques you can use to form a pincurl. You can either begin to form the pincurl at the points of the hair or, alternatively, near the roots. You will discover which technique suits you best and the particular type of pincurling you are doing. There are no firm rules to this — after all, it is the result that is important. Incidentally, any curling that begins at the points of the hair is called *croquignole winding* while if it begins at the roots it is called *spiral winding*. That means that when we put in rollers we are winding using the croquignole technique because the roller is introduced to the points of the hair.

Spiral winding technique

1. Section the hair so that you have a cleanly parted base. Comb the hair thoroughly right through from the roots to the points to free it from tangles and to make it smooth. During this combing you should be positioning the hair in the direction of the pincurl stem. (Remember that a pincurl takes its direction from the roots.)
2. Hold the comb so that it rests in the palm of your hand so that your fingers are free to hold the points of the mesh.
3. Using the index finger of the other hand, begin to wind the ribbon of hair around your finger as in Figure 7.19. You will need to use your thumb to help hold the wrapped hair in place.
4. When you have wound all the hair, carefully slide the curl off your finger and wind it down to the head as in Figure 7.20 so that it can be secured.

Croquignole winding technique

1. Prepare the hair by making a cleanly parted base and comb the ribbon of hair thoroughly in the direction of the pincurl stem that you will be forming.
2. Holding the points of the hair securely between the thumb and index finger, use the thumb and index finger of your other hand to wind the hair towards the head as shown in Figure 7.21.
3. As soon as the pincurl is fully wound, it can then be secured. N.B. If you are doing a stand-up pincurl the hair should be held out from the head as shown in Figure 7.22 so that it sits on its own base when it is secured.

Guidelines for pincurling

1. Use cleanly parted bases that are the correct shape and size for the effect you want to achieve.
2. Make sure the hair is wet because it will be easier to control and the finished effect will last longer.

3. Thoroughly comb the ribbon of hair form roots to points.
4. Remember that all pincurls take their direction from their stem.
5. Make sure that the points of the hair are neatly enclosed within the pincurl to prevent distorted or buckled ends.
6. Secure the pincurl carefully so that the clip or pins do not cause the body or stem of the curl to be misshapen or marked.
7. Use cotton wool or crepe hair to pad and support stand-up pincurls that could collapse and distort during drying.

Questions

1. What is pincurling?
2. How are pincurls secured?
3. What are the two main types of pincurl?
4. What should be used to secure fine hair?
5. How do you position a pincurl?
6. What are the four types of flat pincurl?
7. Describe open pincurling and when it would be used.
8. Describe closed pincurling and when it would be used.
9. Describe reverse pincurling and when it would be used.
10. Describe long stem pincurling and when it would be used.
11. What determines the amount of curl in a stand-up pincurl?
12. How can a stand-up pincurl be supported?
13. How are pincurls secured?
14. What are the three different types of base for pincurls?
15. Draw them.
16. When are they used?
17. What are croquignole and spiral winding?
18. Describe the spiral winding technique.
19. Describe the croquignole winding technique.
20. Make a list of guidelines for pincurling.

Roller setting techniques

Roller setting is the term used to describe wrapping meshes of hair around cylindrical or conical-shaped rollers to produce varying degrees of volume, curl and wave.

Unfortunately, there are far too many hairdressers who think there is only one way to put in a roller — with the roller sitting squarely on a base that is the same size as the roller being used. This is not so! You only have to witness the work of the great competition stylists to see beautiful roller placement that is imaginative and incorporates some of the techniques we will describe. If you can master these techniques you will be able to create varied degrees of volume and movement in hair that will require the minimum of work when you dress it out. Don't fall into the trap of being one of those lazy hairdressers who puts in rollers without giving any thought to the finished look. They are the hairdressers who struggle during the dressing using far too much backcombing and hairspray in an attempt to force the hair in a direction contrary to the way it was set. They have clients with hair that looks shapeless and is difficult for the client to handle because the setting faults have been disguised by the backcombing and hairspray.

There are three considerations to be taken when using rollers and these are:

- The degree of movement you want to achieve (roller size);
- The amount of volume required (base size and roller placement);
- The direction of the intended style (roller direction).

Choosing the right sized rollers

There are several factors to consider when deciding which size rollers to use. First, you will need to think about how much movement you want to see in the hair when it is dressed. A mesh of hair wrapped around a roller six times will obviously produce a tighter curl than if it were wrapped three times around a larger roller. The larger the roller, the fewer times the hair can be wrapped around it resulting in looser movements. You will also need to consider the type of hair you are styling. Is it fine and lank, being susceptible to dropping quickly, or has it been permed too tightly for the look the client is hoping for? Is the client looking for a smooth result or something which is tightly curled? Perhaps it is the right time to mention that you should not ask the client what size rollers she thinks should be put in her hair! This is most unprofessional and signals that you lack the confidence or skill to make this decision yourself. After all, does your dentist ever ask you which teeth you would like to be filled? If he did ask you we doubt whether you would have much confidence in his ability!

If you are unsure of how the hair will respond to setting and you cannot decide between two roller sizes, it is always advisable to use the slightly smaller ones because you can correct an over-tight set more easily than one which is too loose, which will be described later on in this chapter under the heading of 'fault correcting techniques'.

Base size and roller placement

As for pincurling, there are different types of bases that are used when using rollers to set the hair. The size and shape of the base and the position that the roller sits on it will determine how much volume there will be in the dressing by the way the roots have been positioned. If you don't want volume at the roots why put it there in the first place? Doing this means having to work harder getting rid of the unwanted volume when you dress out the hair. Alternatively, not enough volume means you have to resort to copious amounts of backcombing to achieve the necessary lift. Read on, and you will discover the technical art of placing rollers that will never have you fighting with hair during dressing again. By the way, your clients will notice the difference too, because their hair will be so much easier to manage and the set will last longer.

A base for roller setting is the area of the scalp where the roller will be positioned and secured – just as for pincurling. Sometimes the bases you use will correspond exactly to the size of the roller you are using. For other techniques the base will be up to twice the diameter of the roller, but will still be as long as the length of the roller. Finally, you will use bases which are not rectangular but shaped like pie-segments.

On-base roller placement

This is the most widely used rollering technique – but not, unfortunately, for the right reasons! There are a large number of hairdressers who think that this is the *only* way of putting in a roller, and as we said earlier, this is untrue.

As the name implies, the roller is positioned and secured so that it sits exactly on its own base. This produces volume at the roots which depends on the diameter of the roller used. A large roller will produce more volume at the roots than a smaller one because the hair is lifted away from the head much higher. However, if a large roller is used, the curl in the hair will be loose, which is not always what you want.

To put a roller on-base, a base is made which is exactly the same length and diameter as the roller being used. The roller sits exactly on this base as shown in Figure 7.23.

Figure 7.23 On-base roller placement.

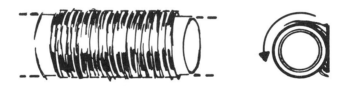

Over-directed roller placement

If you want to achieve maximum volume without necessarily using large rollers the base size you need to use is still the same length as the roller you are using but its width can be up to twice the roller's diameter. The mesh of hair is rolled down so that it sits on the upper part of the base thus creating much more volume at the roots. A diagram of the over-directed roller placement is shown in Figure 7.24(a). You will be able to see that the roller is still sitting within the confines of its own base.

Under-directed roller placement

Sometimes, we want to avoid producing too much volume for certain looks. If you imagine setting a bob, you wouldn't want masses of root lift, but bounce at the ends of the hair. This is an example of when you would use this particular technique. The base is made the same as for an over-directed roller except that the roller is wound down to sit on the lower part of its base. Again you will be able to see that the roller sits

Figure 7.24 (a) Over-directed roller placement. (b) Under-directed roller placement.

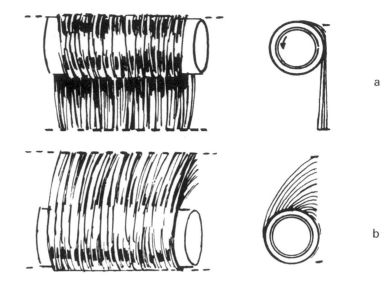

within the confines of its own base in Figure 7.24(b).

N.B. If you use this technique on a hairline the roller will actually sit on the client's skin and is sometimes called an 'off-base' roller. This is quite acceptable providing it does not cause discomfort to the client.

Curvature hairstyling using circular roller placement

Curvature hairstyling is based on the fact that the hairdresser is dealing with a rounded object (the head!), so all partings and sectioning are in a curved form to blend with the curvature of the head. The type of roller placement uses segment-shaped bases, like pieces of pie; conical rollers are used as opposed to the cylindrical type. This roller placement works on the principle that all the bases are made from the same point so is often referred to as 'pivot' setting. It is used to create circular and semicircular movements in the hair that are impossible to achieve using rectangular bases. The point from which the bases are taken (the pivot) enables the hair to be set so that it fans outwards in a curved movement. An example of using this technique on a hairline is shown in Figure 7.25.

Figure 7.25 Rollers placed on pie-shaped bases to create a semi-circular movement. Notice that conical rollers have been used.

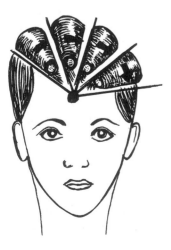

Roller direction

Apart from being able to control how curly to make the hair and the degree of volume that is introduced, the hairdresser also has the ability to control the direction of the movement in the finished style. This is controlled by the way in which the rollers are positioned in the hair. An example of this is the technique of placing rollers in a circular direction as described above. Also, we sometimes want to produce an upwards flick as opposed to the hair being wound under. The way in which rollers are positioned and combined with pincurls and waves requires practice to create styles which have interest and appeal.

We do not preach that you must place the rollers in brick formation nor that straight rows of rollers are unacceptable. What we do say is that *you should place the rollers so that they are in the direction of the finished style*. This might mean putting in rollers in a straight line, or placing them so that they are sitting vertically, or on an angle as opposed to sitting horizontally. It also means *thinking* about what you want the hair to do before you start. This will be more fully explained in the next paragraphs.

Planning a pli

A pli (pronounced as 'plee') is simply the term used to describe a set. People talk about 'first pli' and 'second pli'. 'First pli' refers to the hair in rollers, pincurls etc. ready for drying. 'Second pli' refers to when the finished style after it has been dried and dressed. Incidentally, the word pli comes from the French term used for setting which is 'mise-en-pli' and literally translated this means to 'put into set'.

A good pli does not just happen. Hairdressers must look at the type of hair they are working with, the client's facial and head shape characteristics and also the occasion for which the client is having it done. The natural fall of the hair must be assessed so that the style is not forced against the direction in which the hair grows. Obviously, a lot of this analysis will be done before the hair is even wetted but the hair-dresser should look at the hair again once it is wet. After hair has been wetted, the natural movement and direction of the hair can be seen more easily. The hairdresser does this by combing the hair and carefully watching for the way it moves and responds to being combed in different directions. Once the most suitable style directions have been established (in consultation with the client) the stylist can mould the hair. Moulding is combing the hair into the shape, form and direction of the finished look. It is also very helpful to the hairdresser because it defines areas that will need volume and those that will require movement. By seeing this, it makes the task of deciding which setting techniques to use a lot easier. For example, if the client wants her hair to be very flat at the sides in an upwards movement away from the face, it would be pointless putting in on-base rollers in this area because volume would be created. To achieve this effect, the stylist would find it far better to use flat pincurls as shown earlier. After drying the hairdresser would have a minimum of work to do when dressing out than if rollers had been used.

Figure 7.26 shows an example of a pli which has been carefully planned and will create a style that has movement, shape, volume and indentation.

Styling hair for the individual

The ultimate test of a hairstyle is how well it suits the client. Hairdressers should aim to achieve perfect balance by dressing the hair to compliment

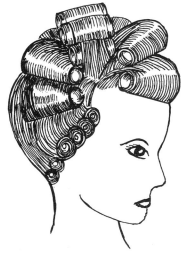

Figure 7.26 Example of a carefully planned pli.

the client's characteristics. That means styling the hair to suit the face shape, lifestyle, stature and age of the client and the occasion for which the hair has been styled. A regular client may request something different from her usual style if she is going to a special function like a ball or party. You may be asked to style a bride's hair for her wedding which may also involve the fitting of her headdress.

Roller practice

To be able to use the techniques described earlier you will need to practise putting in rollers in a variety of ways on all types of hair. Learning roller placement on only one type of hair (like a block) is all right at first, but you must progress to working on different types of hair to appreciate how they respond and behave when dealt with in the same way. Just as a tailor handles certain fabrics in different ways, you as a hairdresser need to learn to handle hair. This experience and skill can only be learnt 'hands on', by actually doing it and feeling the differences yourself.

Whatever size of roller or placement technique is used, there are some fundamental rules about the way you put rollers in. Needless to say, however a roller is put in will determine how the hair will look when the roller is taken out after drying. Do not be misled into thinking that a poorly put in roller will not make any difference to the finished style, or how easy it will be for you to dress. Nothing miraculous happens when the client is under the dryer to change bad setting into good setting! What you put into the hair before the client goes under the drier is exactly what you'll get when the hair is dry.

Guidelines for putting in rollers

1. Mould the wet hair into the shape of the style to help you determine your pli.
2. Use only cleanly parted bases which are the correct size and shape for the technique you are using.
3. Place rollers in the direction of the finished style.
4. Ensure the points of the hair are cleanly and smoothly wrapped around the roller to prevent buckled ends.
5. Make sure that the hair is wrapped around the roller with sufficient, even tension.
6. Do not allow the hair to be bunched on the roller but evenly distributed and smooth.
7. Secure the rollers firmly, but do not cause discomfort to the client or cause marks on the hair by poor placing of the pins.
8. If you are not completely satisfied with your pli, make the changes before the client goes under the dryer.

Drying the hair

Once the hair is in pli, you will need to place your client under a hood dryer so that the hair can be dried. Depending on the type of dryer you have in your salon, you may need to put a hairnet over the rollers to prevent the hair being disturbed by the airflow of the dryer. If you do need to use a net, check that it does not interfere with your pli by pushing down onto pincurls, etc. You will need to place some form of protection over the client's ears to stop the heat from making them too hot. Any form of ear protection used should ideally be disposable to avoid the transfer of germs. Pads of cotton wool are ideal for this purpose. When you place the client under the dryer there are a number of things you should do:

- Make sure there are no pins or clips placed so that, once heated, they could burn the client's skin.
- You should be able to estimate the approximate drying time so that you can tell the client. It is not unknown for the hairdresser to forget about someone under the dryer!
- Check that the dryer you intend to use is in good working order and safe to use.
- Ensure that your client is comfortable and that the hood is correctly positioned so that all the hair will be dried.
- Tell clients how to control the heat themselves if the dryer you are using has this facility.
- Ask clients whether they would like tea or coffee and magazines; ashtrays should be provided if smoking is allowed in your salon and the client smokes.

Checking that the hair is dry

If the hair is not completely dry when you begin dressing it you are heading for disaster. The hair only has to be a little bit damp for the style to collapse in a matter of hours. To check that the hair is dry, always remove a roller at the crown and at the back of the head and feel for dampness at the points. Do not try to do this if you have just had your hands in water as you will probably think the hair is dry when in fact it isn't, because your hands will be very slightly damp. If you are unsure, there is no harm in asking someone to check it with you — it is always worth a second opinion if you are in doubt. If you find the hair is still damp, replace the roller or pincurl and put the client back underneath the dryer until the hair is completely dry.

Removing the rollers

Once you are positive that the hair is dry, you should ideally allow the hair to cool for a couple of minutes before you start removing the rollers and clips. If you remove them when the hair is still hot, the action of removing the rollers could loosen the set. If the hair is long, start taking out the rollers at the nape area first, or the hair could get tangled.

Brushing the hair

Do not be afraid to brush the hair after setting − the set will not come out that quickly. You should brush the hair in the direction that the pli was made (i.e. the direction that the hair will be in the finished look) using a flat brush which has nylon or natural bristle filaments. The purpose of this brushing is to blend the hair and get rid of the partings caused by the rollers and also to get the stiffness out of the hair which the setting aid gives it. When you are brushing the hair at this stage, you should be moulding it into the desired shape. You will be able to see areas that will require backcombing, to give the necessary support and fullness. Do remember that if your pli was well planned, the amount of work you will now need to do will be minimal, and you should not automatically backcomb the hair as it may not need it. You will probably see some hairdressers do this out of habit, but it is not always necessary.

Dressing the hair

If the hair you are dressing does require some support in the way of backcombing or backbrushing, bear in mind that no matter how much of this you put into the hair, there should be no trace of it showing in the finished dressing. Nothing looks more ugly than knotted hair showing through a finished style. If backcombing and backbrushing are done properly in the first place, you should be able to dress the hair so that it looks clean and polished without it showing.

Backcombing

As the name implies this is using the comb to make the hair go back on itself to provide support, height and volume. However, it is often used to disguise a poor pli by redirecting hair into the desired position. Backcombing should always be done in the direction that you want the hair to go and this is often called 'directional backcombing'. The most important factor about backcombing is the size of mesh that you take. It should not be wider than the part of the comb you will be using. For example, if you backcomb using half of the teeth in the comb only, and you take meshes which are wider, it results in some of the hair being missed. Also, you should only use meshes which are slightly deeper than the length of the teeth of your comb. Too deep a mesh will mean that some of the hair will be missed by the teeth, while if the meshes are too narrow, the back-combing will show through the front of the mesh and be difficult to clean out.

When you backcomb, the shorter hairs within the mesh are pushed down towards the roots, providing a supportive padding to the mesh of hair. The comb you use to backcomb should have both close and widely set teeth, but it is the fine teeth that are used to put in the backcombing. Holding the mesh of hair in the direction of the finished style, and at a 90 degrees angle to the part of the head you are working on, your comb should be inserted about two-thirds of the way down its length. It is then pushed down to the roots to take the shorter hairs with it as shown in Figure 7.27. Notice that it is the *underside* of the mesh that is backcombed, so that it does not show when the hair is dressed. Because backcombing should always be done in the direction of the style, you will need to change your position around the client, to be standing directly behind the part of the head you are dealing with at any time. This action is repeated until the required degree of support is achieved but do remember that, by pushing some of the hair down to the roots, the amount of hair at the points will be reduced.

Backcombing should be carried out in a systematic fashion so that areas requiring the support are not missed. After the backcombing has been put in, the hair is dressed using the widely spaced teeth of your comb. This end of the comb is used because the narrow teeth would clean out the backcombing you have worked so hard at putting in. The mesh of hair is gently combed into position ensuring that the support and volume of the backcombing is not removed. When the hair is in position, you should not be able to see any trace of backcombing.

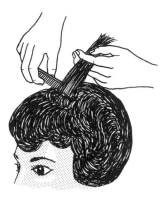

Figure 7.27 Backcombing a mesh of hair.

Backbrushing

Backbrushing is similar to backcombing because although done with a brush, it does increase the apparent volume of the hair. Again it is the shorter hairs on the head that are responsible for adding the support and volume, but backbrushing does not produce as much 'stiffness' to the hair because it does not reach the roots of the hair as backcombing does. However, it is really effective for hair that needs dressing into voluminous curls because it makes the hair separate and increase in width. The brush is used in a turning action so that the filaments of the brush nearest to the client's head meet the hair first with the rest of the brush following. The brush filaments furthest away from your client's head will be the last to have contact with the mesh of hair. If you are doing it properly your wrist will ache! As with backcombing, you need to hold the mesh of hair you are doing firmly between your fingers away from the other hair. This is shown in Figure 7.28.

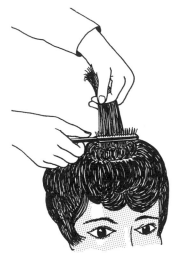

Figure 7.28 Diagram showing how backbrushing requires the brush to move in a turning movement.

Checking the balance of the dressing

When you are actually dressing the hair, you should always be aware of the shape and form you are creating by looking at frequent intervals in the mirror in front of the client. You should be checking that the balance of the style is properly proportioned and as you planned it. You should also be checking that the hair is cleanly finished and that there are no hairs sticking out where they shouldn't be. Not only do you need to check the front view in the mirror but also the profile (side) and back views as well. This might mean that you have occasionally to stand slightly away from your client to see the overall shape. The best styles are those that compliment the natural form of the head as well as the client herself. When you (and your client) are satisfied with the dressing you are ready to apply hairspray, if desired, and show the client the back view of the style. Use a backmirror to display the finished style to the client as previously described in Chapter 6.

Table 7.1 Fault-correcting techniques

Problem	Cause	Solution
Buckled ends.	Points of hair not wrapped properly when set.	As your client will not want you to cut them off, try using a pair of tongs to reshape the ends.
Hair not dry.	Hair not checked properly.	If the hair has not been brushed, replace the client under the dryer. Otherwise, use a blow-dryer on the affected areas in conjunction with a circular brush.
Hair too curly.	Rollers etc. too small	Use a blow-dryer and hairbrush to stretch and relax the hair.
Set too loose.	Incorrect size (too big) of rollers, etc.	Use tongs to curl affected areas.
Hair going in wrong direction.	Incorrect placement of rollers, etc.	Try to redirect hair using either a blow-dryer or tongs.
Hair is flyaway and difficult to control.	Too much shampoo was used or could be the natural characteristic of the hair, especially if it is fine.	Apply some dressing cream or spray to the hair.
Hair is lank and greasy.	Poor shampooing or hair insufficiently rinsed after a conditioner was applied.	No alternative other than re-shampooing and setting the hair.

Fault-correcting techniques

It is important that you are able to identify any mistakes in your work and, once identified, are able to correct them. Such mistakes are usually only seen and identified when the client is taken out from underneath the dryer. In Table 7.1 we have identified the most common faults that occur during setting with suggested methods of correction.

Questions

1. Is there only one way to put in a roller?
2. What points should be considered when using rollers?
3. How is the choice of roller determined?
4. If in doubt, what size rollers is it best to use?
5. What determines volume in the dressing?
6. What is on-base roller placement?
7. How does roller size influence the volume produced?
8. Why is over-directed roller placement used?
9. Why is under-directed roller placement used?
10. What is an off-base roller?
11. What is curvature hairstyling?
12. Draw a diagram to illustrate the type of roller placement used.
13. What does roller direction control?
14. What is a pli?
15. What is the difference between a first and second pli?
16. What is the French term for setting?
17. Why should your analysis be made on both dry and wet hair?
18. What is moulding?
19. What makes a successful hairstyle?
20. List the guidelines for putting in rollers.
21. What can be used for protecting the ears when drying the hair?
22. How should you ensure client comfort under the dryer?
23. How do you check that the hair is dry?
24. Why should the hair be allowed to cool before removing rollers?
25. Where should rollers be removed from first on long hair?
26. What is the purpose of brushing?
27. Does the hair always need to be backcombed?
28. Explain to somebody else in the salon how you would backcomb a head of hair.
29. Make a list of points that are important for successful backcombing.
30. When are the wide teeth of the comb used in backcombing?
31. What is the difference between backcombing and backbrushing?
32. Describe how you would backbrush hair.
33. Make a list of fault-correcting techniques and then get someone to test you on it.

Plaiting or braiding long hair

Plaiting or braiding long hair is a skill which can be used to create interesting and stunning looks for longer hair. In this section, we look at methods of braiding hair with the use of clear, simple diagrams to help you master these techniques. Once you have mastered the various braiding techniques, it is only the limits of your imagination that will determine how intricate and original your designs can be. These can be performed on training heads with long hair, or obliging friends!

How to make a two-strand braid

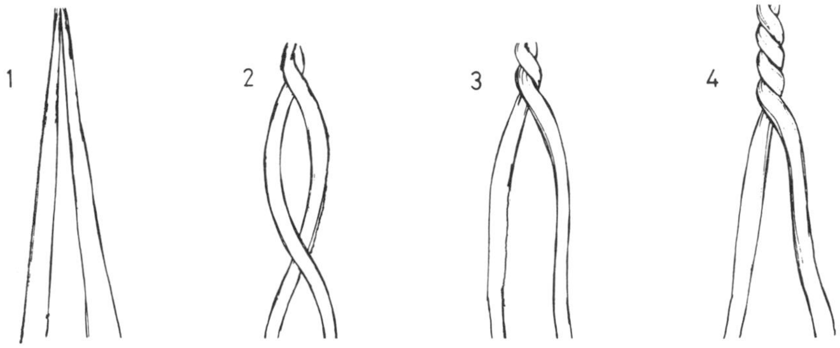

Figure 7.29 How to make a two-strand braid (1–4).

1. Separate the section into two equal parts.
2. Cross the sections over each other.
3. Continue crossing the hair strands over each other, being careful to maintain even tension on the strands.
4. Cross the strands over each other along the entire length. When you reach the ends, secure with a pin, or tie with thread without letting go.

How to make a three-strand braid

This is perhaps the most common of all braiding techniques.

1. Separate the section into three equal parts.
2. Begin by crossing one of the strands on the outside across the one in the centre. Then cross the other outside strand across the centre one. In the diagram, you can see that the strand on the right side is the next one to be crossed over to the centre.
3. In this diagram it is the strand on the left that now needs to be crossed over to the centre. Keep the tension even to produce a regular shaped braid.
4. Continue crossing the outside strands into the centre until you reach the ends. Secure with a piece of thread or a pin.

Figure 7.30 How to make a three-strand braid (1–4).

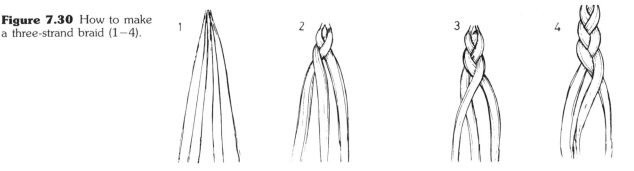

How to make a four-strand braid

The four-strand braid looks very intricate but is really quite easy to master if you study the diagrams carefully.

1. Separate the section into four equal parts.
2. Start braiding with the two centre strands, taking the left strand over the right one.
3. The side strand is then brought to the centre by bringing the one on the right side *above* one of the first two strands, and the strand on the left side is taken *under* the other one.

4–6. These diagrams show how this is continued along the hair length with the two centre strands always being crossed in the same manner as in (2).

7. The finished braid is shown here. It can be fastened by a covered elastic hair band or ribbon. A needle with a large eye can be used to weave coloured thread or ribbon through the braid to create a stunning effect for special occasions. This looks particularly effective if it has a metallic coating.

Figure 7.31 How to make a four-strand braid (1–7).

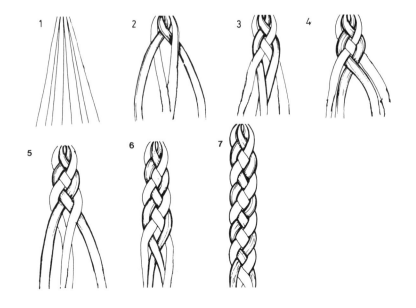

You can keep going on adding more braids once you become adept at this technique. For more details on specialist hair work refer to *Cutting and Styling – A Salon Handbook*.

Machines, tools and equipment used when setting hair

Hood dryers

Hood dryers can be wall-mounted, fitted as part of a bank of dryers, or individually fitted to a pedestal with wheels. Hood dryers require regular dusting to prevent any build-up of fluff affecting their performance. A typical, modern hood dryer is shown in Figure 7.32.

Figure 7.32 A modern hood dryer with its own built in timer. (Courtesy Wella Ltd.)

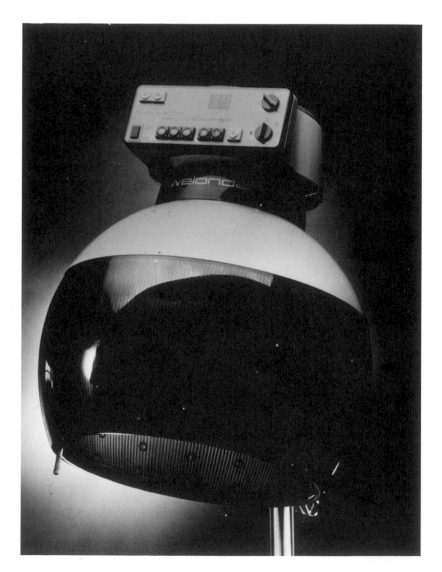

Figure 7.33 A double-prong clip.

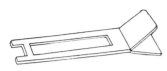

Figure 7.34 A fine wavy pin.

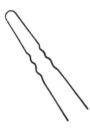

Figure 7.35 A straight prong pin.

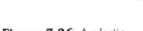

Figure 7.36 A plastic setting pin.

Figure 7.37 A hairgrip.

Clips, hairpins and hairgrips

Double-prong clip: These are usually made of metal but plastic ones are also available. This type of clip is small and is not intended to hold large quantities of hair. They are mainly used to secure pincurls. Figure 7.33 illustrates a double-prong clip.

Fine wavy pins: These pins are made of metal and are available in several shades to match different hair colours. They can be used to hold hair in place in the final dressing because they are fine, and if the right colour is used, can be effectively concealed in the hair. Fine wavy pins can also be used to secure flat pincurls in position and are preferred by many stylists for this because they do not mark the hair as much as metal double-prong clips. Because they are fine, the prongs are very pliable, with a tendency to bend, so are not effective for holding large quantities of hair securely. A fine wavy pin is illustrated in Figure 7.34.

Straight prong pins: Straight prong pins, otherwise known as setting pins, come in various colours to match the hair. They are also available in different lengths, the most common being 6–7 cms (3 inches) long. Apart from being used to hold rollers in place, they can also be effective for holding hair securely in place when dressing the hair. In the latter case, they would normally be used in conjunction with fine wavy pins. A straight prong pin is illustrated in Figure 7.35.

Plastic setting pins: These are often preferred by stylists to the metal pins just described for securing rollers in place. They do, however, have a tendency to distort if they are misused by forcing them into rollers. A plastic setting pin is illustrated in Figure 7.36.

Hairgrips: These are made of metal and come in a variety of colours. In North America they are called Bobbi pins. They are available in both a shiny and matt finish, the latter being preferred for film and photographic work, because they do not glint in bright light. The flat prong is always placed against the scalp as the wavy prong could cause discomfort. The two ends of the prongs are guarded by a plastic covering which resembles a small blob, protecting the client from their otherwise sharp ends. The blobs also make the opening of the grip easier. A hairgrip is illustrated in Figure 7.37.

Brushes and combs

The most frequently used brush for brushing through a set after it has been dried is a flat brush an example of which is shown in Figure 7.38.
    With regard to the combs used when setting, the choice is greater because different combs are available for the job you are doing.

Tail comb: Used for sectioning the hair for rollers and pincurls. The 'tail' of the comb is useful for helping to tuck the points of the hair cleanly around a roller to prevent buckled ends. Tail combs usually only have teeth of one size which are uniformly spaced. The 'tail' can either be

Figure 7.38 A flat brush.

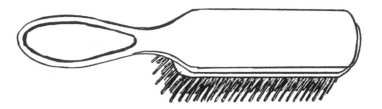

made of plastic or metal. By the way, in the United States, these combs are often referred to as 'rat-tail' combs.

Straight comb: This type of comb is used for finger waving and also dressing the hair. It has two sizes of teeth that can clearly be seen in Figure 7.40.

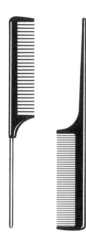

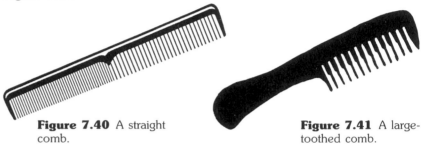

Figure 7.40 A straight comb.

Figure 7.41 A large-toothed comb.

Figure 7.39 A tail comb.

Large toothed comb: This type of comb is used for disentangling wet hair after shampooing because the wide spaces between the teeth allow the hair to be combed free of tangles with the minimum of stress being put on the hair.

Figure 7.42 Cylindrical and conical rollers.

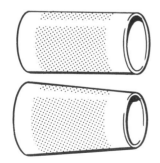

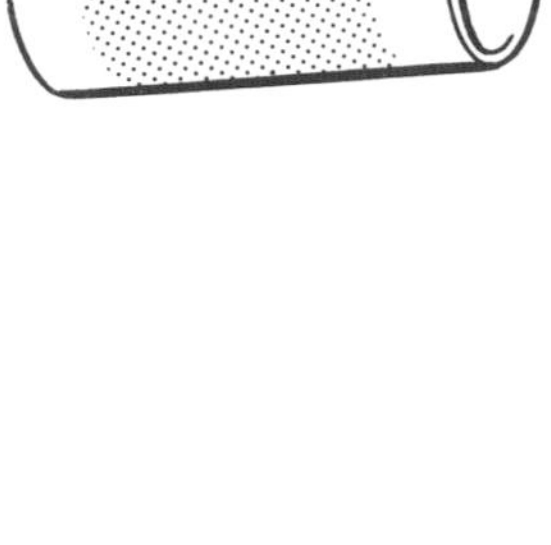

Rollers

There are a wide range of rollers available to the hairdresser which can make it confusing when choosing which ones to purchase or use. They will vary in diameter and sometimes also in length. The other main differences are their shape and the material of which they are made. The best results are produced from rollers which have a smooth finish but these are more difficult to put in than rollers which have little spikes on them, because the hair has nothing to cling on to. Rollers are available in cylindrical (the most common) and conical shapes. Examples of these are shown in Figure 7.42.

Hairnets

There are two main uses for hairnets; they are used either to prevent disturbance from the airflow of a hood dryer during drying or to keep the hair in place after it has been dressed.

Setting nets: This type of net is generally made of nylon and is triangular in shape. Setting nets are placed over the pli and tied at the nape of the neck before the client is placed under the dryer. Some models of modern hood dryers do not require the use of a net because the airflow is filtered through tiny perforations in the hood instead of the airflow coming directly from a fan which is directly situated above the client's head.

Hair nets: This type of net is not used as widely as they were during the 1940s and 1950s but are still available and can be very useful for show and theatre work. They are made from real hair, are available in all colours and are extremely fine and delicate. They should be very carefully positioned over the finished dressing to help keep it in position and, if necessary, gripped in place at an unnoticeable point (such as the nape) to take up any excess or slack.

Questions
1. What types of hood dryer are available?
2. What are double prong clips used for?
3. Why are wavy pins available in different colours?
4. What are they used for?
5. When are straight prong pins used?
6. What are plastic setting pins used for?
7. How do you use a hairgrip?
8. What is a tailcomb used for?
9. What are straight combs used for?
10. When would you use a large toothed comb?
11. How do rollers vary?
12. What are the two main uses of hairnets?

Chapter Eight
Permanent Waving

Introduction to perming

People are never satisfied with what they have naturally! Thus those of us with straight hair generally wonder what we would look like if our hair were curly. As a hairdresser, you can impart curl to a client with straight hair by the process of permanent waving.

As a definition, permanent waving is a chemical process that permanently alters the curl pattern of hair by changing the internal structure of the hair shaft. It is described as permanent, because the change is not removed when the hair is wetted or styled in different ways. However, because hair grows, falls out and then is replaced by new hair, it is obvious that the term 'permanent' is not totally an accurate or exact description. Before we go any further, however, there are a number of things that you should know about the chemistry of the hair.

The bonds in the hair

Figure 8.1 The different cross-linkages of hair. The most important of these are the disulphide bonds because they maintain the structure of the hair and are difficult to break. The hydrogen bonds and salt linkages are much weaker but there are more of them. Hydrogen bonds are broken during setting but are easily reformed.

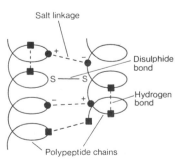

If you think back to earlier in the book you will remember that all proteins are made up of amino acids, and these are held together by peptide or end-bonds. These strings of amino acids, held together by their peptide bonds, are known as polypeptides (the prefix 'poly' on a word means many). Polypeptides in long coiled chains may contain many hundreds of amino acids and are sometimes referred to as 'simple' proteins. More complicated proteins are formed when adjacent spirals of polypeptides are cross-linked by other bonds. Human hair is called a 'fibre' protein and it possesses an exceptional number of cross-bonds or linkages. These are of three types, illustrated in Figure 8.1:

(1) Disulphide linkages: These are the most important bonds as far as perming and straightening are concerned as it is these that are broken to allow the alteration of the hair shape. They are found on the amino acid cystine, forming a link through the central disulphide bond between two polypeptide chains, rather like the rungs of a ladder. They are very strong bonds which are only broken down by chemicals.

Normally hair contains between 4–5 per cent sulphur, but natural red hair may contain up to 8 per cent sulphur. Because this is about twice as much as normal hair, red hair, with its higher sulphur content, is more resistant to perming.

(2) Salt linkages: The amino acids that form polypeptides may have free acid (negative) or basic amino (positive) groups. If a free negative group in one polypeptide chain lies opposite a free positive group in an

adjacent chain there will be an attraction between them. Opposite electrical charges attract, rather like the North and South poles of a magnet. If you have two strong magnets try this; they can take a lot of effort to separate. These salt linkages are also called ionic or electrostatic charges. Because they are weaker than the disulphide linkages they can be easily broken by weak acids or alkalis. If you quickly run a nylon comb through your hair for a minute it will be able to attract and pick up a small piece of paper. The comb has picked up a charge from the hair and an opposite charge has been induced in the piece of paper, attracting the two together.

(3) Hydrogen bonds: These weak bonds are due to the attraction between hydrogen atoms and oxygen atoms (like the salt linkages, this is an electrostatic attraction). This kind of bonding can occur in a polypeptide chain (between the coils) or between adjacent polypeptide chains. Since they form cross-bonds, they help the disulphide bonds to keep adjacent polypeptide chains together, giving 'body' to the hair. Although the hydrogen bonds are very weak, many more of them are present than any other bond in the hair. Hydrogen bonds can be broken by water and most weak chemicals and are important in temporary changes of hair structure such as setting.

Questions sections
1. What is permanent waving?
2. Is the wave actually permanent?
3. How are amino acids joined together?
4. What is a polypeptide?
5. What is a simple protein?
6. How do more complicated proteins differ?
7. Which type of linkage is strongest?
8. Why is red hair more resistant to perming?
9. How are salt linkages formed?
10. What breaks them?
11. How are hydrogen bonds broken?

What are the reasons for curl?

In the past many hairdressers believed that curl in the hair was due to the shape of the hair follicle. The theory was that a straight hair came from a straight follicle, while a curly hair came from a curved follicle. This could not explain how an individual's hair could change from being curly to straight, or vice versa. There are many examples of this – the child with curly hair which suddenly becomes straight after the first haircut!

Hair growth depends on cell division in the papilla which is found at the base of the hair follicle. If you think of the growing hair as a clockface, and if the cells dividing at each hour divide at an equal rate, the hair will grow straight upwards. If the cells at 3 o'clock are dividing faster than the rest, the hair will bend towards 9 o'clock as it grows. If the cells then began to grow faster at 9 o'clock the hair would bend back towards 3 o'clock. If this example were actually to happen in a hair follicle, the hair would be wavy. Tight curls are formed when the hair cells divide faster in a cycle 'round the clock'. If the cells in the follicle of someone with curly hair suddenly started to divide at an equal rate, the hair produced would become straight. This kind of thing occurs with illness.

Questions

1. Why does the shape of a hair follicle not explain the reason for a hair being curly or straight?
2. What does hair growth depend on?
3. How can this explain the hair being curly or straight?
4. If cells were growing faster on the left side of the papilla, in what direction would the hair bend?

What is the sequence and procedure for a perm?

Permanent waving is a fairly straightforward process. Here, we aim to list this process in a concise and easy to understand way so that if perming is new to you, it will enable you to have a basic idea of what it entails before we go into the chemistry of perming.

We will presume that the client has been consulted about the type of perm that is required and all precautionary tests have been carried out. If your memory needs refreshing on these aspects, please refer back to the sections dealing with the consultation of clients and precautionary diagnostic tests. Also, we will presume that the hair has been shampooed in preparation for a perm (see Chapter 4) and that any cutting has been carried out. You need to imagine that your client is sitting in front of you, gowned and protected, with disentangled, towel-dried hair, ready for their hair to be permed.

(1) Preparation

Set up your trolley with the materials and tools you will need:

- End papers and rods
- Perm lotion (and applicator bottle if necessary)
- Cotton wool strips
- Protective gloves for your hands
- Tail comb
- Sectioning clips
- Water spray
- Timer
- Plastic cap
- Matching neutraliser (plus applicator or bowl and sponge)

Optional extras:

- Pre-perm lotion
- Flexible plastic strips

Once you have everything ready that you will need you are ready to start work on the hair.

(2) Sectioning

With the popularity of winding the perm rods in the direction of the finished style (directional winding) and improved product formulae that enable the lotion to be applied once the hair has been wound (post-damping), many hairdressers do not section the hair for perm winding any more. However, this book is aimed at basic techniques, and so we will suggest that the hair is sectioned before winding commences. (For those who are interested, more advanced perming techniques are described in *Perming and Straightening – A Salon Handbook*.)

To section the hair for perming, it is divided into nine divisions that are carefully measured and parted. Winding then follows in a specific order according to the position of these sections. A detailed description of how these sections are made is covered later on in this chapter.

(3) Winding

After the hair has been sectioned, you are ready to start wrapping the hair on the perm rods. If you are using the pre-damping method of applying your perm lotion, you will be applying the product to each of the nine sections as you begin winding in that area. Alternatively, if you are post-damping, the perm lotion will not be applied until all the sections have been wound. We will be going into these methods of application in greater detail later on but let's imagine that you will be using the post-damping technique for this list outlining the sequence of perming.

(4) Application of perm lotion

Before the perm lotion is applied, you should offer the client additional protection. This is done by placing a strip of slightly dampened cotton wool around the entire hairline. Because the strip is damp, it will not be able to absorb the perm lotion so easily. Using an applicator bottle, the lotion is carefully applied to each rod ensuring that all the hair is treated. A small pad of cotton wool held in your other hand underneath each rod that you treat will help to catch any drips. If you wish to leave the cotton wool strip in place during the processing, you should now replace it with a fresh strip if it is saturated.

(5) Processing

The majority of perms require the use of a plastic cap to serve as an insulator during processing. Some products, however, may have to be processed with the addition of heat from a hood dryer or other machine. The manufacturer's instructions will guide you in this and must be strictly obeyed. Usually, the product instructions will give you an idea of how long the processing is likely to take and at what intervals you should check what is happening. Most manufacturers will recommend that you take a curl test every five minutes.

(6) Rinsing

When the hair is sufficiently processed, the lotion must be thoroughly rinsed from the hair. The action of rinsing stops the perm lotion from affecting the hair any more. Technically speaking, this is now the end of the perming process but the neutralising stage immediately follows the rinsing. You may now wish to turn to Chapter 10 to read about neutralising.

Questions
1. What do you need to prepare for a perm?
2. What is directional winding?
3. How many sections is the hair divided into?
4. What is the difference between pre- and post-damping?
5. How do you protect the client when perming?
6. How is perm lotion applied to wound rods?
7. How can heat be supplied during processing?
8. Why do you rinse the hair?
9. How do you know when to do this?

What effect does pH have on the hair?

What is pH?

The term 'pH' is simply a way of indicating how acid or alkaline something is. pH is expressed on a scale from 0 to 14, with 7.0 in the middle being the neutral point, where something is neither acid nor alkaline.

Acids contain hydrogen ions (positively charged hydrogen atoms). The stronger an acid is, the greater the concentration of hydrogen ions it contains. A pH of below 7.0 is acid; the smaller the number, the stronger the acid. A pH of 2 is a stronger acid than 3, and 0 indicates the strongest acid.

Alkalis contain hydroxide ions (oxygen and hydrogen atoms joined together with a negative charge). The stronger an alkali is, the more hydroxide ions it contains. A pH of above 7.0 is alkaline; the larger the number, the stronger the alkali. A pH of 10 is a stronger alkali than 8, and 14 is the strongest alkali.

Therefore, if a chemical contains more hydrogen ions than hydroxide ions it is acid, whereas if it contains more hydroxide ions than hydrogen ions it is alkaline. So, what happens if it contains the same amount of each type of ion? It can be neither acid nor alkaline. When this happens the chemical is neutral. This is exactly what happens with pure water as is shown below:

$$H_2O \quad gives \quad H^+ \quad + \quad OH^-$$
$$water \quad \longrightarrow \quad \underset{\text{ion}}{hydrogen} \quad \underset{\text{ion}}{hydroxide}$$

Remember, if a solution contained more hydrogen than hydroxide ions it would be acid, and alkaline if it contained more hydroxide than hydrogen ions. Also, if 7.0 is neutral (neither acid or alkaline) the nearer a number is to 7.0 the weaker an acid or alkali is.

How do I test for pH?

If you look at Figure 8.2, a diagram to show how hairdressing chemicals affect the hair, you will see two ways of testing pH. One is litmus, which will be red in acids and blue in alkalis. This is available as paper or a liquid. It has the disadvantage that it can only tell you whether a chemical is acid or alkaline, not how weak or strong it is. The second product is called universal indicator, and this changes over a range of

Figure 8.2 pH chart showing how hairdressing chemicals affect the hair.

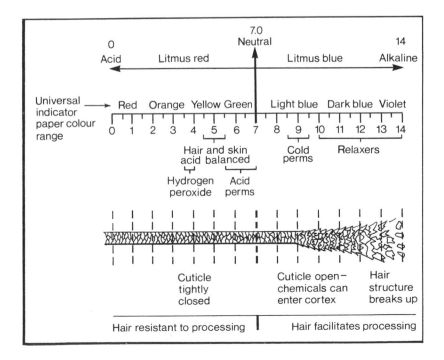

colours which correspond to different pHs. The colour is simply matched up to a chart. This is available as paper or liquid. When the product manufacturers make their various products they use delicate electronic pH meters to make sure that the pH is correct.

Just how strong is a particular chemical?

If you take two particular hairdressing chemicals and find that they have a pH of 8.0 and 9.0, the latter is the stronger alkali. The difference of one unit on the pH scale means that it is 10 times stronger or more alkaline. If you had another chemical with a pH of 10.0, this would be 100 times stronger than a pH of 8.0 ($10 \times 10 = 100$). You can see that a small difference in pH number can mean a lot in terms of strength. If you took an acid product with a pH of 6.0 and another with a pH of 3.0, the latter would be 1000 times more acid than the product with a pH of 6.0 ($10 \times 10 \times 10 = 1000$).

Why is pH important to hairdressing?

pH is important for a number of reasons. Acids close the cuticle of hair, making it reflect light and appear shiny (remember the *c* in acid for *close*). The cuticle is closed tightly so will resist chemical processing, as the chemicals cannot pass through the cuticle into the cortex. A closed cuticle is also less likely to get damaged in brushing or combing.

Alkalis open the cuticle, making the hair appear dull as light is scattered rather than being uniformly reflected. Many hairdressing chemicals are alkaline because they will open the cuticle and allow the chemical to enter the cortex. Porous hair with its open cuticle will thus facilitate processing so that hairdressing chemicals work more quickly. To counteract this hairdressers either use weaker products or put barriers on the hair to slow down the penetration of chemicals through the cuticle.

A strong alkali can cause more damage than a strong acid because it gets into the cortex easily where it can break the various bonds that hold together the structure of the hair. An acid will close the cuticle so that the chemical cannot enter the cortex very quickly. From Figure 8.2 it can be seen how the hair swells and eventually breaks up. Chemicals that destroy hair are called depilatories. Most alkaline hairdressing chemicals can act as depilatories if they are left on the hair for too long!

Questions sections
1. What is pH?
2. Draw a simple pH scale.
3. What is the strongest acid and alkali available?
4. What do chemicals contain that make them acid or alkaline?
5. What makes a chemical neutral?

6. How can pH be tested?
7. How much more alkaline would a perm lotion of 9.0 be than 8.0?
8. What effect has an acid on the cuticle?
9. What effect has an alkali on the cuticle?
10. Why do alkalis do more damage to the hair than acids?

What is the chemistry of permanent waving?

(Read in conjunction with Figures 11.1a and b.)
Figure 8.3 shows normal hair. It contains an amino acid called *cystine*. While cystine is the most predominant *sulphur*-containing amino acid of keratin the hair structure will remain stable.

Figure 8.4 shows the application of the cold wave lotion. When the perm lotion is applied to the hair the reducing agent, *ammonium thioglycollate*, adds *hydrogen*. The hydrogen attacks and breaks down the disulphide bonds of the cystine molecules in the cortex of the hair.

In Figure 8.5, the hair is divided into sections and wound onto the perm curlers. This is done so *evenly, without tension* (the hair is much more elastic with perm lotion on and could be easily damaged). Curler size will determine the final curl size. As the disulphide bonds are broken by reduction each cystine is reduced to form two *cysteines*. The softened hair now takes on the shape of the curlers.

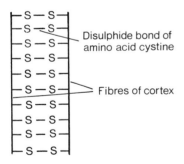

Figure 8.3 The disulphide bonds of the cortex in hair before perming.

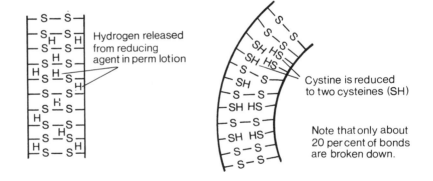

Figure 8.4 Perm lotion is applied to the hair.

Figure 8.5 The hair is wound onto rods and starts to take on their shape.

If too many of the disulphide bonds were broken down during processing the structure of the hair would break up and the hair would be destroyed. Most cold wave lotions break down an average 20 per cent of the disulphide bonds in hair (about one in five). The diagrams here therefore exaggerate this number to show how the lotion works. Once processing is complete the perm lotion is rinsed from the hair to stop further processing.

Questions

1. Draw diagrams to illustrate how perming works chemically.
2. What happens to the hair if too many bonds are broken down?
3. What percentage of the bonds should be broken down?

Permanent waving products

If you aim to offer each of your clients a complete and professional consultation before a perm, you need to have a sound product knowledge. How can you talk to clients about the various perms that are offered by your salon if you don't know about them yourself? For example, clients will often ask these kinds of questions and you must be able to provide truthful, factful answers. For example;

'Why is that perm more expensive than this one?'
'How long will it last?'
'Which will be the best perm for my hair?'
'How much will the perm cost me?'
'Will the perm make my hair dry?'
'What's the difference between the perms you are recommending?'
'Who makes this perm?'
'Do you do the perm I've seen advertised in magazines?'

Until you are able to give answers to these type of questions you will be unable to offer a complete service. If you found any of the questions difficult to answer, make it your priority to go and find out about the perms in your salon. Other hairdressers in your salon will be able to help you as well as product literature that is readily available from manufacturers. Once you have done your research try to classify this information under the following headings:

- Cost to client.
- Manufacturer.
- Product formulae (i.e. different strengths).
- Benefits and suitability.

An example of how you might set out this information is given below. (Remember that you will need to look at your salon's price list for the cost of each perm.)

Product: Opta Form
Manufacturer: Wella
Formulae: Available in three variants
　　　　　　0 – For difficult-to-perm hair
　　　　　　1 – For normal hair
　　　　　　2 – For tinted hair
Cost to client: £25.00 (excluding cut and finish)
Suitability: Suitable for all hair types except bleached.

Benefits:

Has a 'no wait' neutraliser which saves time and increases client comfort.

The perm is individually packaged and contains instructions, lotion, matching neutraliser, finishing rinse and plastic cap and gloves.

The finishing rinse is acid-balanced so restores the hair back to its natural pH.

How can wastage be controlled when perming?

The greatest amount of wastage in salons is caused by misuse of products, resulting in products being discarded or clients returning to the salon for corrective treatment to services that have been unsatisfactory. As you will appreciate, this wastage can be attributed to salon staff's lack of knowledge of the products they are using. Too often, less scrupulous hairdressers blame poor results on the client's hair, when they are at fault for failing to analyse the hair or client's requirements properly. They say things like 'She should have told me that she had henna on her hair' or 'How was I to know her hair was resistant? She should have told me if she'd had a perm drop out before'. Can you see from these examples that the hairdresser is the one at fault and not the client? Such information should be elicited from the client in the initial consultation, by carrying out precautionary tests on the hair.

Here is a list of examples of how wastage can be minimised:

- *Knowing your products*: their capabilities and limitations, chemical contents, instuctions, quantities to use, etc.
- *Carrying out precautionary TESTS*: to avoid mistakes and the need for clients returning to the action for corrective treatment. For perming, these tests will include:

  - test curl;
  - porosity test;
  - elasticity test;
  - examination of the scalp;
  - incompatibility test (check back to Chapter 2 if you have forgotten how to do these).

- *Correct gowning and protection*: If a client's clothing is spoilt it is *Your* fault and the client can claim for damages.
- *Working efficiently*: By organising all the materials and equipment you will be needing, time will be saved because you will not be leaving your client every time you realise that what you need is not on your trolley.
- *Controlling application of products*: Products that are applied with care do not end up on the floor or the towel around the client's shoulders.
- *Controlling the flow of water*: Do not leave the water running when you are not actually using it to rinse the hair. If your salon water is supplied from a boiler, wasting water could result in the salon running out of hot water.

Giving a permanent wave on non-colour treated hair

To begin this section, let us first consider exactly what we mean by the term 'non-colour treated hair'. When hair is subjected to hair colorants that work by affecting the internal structure of the hair, the hair will respond differently to further chemical processing. Hair colorants that affect the hair in this way are permanent tints, bleaches and henna. Semi-permanent and temporary colorants do not affect the hair structure in the same way so can be included when we talk about hair which is not colour treated. (If you are now interested in how colorants affect the hair, you may wish to turn to Chapter 9 for this information.)

A special note on perming hair which is treated by bleaching and other forms of colorants is covered at the end of the text.

Towel-drying the hair for perming

Most perm products require that the hair is shampooed and then towel-dried before the actual perming process begins. You should heed the manufacturer's instructions with regard to how much moisture should be present in the hair after the shampoo. If the hair is left too wet, the effect of perm lotion will be reduced because it would have been diluted; while if it is allowed to dry out too much, the lotion could be too active for the hair.

An average head of hair can hold up to 60 mls of water before it even drips – if this amount of moisture is left when the instructions advise towel-drying, just imagine how much the lotion will be diluted. To towel-dry hair, use a dry towel, and squeeze the hair gently between it. This should be done in a movement that begins at the front hairline and ends at the points of the hair at the back of the head.

Remember that the hair will be losing moisture all the time you are working because it will be evaporating into the atmosphere. Keep a water spray close by so that parts which are too dry can be easily dampened.

Sectioning the hair for perming

When perming, it is important to work in a methodical manner which not only makes you look professional, but also helps you to wind more

Figure 8.6 Top section secured with clip.

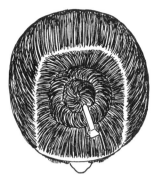

Figure 8.7 Sections taken at the crown and occipital regions.

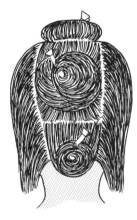

quickly. Working in a methodical fashion is achieved by sectioning the hair so that it allows you to take meshes for winding more easily while following a particular order which begins at the nape.

Method of sectioning for a basic perm

1. Begin by measuring with a perm rod the width of the first section and make two partings that run parallel to each other along the top of the head. This section should go as far as the crown and is secured neatly in position with a sectioning clip as shown in Figure 8.6.
2. To make the next sections, continue the two parallel partings down the back of the head to the nape. Divide this long section into two, horizontally, at the occipital region (the protruding bone of the skull situated, just above the nape) as shown in Figure 8.7.
3. Now make a vertical parting that runs from the first section you made to just behind the ear as shown in Figure 8.8. This parting needs to be slightly angled so that it runs parallel to the front hairline and is not wider than the length of the perm curler.
4. Directly behind the front section you will have formed another long section of hair as shown in Figure 8.9. This is divided into two horizontally level with the back sections.
5. This sectioning technique is then repeated on the other side of the head to give you nine sections in all, as shown in Figure 8.10.

Although the sections have been made in this order, the actual winding of the rods, if pre-damping, begins at the least receptive (most resistant) area of the head, which is the nape. This allows the resistant area to be in contact with the lotion for longer than the more receptive areas. The order that the sections are wound for pre-damping is shown in Figure

Figure 8.8 Making the section at the side.

Figure 8.9 The long section that requires dividing.

Figure 8.10 The completed sections which are the same on the other side of the head.

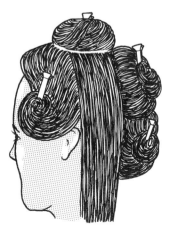

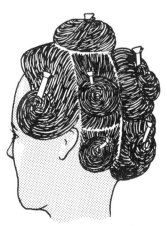

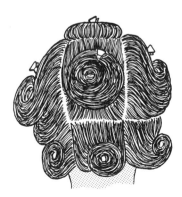

Figure 8.11 Order of winding the nine sections. (Courtesy L'Oréal.)

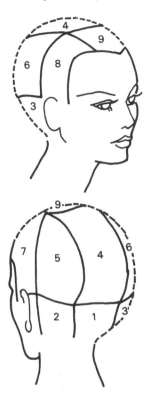

8.11. However, if you are post-damping, where you begin your wind has no effect on the final curl result, because all the hair will be treated with the lotion at the same time.

How are perm rods wound?

A mesh of hair for winding should not be wider or longer than the rod you are using. In other words, for a basic perm, all the rods should be sitting on-base (please refer back to Chapter 7 if you are not sure of what on-base means). If winding is done without making the meshes the same size as the rods, you will be left with a poor result and a dissatisfied client. The winding should be even so that the hair is wrapped smoothly around the rod. The points of the hair should be carefully wrapped around the rod with the aid of an end paper to prevent buckled ends. Too much tension by the operator or by the way the rod is secured can cause damage to the hair and scalp. Have a look at the following diagrams of common winding faults:

In Figure 8.12 the mesh is too wide which will result in an uneven curl.

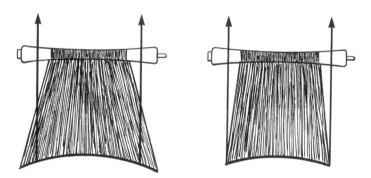

Figure 8.12 Mesh too wide which will result in an uneven curl.

Figure 8.13 Points of hair incorrectly wrapped around the rod will result in buckled ends which stick out.

In Figure 8.13 points of hair have been incorrectly wrapped around the rod. The result will be buckled ends that will stick out.

In Figure 8.14 incorrect positioning of a tight rubber shows how a fracture mark is caused which can lead to breakage.

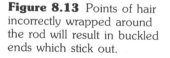
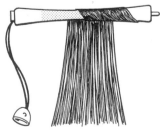

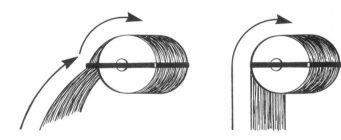

Figure 8.14 Incorrect positioning of a tight rubber showing how a fracture mark is caused which can lead to breakage.

Figure 8.15 shows how failing to hold mesh at a 90 degrees angle to the part of the head you are winding will also result in a band mark on the hair.

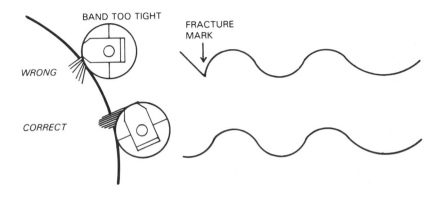

Figure 8.15 Failing to hold mesh at a 90 degrees angle to the part of the head you are winding will also result in a band mark on the hair.

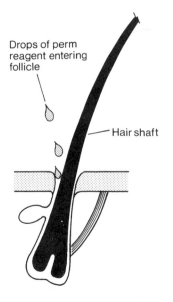

Figure 8.16 Excessive tension on the hair can permit lotion to enter the hair follicle causing a 'pull-burn'.

Figure 8.16 shows how excessive tension on the hair can permit lotion to enter the hair follicle causing a 'pull-burn'.

To summarise the pointers to successful winding, let's now list the important 'dos':

DO section the hair carefully before perming.
DO take meshes that are not longer or wider than the rod you are using.
DO make sure that all your partings are clean when taking a mesh.
DO fasten the rubber band of the rod so that it will not cause excessive tension on the hair or scalp.
DO keep rubbers as flat as possible on the rod without twisting them.
DO keep the tension even without causing stress on the hair.
DO hold a mesh for winding at a 90 degrees angle to the part of the head you are winding so that all rods sit on their own base.
DO use end papers on the points of the hair to assist you in preventing buckled ends caused by bad winding.

Bearing all the above points in mind, you will appreciate the necessity of practising your perm rod winding before attempting to do a perm on a client. Practice does make perfect and helps to increase your speed and control over different hair types and lengths. We suggest you practise the following winding exercise.

Rod winding exercise

You will need:

- a training block and clamp;
- a wide toothed and tail comb;
- clips;

Figure 8.17 Training block sectioner ready for winding exercise.

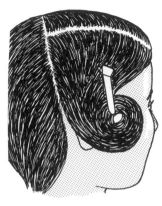

- trolley;
- perm rods and end papers.

Preparation:

- Lay out what you will need on your trolley.
- Wet the training block then towel-dry the hair.
- Disentangle the hair using the wide-toothed comb.
- Section the hair as shown in Figure 8.17.

Sectioning:

- Using a rod as a guide, make two partings that run parallel to each other from the crown to the nape as shown in Figure 8.18. Remember that this panel of hair must not be wider than the perm rod.

Taking a mesh of hair:

- Using your tail comb, slide your comb through the hair, along the scalp, to get a cleanly parted mesh of hair as shown in Figure 8.19.

Figure 8.18 Sectioning a panel of hair for winding practice.

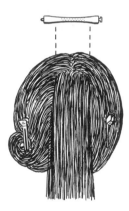

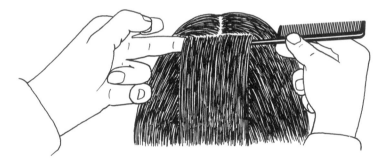

Figure 8.19 Taking a mesh of hair to wind a perm rod.

Combing the mesh:

- Comb the mesh through from roots to points until you are satisfied that it is tangle-free and smooth.
- The mesh should be combed and directed at a 90 degrees angle to the head. For winding at the crown, the mesh is therefore directed upwards as shown in Figure 8.21.

Positioning the end paper:

- Place the end paper around the points of the hair and fold it so that it lies both sides as in Figure 8.22.
- Try not to bunch up the points of the hair when you do this.
- Sliding the end paper up towards the points should ensure that the longest ends are enclosed inside.

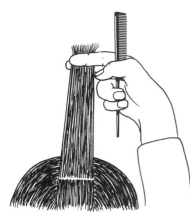

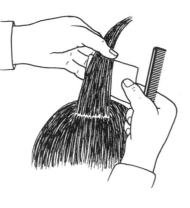

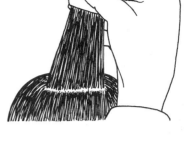

Figure 8.20 Lifting the hair ready for winding.

Figure 8.21 Combing and positioning the mesh of hair.

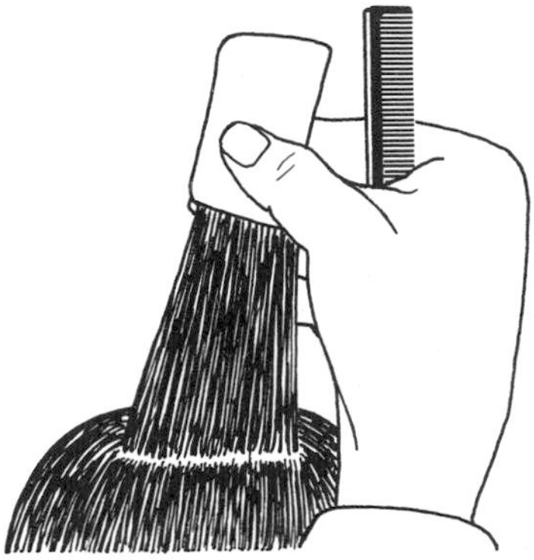

Figure 8.22 Positioning the end paper.

Introducing and winding the rod:

- Holding the rod parallel to the scalp place the rod on the underneath of the mesh against the end paper as shown in Figure 8.23.
- Begin to wind the rod towards you, making sure the points of the hair are wrapped smoothly around the rod.
- Continue winding the rod until it sits on the scalp.

Securing the rod:

- Fasten the rod by pulling the elastic band to the other end and hook the band on its place at the tip of the rod. This is shown in Figure 8.24.
- Make sure the band is properly positioned so that it will not mark the hair.

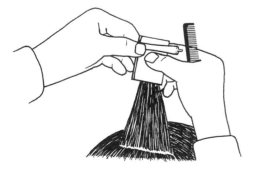

Figure 8.23 Winding the rod.

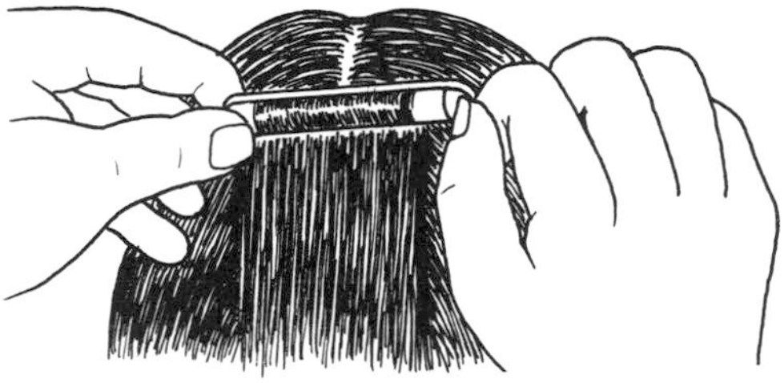

Figure 8.24 Fastening the rod in position.

Figure 8.25 Plastic strips can be used to prevent any chance of the bands marking the hair. (Courtesy Goldwell Hair Cosmetics Ltd.)

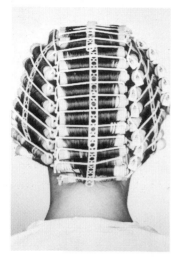

Continue with this exercise all the way down the panel of hair, making sure that all the meshes are the correct size and are held at the correct angle, according to the part of the head you are winding.

It is possible to eradicate any possibility of the elastic bands on perm rods causing any marks on the hair. This is achieved by the use of flexible plastic strips as shown in Figure 8.25.

How are different hair lengths controlled when winding?

It is much easier to wind hair which is 'average' in length compared with very long or very short hair. Long hair needs special care because if your tension changes during winding, there will be noticeable unevenness of the wrap around the rod. Very short hair can create the problem of slipping out of the rod and generally being difficult to wind. When this happens, hairdressers often put too much tension on the hair as they try to get more control over it. Sometimes it is impossible to wind really short hair successfully on perm rods and the hairdresser may need to use pincurls instead of rods to achieve the movement. Please refer to *Perming and Straightening – A Salon Handbook* for details of pincurl perms.

Another problem that a hairdresser might face when winding, is the realisation that the client's hair is all different lengths. This is a fearsome experience to encounter, especially on a busy Saturday afternoon in the salon. If every mesh of hair you take results in the points of the hair ending at vastly different levels, there is no use pretending that you will not have problems. Again, try not to use excessive tension in the attempt to control the hair as this will cause damage. Some hairdressers find that using more than one end paper helps because the second paper can be placed lower down the mesh of hair to keep stray hair in position while it is wound. If you have a mesh with one really long area of hair, we suppose you could always cut it off! However, this can look unprofessional and could upset the client if you are not responsible for the haircut. In such a case, try winding the really long strands around the rod first and then introduce the rest of the hair to the rod. Practising on badly cut training blocks does have its purpose!

How should the client's head be positioned and where should you stand when winding a perm?

When you are winding, you will need to position yourself so that you are standing directly behind the part of the head you are winding. This will mean that you will not be standing in the same place throughout the winding process. Also, you may need to ask the client to move the head to give you better access to that particular area. If you do need to do this, always ask the client to move the head, while at the same time, using both hands to gently position it where you want it to be. Never get into that awful habit of just pushing the client's head into position with no regard for their comfort or feelings.

How is perm lotion applied?

As we said earlier, there are two techniques for applying perm lotion to the hair. These two techniques are:

Post-damping: applying the lotion to the rods after the wind is completed, and

Pre-damping: applying the lotion as you are winding.

Post-damping technique

This is probably the most popular of the two techniques and is preferred by many hairdressers for the following reasons:

- The time it takes to wind the hair will not affect the end result because the hair is wound without the lotion.
- Some hairdressers do not like winding with gloves on. If there is no lotion on the hair there is no need to wear gloves.
- Clients often prefer not to have the sensation or smell of the lotion on their hair during the winding.

The lotion can be applied using any of the following methods:

- an applicator bottle;
- from a bowl with a pad of cotton wool (not coloured cotton wool);
- from a bowl using a brush (but can splash).

Many lotions are now packaged as individual treatments and come in their own applicator bottle.

Pre-damping technique

This technique was once the most popular of the two ways to apply perm lotion to the hair, but is now in decline due to improved product formulae and uniformity of results. Also, various winding patterns used for fashion looks need to begin at the front hairline where the hair is most receptive to the lotion. If the lotion was applied as the winding commenced at the front, this area would be processed before the back of the hair was wound.

To pre-damp, the application of the lotion is done using any of the methods described above but usually begins at the nape where the hair is more resistant. By the time the hairdresser reaches the receptive areas of hair at the front hairline, the nape hair is partly processed, resulting in an overall even processing time which is consistent with the varying degrees of the hair's porosity on the head.

As each section of hair is wound, lotion is applied to within half an inch of the scalp. This ensures that the lotion will not settle on the scalp and that the hair nearest the warmth of the head will not process too quickly. The section of hair to be moistened with the lotion should be held in the palm of the hand to prevent drips and to ensure an even application. After the lotion is applied, the mesh of hair is combed through to distribute the lotion along the length of the hair. Even though the lotion is applied to the hair during the winding, more lotion is applied when the wind is completed.

How is the curl development (processing) monitored?

As soon as perm lotion comes into contact with hair it will begin to penetrate through the cuticle and start to break down disulphide bonds in the cortex (hairdressers often refer to this as 'softening'). To help speed up this process, manufacturers' instructions may tell you to cover the rods with a plastic cap (which acts as an insulator) or use external heat supplied by a hood dryer or infra red appliance such as a Climazon.

It could only be a matter of minutes between a head of hair being processed or over-processed, so you must never forget that the client is there! This does not mean you have to hover around them, but we can recall instances of how easy it is to forget the client is there!

Never use additional heat to accelerate the processing of a perm if it is not advised by the product manufacturer. Failing to follow such instructions can result in ruined hair and a damaged scalp. It might be worth mentioning at this point that the majority of cases taken to court against hairdressers are ones which are related to damage caused by perming done in 'professional' salons. Heat can speed up any hairdressing chemical reaction, so be aware of this on a hot day and check processing more often.

Some perms require the addition of heat to achieve the best results. Heat is often required for acid perms to assist the penetration of the lotion through to the cortex. This may be supplied by a chemical reaction when the perm lotion is mixed with an activator. Remember that as an acid will not open the cuticle, heat must be supplied to do so instead.

When you check a perm to see if it is sufficiently processed it is necessary to assess the degree of curl that has been formed in several areas on the head. If you used the pre-damping technique for applying your lotion, you should check the first and last rods that were wound. If you applied the lotion to the hair after all the rods were wound, you should check a rod in the front, sides, crown and nape areas. The method of taking a curl test was shown in Figure 2.27, from A − D. If the hair is not yet ready for rinsing, the S-shape will appear too loose and large when compared to the rod the hair was wound around. As an example of how the curl formations will vary according to the diameter of rod used, see Figure 8.26.

If you have made a mistake and used a rod which is too large for the desired curl pattern, an extended processing time will not make the curl the size that is desired. All that will happen is the hair will become over-processed, causing irreparable damage. If you have chosen rods that are too small, the resultant curl formation will be too tight. Both of these examples show that you have either misinterpreted what was required or not properly considered which size rod to use.

Figure 8.26 Rod size and the effect on the resultant curl formation.

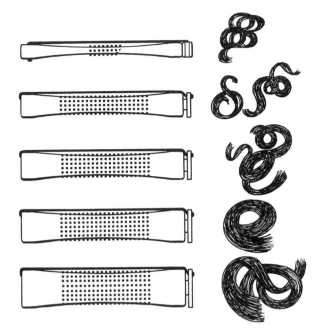

How is the water tested for rinsing?

After the hair is sufficiently processed, the lotion must be thoroughly rinsed from the wound rods. The rinsing stops the action of the perm lotion and is the final part of the actual perming stage.

The water used for this rinsing should be neither too cold nor too hot. A comfortable temperature to use is tepid, which is slightly warm. Remember that hot water on a scalp which has been subjected to a chemical will be sensitive and easily irritated. Cold water is never pleasant on the hair and most uncomfortable on a winter day.

To test the temperature of the water, allow it to run on the inside of your wrist. This area is sensitive to heat and is good for assessing the heat of the water. Obviously, gloves cannot be worn for the rinsing unless you can trust a colleague to adjust the water temperature for you. If the water supply in your salon has the common problem of altering in temperature every time another basin is used, try to hold your little finger in the flow of water so that you will be aware of any temperature changes.

How is the perm lotion rinsed out of the hair?

After the perm is sufficiently processed (i.e. enough disulphide bonds have been broken) the hair is thoroughly rinsed to stop the action of the perm lotion. Failing to rinse all the lotion out of the hair can affect the curl result. The rods should be rinsed with tepid water for a *minimum* of 3–5 minutes. It takes at least five minutes to thoroughly rinse hair that is

15 cms (6 inches) long and an extra minute should be added to this time for every additional 2.5 cms (1 inch).

Rinsing is made easier if the water pressure in your salon has force because it helps to flush out the lotion. Remember to hold the hose close to the rods to prevent unnecessary splashes and shield your client's face with your other hand. There is no need to rub the rods to help flush out the lotion – all this does is to disturb the hair that is around the rods.

It is far safer to use a backwash for rinsing perm lotion out of the hair because it reduces the chance of chemicals entering the eyes. If you have no other choice than to use a forward basin, do make sure that you give the client a small towel to protect the eyes and replace this as soon as it becomes saturated.

Some salons train their staff to check that all the lotion is out of the hair by making them taste the hair! They are taught to wipe their finger along a rod and then taste their finger. If they taste salt, it tells them there is still lotion in the hair. An alternative method is to use litmus paper which will change colour when the pH changes and the alkaline perm lotion is removed.

Blotting the hair after rinsing

The excess moisture in the hair must be removed before the neutraliser is applied. If this is not done, the water in the hair will dilute the neutraliser and stop it from working effectively. To do this, first place a towel over the rods and press against it to blot the rods. Next, take a wad of cotton wool and press this onto each rod to remove more water. You will be amazed how wet the cotton wool will be by the time you have finished.

REMEMBER: Fill in the client record card.

Questions

1. What do we mean by non-colour treated hair?
2. How and when should the hair be towel-dried?
3. Why is it important to work methodically?
4. Describe how you should section a head of hair for a perm.
5. Practise this on a block.
6. Why does the order of winding not have to be followed for post-damping?
7. How should you wind a perm rod?
8. Describe some of the common winding faults listed.
9. Make a list of 'Do's' for winding.
10. Follow the suggested rod winding exercise.
11. What problems does long hair present on winding?
12. Where should you stand when winding?

13. Give reasons for post-damping.
14. How can lotion be applied?
15. Why has the popularity of pre-damping declined?
16. Explain why different areas of the head process at different rates.
17. When is heat used on a perm?
18. How do you check processing?
19. Why is the diameter of the rod so important to final curl size?
20. What temperature should the water be for rinsing?
21. What determines how long rinsing should go on?
22. How do you know when rinsing is complete?
23. Why is the hair blotted after rinsing?

Perming colour treated hair

When you are perming colour treated hair, the actual process is the same as when you perm natural hair, but you do need to consider the fact that the hair is already chemically treated and is therefore more porous.

Choice of lotion: The lotion you choose will have to be weaker than one you would use on natural hair. That means, it contains a lower percentage of ammonium thioglycollate than a lotion for, say, natural hair in good condition. Each manufacturer uses a code on the packaging which tells you for which hair type the lotion has been made. If you use a lotion which is too strong for the hair you are perming (i.e. it contains a higher percentage of ammonium thioglycollate than is necessary to process the hair) it will be over-processed. Many hairdressers prefer to use an acid perm on colour treated hair because these lotions cause less damage to the hair than their alkaline counterparts.

Protection: Hair that has been colour treated will be more porous than hair which has not been chemically processed. This means the cuticle scales will be open instead of lying flat as in the case of hair in good condition. How much the cuticle is open and damaged will depend upon other factors apart from the coloration, but porosity is never even along the hair shaft nor uniform over the head. This uneven porosity results in the perm lotion being able to penetrate the hair shaft far more rapidly where the cuticle scales are open or damaged. If perm lotion is allowed to penetrate the hair shaft at different rates, the hair will process more quickly in some areas than in others, resulting in an uneven curl pattern. To prevent this from happening, you can apply a pre-perm lotion that will actually regulate the hair's porosity, so that the processing will be controlled. An example of a product that does this is shown in Figure 8.27.

These types of lotions are specially formulated so that they do not cause a barrier on the hair shaft that might prevent the perm lotion from penetrating the hair. Ordinary conditioners should not be used for the same purpose as pre-perm lotions because their contents will form a non-penetrable coating on the hair shaft.

Figure 8.27 'Pre-curl' lotion by Goldwell. (Courtesy Goldwell Hair Cosmetics Ltd.)

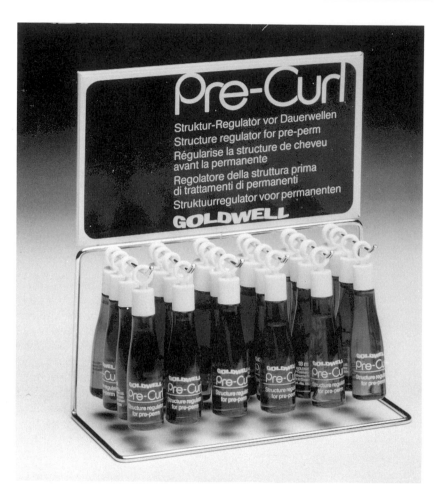

How is a pre-perm lotion applied?

The hair should be shampooed and towel-dried, ready for perming. The lotion is carefully sprinkled through the hair, ensuring that it treats the more porous areas and is evenly distributed by combing. Applying too much of the lotion could interfere with the ability of the perm lotion to work effectively, so do read and follow the instructions on the product carefully. With certain types of perm lotion, manufacturers may instruct you not to use a pre-perm lotion, because they may already have chemicals added to the lotion to help even out the porosity. After the pre-perm lotion has been applied, winding is then done in the normal way. You don't usually have to rinse the pre-perm treatment out of the hair but do check the product instructions. Incidentally, when you have applied a pre-perm lotion and wound the hair without the perm lotion (post-damping technique), if the hair should dry out, re-damp the hair with water and not more pre-perm lotion. Too much pre-perm lotion can create a film on the hair which may inhibit the penetration of the perm lotion.

Tension

Hair that has previously been chemically treated will always be more elastic than untreated hair because the internal hair structure (the cortex) will have been affected. Such hair will have less resistance to tension and, just like an old elastic band, will easily over-stretch, and not return to its original length when the tension is released. If you put too much tension on an old elastic band it will break. The same will happen to hair if it has poor elasticity. Therefore, when you are winding weak hair, you should never use unnecessary tension.

Test curl

As a safety precaution, it usually recommended that highly colour treated hair is first tested to assess its suitability for perming. This is especially true for whole head bleaches, and also partially bleached hair, as in the case of highlights. For information about test curls and why they are necessary, see Chapter 2. Bleached hair will have lost a lot of its disulphide bonds because they will have been oxidised, and therefore tends to be damaged more in perming. Bleached hair will also not hold the curl as well as it should do. Henna can bind with disulphide bonds, making them unavailable for breaking down; again it may be difficult to get a result.

Trouble shooting!

Figure 8.28 is a quick guide to technical problems in perming showing common problems, their causes, and solutions.

Questions
1. Why must colour-treated hair be permed with weaker perm lotions?
2. What ingredient is there less of in the lotion?
3. How does the pre-perm treatment help in obtaining a good perm result?
4. Should you always use a pre-perm treatment?
5. What should be used to re-damp the hair?
6. What is the rule about tension when winding chemically treated hair?
7. Why should you carry out a test curl on colour-treated hair?
8. Get someone to test you on the problems listed in Figure 8.28.

Problem	Possible causes	Solution
Too curly	Curlers used were too small	If the hair is in good condition, it could be gently relaxed using perm lotion *not* a relaxer.
Straight frizz	Either: (a) perm product used was too strong: (b) hair was over-processed; (c) too much tension was used.	Nourish the hair with a course of deep penetrating conditioning treatments or hair restructurants. The hair could be set to 'smooth' the hair temporarily. Suggest the client has regular haircuts.
No result	Either: (a) perm product was too weak; (b) insufficient product was applied; (c) insufficient processing; (d) curlers used were too large; (e) insufficient tension was used; (f) incorrect neutralising.	Re-perm the hair using a weaker product.
Good result when wet, poor result when dry	Either: (a) the hair has been overprocessed; (b) the hair is being stretched too much when drying.	If the hair has been overprocessed; follow the same advice as given for dealing with a straight frizz. If the problem is caused by the way the hair is dried, change the method, i.e. natural dry, scrunching, etc.
Result quickly weakens	Either: (a) incorrect neutralising; (b) too much tension on hair immediately after perm (e.g. over-stretching when the hair was dried).	Re-perm the hair using a weaker product.
Breakage	Either: (a) too much tension was used; (b) the perm product was too strong; (c) the hair was been overprocessed; (d) the rubber bands on the curlers were either too tight or badly positioned.	A series of deep penetrating conditioning treatments or hair restructurants should be given.
Reddening around hairline or sore scalp	Perm reagent allowed to come into contact with skin, causing irritation and discomfort.	Apply a moisturising cream to hairline and treat scalp with nourishing cream. Remember that a sore scalp should be rinsed with cool water and *gently* massaged.
Pull-burn	Perm reagent allowed to enter hair follicle causing discomfort and possible infection, i.e. folliculitis	Apply a nourishing cream to scalp and massage scalp gently. If condition is serious, suggest client visits a doctor or trichologist.
Straight ends or fish-hooks	Failing to wind the hair points evenly around the curler.	Remove the affected parts by cutting.
Straight pieces of hair	Either: (a) incorrect angling and placing of curlers; (b) sections too wide; (c) curlers too large length of hair; (d) carelessly leaving pieces of hair out of curler.	Re-perm affected parts making sure other hair is securely clipped away to prevent reagent from coming into contact with it.
Discoloration of hair	Either: (a) metal tools or containers have been used which cause a reaction which discolours the hair; (b) the hair has been treated with a colorant which is lightened by the perm agent.	Disguise discoloration with a temporary or semi-permanent colorant.

Figure 8.28 Technical problems in perming at a glance.

Machines, equipment and tools

Perm rods

Perm rods are available in a variety of sizes and are colour coded so that the correct size to use can be easily found. This code is not standardised, which means manufacturers will colour code their rods differently from other companies. A selection of perm rods are shown in Figure 8.29.

Figure 8.29 An assortment of perm rods. (Courtesy Goldwell Hair Cosmetics Ltd.)

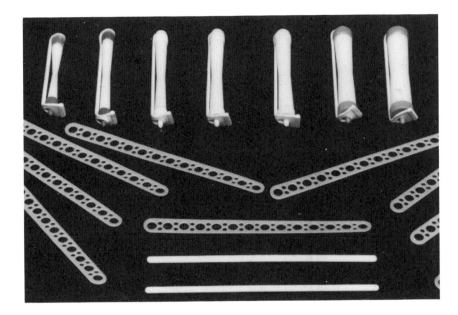

Also, you will be able to see plastic flexible strips that are used to prevent the rubber straps from marking the hair when the rod is fastened. The rubber straps on the rods in this photograph are round instead of flat. This has the advantage of putting less stress on the hair when the rod is secured; flat bands tend to mark the hair more easily. After perm rods have been used, they should be rinsed and patted dry in a towel. Applying a little talcum powder to the rubber straps will prevent them from perishing and extend their life.

Other perm 'rods' are popular to create different looks and to increase client comfort. An example of an alternative to conventional perm rods are Molton Permers. These are flexible and made of foam, with an internal wire which allows the Permer to be bent to hold it in position. In Figures 8.30 and 8.31 Molton Permers are shown being used for a conventional and spiral wind.

Miscellaneous materials

You require a number of things for carrying out a perm. Figure 8.32

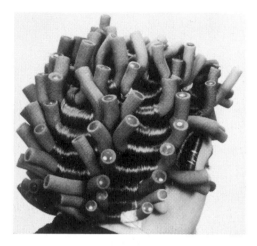

Figure 8.30 Conventional wind using Molton Permers. (Courtesy Wella Ltd.)

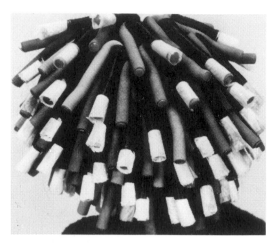

Figure 8.31 Spiral wind using Molton Permers. (Courtesy Wella Ltd.)

shows a variety of materials; from left to right these are: boxed perm papers, litmus testing papers, timer, neutralising sponge (see Chapter 10), water spray and towels.

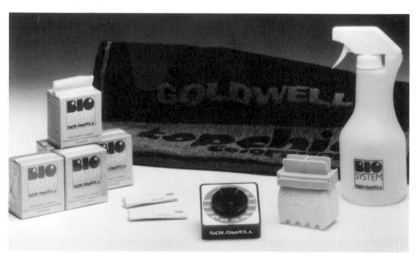

Figure 8.32 Perming materials. (Courtesy Goldwell Hair Cosmetics Ltd.)

Machines

Depending on the perming system you are using, you may need to use machines as part of the process:

- *Hood dryer*: A hood dryer provides moving air that can be adjusted in both force of the airflow and temperature. Some perms require the use of a hood dryer for processing, but do check the product instructions to see if this is recommended. A modern hood dryer was shown in Figure 7.32.

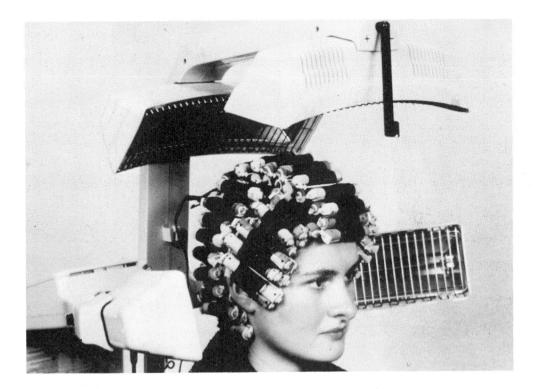

Figure 8.33 A Climazon in use to speed up perm processing. (Courtesy Wella Ltd.)

- *Climazon*: A Climazon provides infra red heat. There is no airflow from this machine because the heat is radiated from the 'arms' which have heating elements. A Climazon being used to process a perm is shown in Figure 8.33.

  When using a Climazon for perm processing, a special sensor clip is attached to one of the rods at the crown of the head and the hairdresser keys in data about the hair on the control panel. This data includes the hair's texture, condition, length and the desired result (i.e. soft, medium, firm). The hairdresser then keys in the special number code for the Wella perm being used and the Climazon will automatically display how long the processing time should be. For perms other than those manufactured by Wella, the correct processing time is keyed in and the perming start button is pressed.

- *Airboy Mobil*: If you are using the Bio-Control perm system by Goldwell, you will need to use the machine that is shown in Figure 8.34.

  The machine, powered by electricity, pumps air into the perm lotion to aerate it into a foam that will not drip once on the head. You will see from the photograph that there are two guns; one is for the perm lotion and the other is for the neutraliser. Applying the foam to the hair using this machine is shown in Figure 8.35.

- *Uniperm Machine*: 'Uniperm', by Clynol, is a perming system which

Figure 8.34 Airboy Mobil. (Courtesy Goldwell Hair Cosmetics Ltd.)

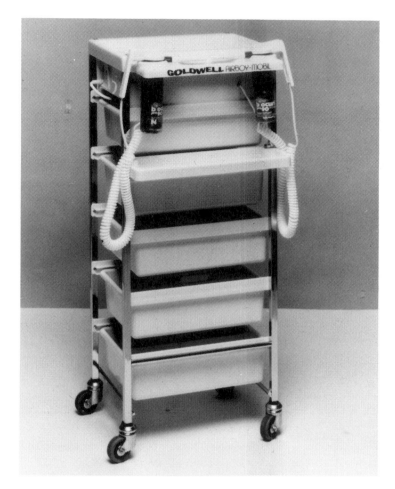

Figure 8.35 Applying a foam perm. (Courtesy Goldwell Hair Cosmetics Ltd.)

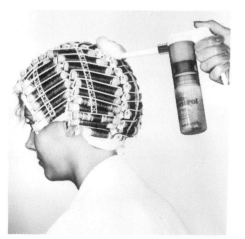

uses a controlled form of heat to process the hair. The source of this heat is the bars on the machine shown in Figure 8.36. Special clamps are heated on the bars of the machine and are then positioned on

Figure 8.36 Uniperm machine by Clynol.

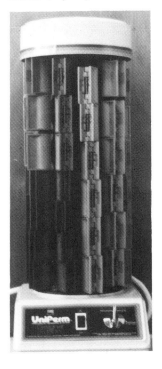

the wound perm rods. Once the lotion is applied and the rods positioned, the timer on the machine is set and the processing time begins.

When using the Uniperm system it is important that the clamps are correctly positioned to allow for the hair to be properly heated. An illustration of how the clamps are positioned on the rods for the best results is shown in Figure 8.37.

Figure 8.37 Placement of Uniperm clamps onto wound rods.

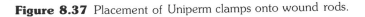
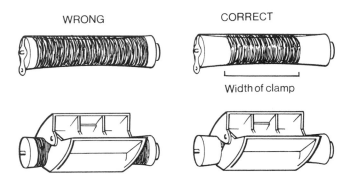

WRONG   CORRECT

Width of clamp

Questions
1. How are perm rods coded for size?
2. Why are rounded bands better than flat bands on perm rods?
3. How should you look after perm rods?
4. What are Molton Permers?
5. What machines might be required to carry out a perm?

For further reading see *Perming and Straightening – A Salon Handbook.*

Chapter Nine
Colouring

Colouring our hair is by no means a new idea. The Egyptians were applying henna and other vegetable dyes to their hair over 2,000 years ago! Obviously we will be looking at the more current colouring techniques that are in use today, which will not include henna. If your interest in colouring techniques grows, we suggest you look at our book *Colouring – A Salon Handbook* which is a comprehensive guide to hair colouring and background information.

Colour

We can all look at an object and say what colour it is, but just what is colour? Natural daylight is technically 'white light', but is itself made up of seven colours – red, orange, yellow, green, blue, indigo and violet. You see these seven colours in this order when you see a rainbow. You can remember the colours by the phrase 'Richard of York gave battle in vain' – the first letter of each word being a colour.

If something appears white it is because all seven of these colours are being reflected off it to your eyes. However, if an object appears as any one of the seven colours, it is because that colour is being reflected to your eyes, while the other six colours are being absorbed. So if you see red, it is because red is reflected, while the other colours are absorbed. Black is slightly different. If an object appears black it is because all the colours are being absorbed, so no colour is being reflected. Thus black is an absence of colour. The colour spectrum is shown in Figure 9.1.

Figure 9.1 The colour spectrum.

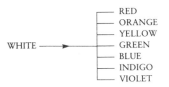

WHITE →	RED
	ORANGE
	YELLOW
	GREEN
	BLUE
	INDIGO
	VIOLET

Primary and secondary colours

A primary colour is a colour which cannot be produced by mixing other colours. In hairdressing we use pigments to colour hair, so our primary colours are red, yellow and blue. This is because we cannot make pigments of these three colours by mixing other pigments.
Secondary colours are the colours which can be obtained by mixing primary colours together. For example:

Primary colour	gives	secondary colour
Red + yellow	⟶	orange
Blue + red	⟶	violet
Yellow + blue	⟶	green

Figure 9.2 The colour triangle.

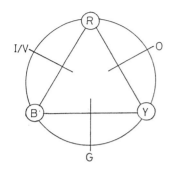

Complementary colours

These are colours which are opposite each other in the colour triangle, illustrated in Figure 9.2. They may also be called contrasting colours. We will talk about them at the end of the chapter as they can mask unwanted colour. From the example above, you can see that it would be possible accidentally (we hope!) to produce green on a head by putting a blue rinse on hair with a lot of yellow in it. As red is opposite green in the colour triangle, the unwanted green can be removed by applying a red toner.

Salon lighting

It is important to remember that most salon light is artificial because we cannot always have natural daylight. Artificial light can have colour in it; for example, light from most normal light bulbs has a yellow tinge. Thus you may not see the real colour created because of this. Have you noticed how some people ask to take clothes into the street to look at them before committing themselves to buying? Although fluorescent tubes are available called 'daylight', the nearest tube to natural daylight is 'warm white'. Look for this if ever you buy a fluorescent fitting. Spotlights in the salon will give hair colour the chance to 'shine', whereas fluorescent lighting will make it appear 'flat' but more like the real result. One international colourist we know pulls models into corridors with fluorescent lighting so that she can see the real result! Salons should not have too many colours on walls as these can leave an after-image in the eyes. This is why pastel colours with matt finishes are seen in the colouring areas of many salons. If ever you are matching colours, rely on your first impression. The longer you look at two colours the more they will blend together.

Safe working guidelines for colouring

- Always read and follow the manufacturer's instructions.
- Check that all necessary precautionary tests have been carried out before the colorant is applied.
- Ensure that you and the client have agreed on the final colour result *before* starting.
- Apply barrier cream carefully to the hairline before tinting or bleaching but ensure it does not get on the hair.
- Accurately measure all colouring products.
- Gown and protect your clients so that there is no chance of any colorant staining their clothes.
- Wear rubber or plastic protective gloves during colour application.
- Avoid inhaling the fumes given off by some types of bleaches or other colorants as these can irritate the nose or lungs.
- Keep record cards up to date.
- Always clean up any spillages of bleach, tint, peroxide, etc. immediately.

- Thoroughly flush out the eyes with tepid water if colorant should accidentally splash or drip into the eyes. If the irritation continues, seek medical attention.
- Never use anything other than proprietary stain removers to remove stains from the skin. If it is necessary to use stain remover, follow the instructions exactly.

How can wastage be controlled?

Far too much wastage occurs in many salons due to lack of product knowledge and careless preparation and use of colorants. Here are some useful hints on how such wastage can be minimised:

- Do not mix products until you are satisfied that your client is in full agreement with the colouring treatment you intend carrying out.
- Estimate how much product you will need for the head of hair you are treating, so that when possible, you are not left with a lot of product that has to be disposed of down the basin.
- Mix products accurately and carefully. Too much product is wasted when too low a concentration results in the wrong ingredients being incorrectly prepared.
- Avoid spillages, drips and careless applications. Colorants are designed to colour hair – *not* the skin, floor, work surfaces, trollies or the client's gown and towel!
- Never mix products before they are needed because they will lose their strength and their performance will consequently be affected.
- Make sure all the product is emptied out of sachets, tubes and bottles when using the entire contents. Squeeze tubes from the bottom to get all the product out and always check you have completely emptied bottles and sachets.
- Store all colouring products as directed by the manufacturers, as failure to comply with these recommendations can result in products 'going off'. This includes replacing caps and stoppers properly to help prevent oxygen from affecting the contents.

Natural and artificial hair colours

Natural hair pigment is contained in the cortex layer of the hair and is seen because the cuticle scales which protect the internal structure are translucent and colourless. Hair which does not contain pigment is completely colourless, and is referred to as being white. Although hair might appear grey, it is the mixture of coloured and white hair that gives the illusion of it looking grey. We challenge you to pluck out a grey hair from somebody's head! Hair can turn white at virtually any age although it is often linked to a person's age. Also people refer to their worries as giving them white hair. This is not too far from the truth because stress and trauma can result in white hairs appearing. However it is *totally* untrue that a person can 'go white overnight'. This is because the pigment is injected into the hair as it is growing, so it cannot therefore miraculously disappear once it is present. Nobody knows why hair should grow colourless, but we can tell you how it happens. The pigment is produced by cells called melanocytes and they inject a newly developing hair in the follicle with colour. Sometimes this process will suddenly cease and the melanocytes stop producing the pigment so have no colour to inject the hair with. This phenonemon usually happens once the old coloured hair has been shed, and the new hair that grows in its place consequently has no colour. You may have heard of the story which tells how Marie Antoinette's hair went white the night before her execution by guillotine during the French Revolution. What we suggest happened is that she already had grey (and therefore some white) hair, and the trauma of knowing her head would be cut off the following day caused her coloured hair to fall out, leaving a sparser head of white hair. Incidentally, there is also no truth in the belief that if you pluck out a white hair that two will grow in its place! Old wives have a lot to answer for!

So, now that you are aware of how hair gets its colour we will explain the reason for all the different natural hair colours that you see around you. The melanocytes that inject the pigment into the cortical cells as the hair is growing produce two types of pigment: melanin and pheomelanin. Melanin is the black and brown pigment and pheomelanin is the red and yellow pigment. Differing amounts of these two pigments in a single hair produce the various hair colours we see from very dark to red or blonde. All coloured hair has a combination of these pigments in each hair; obviously dark hair will contain more melanin than pheomelanin, while red or blonde hair will have more pheomelanin. You will also see that natural hair colours are usually not uniform throughout the whole head. On naturally blonde hair you will often see single, much darker hairs or hairs which glint because they are more golden than the overall colour we see.

All hair (whether it is natural or artificially coloured) has colour except white hair which is colourless. Therefore all hair colours can be described in terms of how light or dark they are and also the tone (or colour) that we actually see. The descriptive terms used to classify hair colours are 'depth' and 'tone'.

Depth = How light or how dark the hair colour is − the intensity of the pigment.

Tone = The colour we actually see − the varying amounts of pigment that produce the overall colour.

The International Colour Chart System (ICC)

There is an International Colour Chart System (ICC) which has classified all hair colour using numbers to discriminate between different depths and tones. The number codes may vary slightly, but the principle remains unchanged from country to country.

Depth

How light or how dark the hair is can be described on a numerical scale that ranges from number one (the darkest) to ten or eleven (the lightest).

Tone

The varying quantity of pigment that is responsible for all the different hair colours that we see is also expressed in a numerical fashion with each number representing a particular colour characteristic.

If you look at Figure 9.3 you will see a manufacturer's depth and tone chart showing how L'Oréal has classified hair colours in its Majirel colorant range. Not all colouring product manufacturers will use the same numerical code to describe the various colours. In fact, some companies will use letters instead, with G standing for a gold tone and R representing a colour which has a red tone. Try to find out as much as you can about the different ways in which companies classify their colours, so that when you work in another salon with unfamiliar products, it will be easier for you to adapt to a different coding system.

Virtually all hair colorant ranges include a special selection of concentrated colours that are designed to be used in conjunction with the other products within that particular range, to increase the tonal vibrance and intensity of the colours. An example that you may come across is a client who wants a colour that is more vibrant than it is shown on the manufacturer's shade chart. By adding a measured amount of the concentrated tone, extra vibrance is achieved.

How are shade charts used to assess colour?

Shade charts are produced by manufacturers to display their colour ranges on swatches of hair. Some of these charts are client-orientated, which means there will be a separate guide for the hairdresser's use. Those shade charts which are client-orientated will have attractive photographs and illustrations to help the clients picture different colours on themselves and help 'sell' the idea of having hair colour. The hairdresser on the other hand just needs a guide which shows the depths and tones of the different colours, with hints on the selection and mixing of the colours.

There will always be a part of the shade chart which displays the natural bases and this might be on a detachable page for ease of use. This page is used to help the hairdresser assess the natural base of the client's hair by comparing the swatches of hair to the client's natural hair colour. It is very important that this analysis is done in a good natural light so that you are not misled by the way the salon lighting alters the apparent appearance of hair colour. Holding the shade guide close to your client's hair will assist you when making the discerning decision about the depth of their natural base.

Depth and Tone Chart

Depth	Tone Basic Shades	.01 Soft Ash	.1 Ash	.2 Mauve	.3 Golden	.4 Copper	.5 Mahogany	.6 Red
Lightest Blonde	10 Lightest Blonde	10.01 Lightest Natural ash blonde	10.1 Lightest ash blonde 10½.1 Sea spray 10.13 Ocean Dawn	10.21 Raindrop	10.31 White sand			
Very light blonde	9 Very light blonde	9.01 Very light natural ash blonde	9.1 Very light ash blonde 9.13 Sirocco	9.22 Mother of pearl	9.03 Sahara 9.33 Gold dust	9.04 Beachcomber		
Light blonde	8 Light blonde	8.01 Light natural ash blonde	8.1 Light ash blonde		8.33 Sunshine gold 8.3 Light golden blonde 8.31 Chamois	8.04 Golden sands 8.43 Marigold 8.45 Wild fox		
Blonde	7 Blonde		7.1 Medium ash blonde	7.2 Mink 7.23 Capuccino	7.3 Medium golden blonde 7.31 Sandstone 7.35 Sandlewood	7.4 Aztec 7.43 Terracotta 7.40 Ultimate copper	7.52 Honeycomb	
Dark blonde	6 Dark blonde	6.01 Dark natural ash blonde	6.1 Dark ash blonde	6.23 Mocca 6.26 Claret	6.34 Bronze gold 6.35 Cherrywood	6.45 Bronzed beech	6.52 Burnt toffee	6.62 Berry
Light brown	5 Light brown			5.2 Truffle	5.3 Light golden brown		5.52 Wild sorrel 5.5 Fire opal	5.62 Ultimate auburn
Brown	4 Brown			4.20 Ultimate burgundy 4.26 Raisin	4.3 Medium golden brown	4.45 Teak 4.4 Cinnabar	4.51 Praline 4.56 Bramble	
Dark brown	3 Dark brown							
Very dark brown								
Black	1 Black							

Figure 9.3 Majirel depth and Tone Chart.

There are many clients who are attracted by the names of particular colours (a reason why manufacturers name their colours) and will choose unsuitable colours based on the attraction of the colour's name. If you don't believe this, try giving a client the shade chart upside down! They will complain that they can't read the names when it is supposed to be the colours they are looking at!

Shade charts can be used to very good effect. For example, a client may select three colours that they think would be suitable, and one of these is impossible to achieve on their particular base colour without pre-lightening (bleaching). You can effectively use the chart to ask questions that will elicit information from your clients that will assist them in their choice of colour. For example:

'Why do you like that colour more than this one?'

'What do you like about this particular colour as opposed to that one?'

'This colour is much lighter than that colour. You would need to have your hair pre-lightened to get the colour but that wouldn't be necessary for the other one. How do you feel about having your hair bleached?'

Questions

1. How long has hair been coloured for?
2. What is white light?
3. How many colours make it up?
4. How can you remember these colours?
5. Why does something appear white?
6. Why does something appear blue?
7. Why does something appear black?
8. What is a primary colour?
9. Name them.
10. What is a secondary colour?
11. Give examples of how they are produced.
12. What are complementary colours?
13. How can we use them in the salon?
14. What type of salon lighting is nearest to daylight?
15. What rule should you remember when matching colours?
16. List the safe working guidelines for colouring.
17. List the ways in which wastage can be minimised.
18. What is responsible for the natural colour of hair?
19. What is grey hair?
20. What is white hair?
21. Can hair go white overnight?
22. What are depth and tone?
23. What is the International Colour Chart System?
24. How are products coded for colour in your salon?
25. What are concentrated tones used for?
26. How are shades charts used to assess colour?
27. Why are clients attracted to certain colours on shade charts?

Lightening hair by bleaching

When the client's natural hair colour is too dark for the target colour, it is necessary to lighten the hair using bleach. Often, a toner is applied after the hair has been pre-lightened to achieve the desired colour, while at other times, it is possible to omit the application of a toner. The word bleaching simply means removal of colour.

Bleaching is a chemical process using products which have a pH of between 8.0 and 10.0, so they are alkaline. If you are unsure of what this means, refer back to Chapter 8 which fully explains pH and the effect that alkaline products have on the hair.

Bleaching hair to the desired depth

If you are pre-lightening the hair in preparation for a toner you will need to lighten the hair exactly to the correct depth so that it acts as the best 'undercoat' for the toner you intend to apply. If you fail to do this, the toner will not achieve the desired target colour. Examples of recommended bleach bases for applying toners are shown in Figure 9.4.

Figure 9.4 Bleach bases and their depths.

	Bleach bases	Corresponding depths
Progressively lighter	reddish	5
	reddish/orange	5–6
	orange/red	5–6
	orange	6–7
	orange/yellow	7–8
	yellow/orange	7–8
	yellow	9
	pale yellow	10
	very pale yellow	10+
	*Destruction of hair!	

How does hydrogen peroxide affect the hair and hair colour?

Bleaches and tints are prepared by mixing them with hydrogen peroxide. Sometimes additional ingredients are also added to bleaches to boost the lightening power of the product.

Hydrogen peroxide is the most common chemical used in hairdressing to provide oxygen. When colouring hair, it is used to lighten the hair's natural pigment and to provide the necessary oxygen for the colorant to work effectively.

Chemically, hydrogen peroxide is similar in structure to water, except that it has an extra oxygen atom which is loosely attached.

$$H_2O \qquad\qquad H_2O_2$$
water   hydrogen peroxide

Hydrogen peroxide is available in different strengths and the higher the strength, the more oxygen will be provided. Strong peroxide can be extremely damaging to the skin and hair. Care should be exercised when working with strong peroxide because it can easily burn the skin and cause irreparable damage to the hair structure. *Never* use a higher strength than the product manufacturers recommend. Many salons use very strong peroxide to mix with bleach because the hair lightens far more quickly. It is true that the hair will lighten a lot faster, but the condition of the hair will suffer as a result. It is far kinder to the hair for a milder bleach mixture to be applied for a longer period, than a strong mixture for a shorter time. If tints are mixed with peroxides that are stronger or weaker than the manufacturers advise, the subtle tones or depth of the colour will be lost.

The strength of peroxide can be described in two ways. You will see that the bottle is marked as showing either a percentage or volume strength. It is important that you know what these readings mean because different manufacturers will label their peroxides in either percentage or volume measurements. If you remember that 3 per cent peroxide is the same as 10 volume it is a very simple method for working out equivalent strengths as shown below:

3 per cent is the same as 10 volume
6 per cent is the same as 20 volume
9 per cent is the same as 30 volume
12 per cent is the same as 40 volume
18 per cent is the same as 60 volume

Volume strength refers to the amount of oxygen that can be released by peroxide. If you had a litre of 20 volume peroxide it could release 20 litres of oxygen. This is why 40 volume peroxide would be considered twice as strong as 20 volume, as it would give off twice as much oxygen. Percentage strength is much more of a chemist's term. It tells you how much of the solution is peroxide, and how much is water. Thus 100 g of a 6 per cent solution contains 6 g of peroxide and 94 g of water (6 + 94 = 100). The strength of liquid peroxide can be checked with an instrument called a peroxometer. This is simply placed in the peroxide in a narrow glass container, and the point on its scale that is against the surface of the peroxide is the strength in either volume or percentage.

Liquid peroxides can be diluted with distilled water if you run out of stock (tap water may cause loss of strength if the peroxide were to be stored). For example, if you had some 40 volume but needed 30 volume, use the following equation to work it out:

A (stronger peroxide) − B (peroxide that you want) = C
Therefore B:C is the ratio to dilute in.

In the example given:

$$40 - 30 = 10$$
$$30:10 \quad \text{(cross off the noughts)}$$
$$3:1$$

Thus if you took 3 measures of 40 volume peroxide and added 1 measure of distilled water, you would have 30 volume peroxide.

Hydrogen peroxide is available in either liquid or cream forms. The liquid types are the same consistency as water and will either be clear (like water) or slightly coloured so that they are a milky colour. Cream peroxides are more expensive than the liquid types because they have added conditioners which help to reduce damage to the hair during the colouring process. Cream peroxides are often preferred by hairdressers because they blend very easily with tints and bleaches. Cream peroxides cannot be accurately diluted like liquid peroxides.

All peroxides are slightly acidic because the addition of acid stabilises the peroxide which helps to prevent it from losing its strength. The acids which are generally used to stabilise peroxides are phosphoric and salicylic acids. Although peroxide will be stabilised, you must still store it properly to prevent it from decomposing. There are three main causes of peroxide going off − dust, alkalis and sunlight.

Guidelines for storing hydrogen peroxide

- Keep containers tightly closed and replace lids as soon as possible.
- Store peroxide in a cool, dark place.
- Measure the amount of peroxide you need but *do not* pour left over peroxide back into the bottle as it could have picked up dust.

What effect do bleaching products have on the hair?

Hydrogen peroxide by itself will lighten the hair but when it is mixed with a bleaching product the lifting power is increased. Bleaches are alkaline and so have the effect of opening the cuticle scales on the outside of the hair shaft. Once the cuticle scales are open, the bleach is able to penetrate the hair and reach the cortex where the natural colour pigment is found. The bleach has no effect on the cuticle other than opening it and making it more porous because the cuticle scales are in fact colourless. However, it is a different story when the bleach reaches the cortex. There are two types of pigment in the cortex and it is differing amounts of these pigments that create the various natural hair colours of individuals. Pheomelanin is the red and yellow pigment and melanin is the black and brown pigment. A person with very dark hair has more melanin than pheomelanin whereas somebody with red hair has more pheomelanin than melanin. An understanding of this concept is important because it will give you an understanding of the way in which bleach lightens hair. Melanin pigment is described as granular, which means the colour molecules are large and spaced out, enabling

Figure 9.5 The lightening effect of bleach on natural pigment.

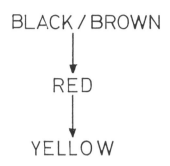

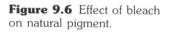

Figure 9.6 Effect of bleach on natural pigment.

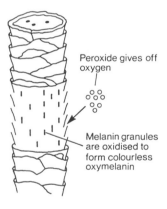

Peroxide gives off oxygen

Melanin granules are oxidised to form colourless oxymelanin

the bleach to reach it easily in the cortex. Pheomelanin, on the other hand, is described as diffuse, meaning that it consists of a larger number of smaller molecules, making it more difficult for the bleach to work on them. This theory explains why naturally red hair is so difficult to bleach to a pale yellow.

If we look at the table in Figure 9.5 which shows the lightening effect of bleach on the hair you will see that it is the black and brown pigment (melanin) which is lost first, followed far more slowly by the red and yellow pigment (pheomelanin). Incidentally, it is *impossible* to bleach the hair to white. We can however create the illusion of white hair by bleaching the hair to a very pale yellow and then applying a toner to subdue the unwanted yellow.

The bleach lightens the natural pigment by changing the melanin granules to a colourless molecule called oxy-melanin. It affects the pheomelanin in a similar way to give oxypheomelanin. Although hairdressers often talk about bleach removing natural pigment, it is not technically taken out of the hair. It simply changes from being a coloured molecule to a colourless molecule. We don't see colour being washed down the plughole when we rinse bleach out of the hair! Figure 9.6 shows how the bleach affects the pigment in the cortex.

Due to the alkalinity and strength of bleaching products oxidation damage to the hair is inevitable. The cuticle will become more porous and the internal structure of the hair will be weaker. This results in the hair shining less (because of the damaged cuticle) and the internal damage will lessen the hair's elasticity and strength. Severe over-bleaching can result in such weakening of the hair that it will actually break off. This is dealt with in the next chapter.

What types of bleaches are available?

Modern bleaches are available as emulsions and powders and both types are mixed with hydrogen peroxide.

Emulsion bleach

This type of bleach is usually made up of three separate parts: oil, hydrogen peroxide and special powder which boosts the release of oxygen, increasing the lightening power of the mixture. The amounts and order of mixing of these ingredients is important and manufacturers' instructions must be precisely followed. The 'boosters' or 'controllers' are sachets of a special powder, usually either potassium persulphate or ammonium persulphate, which are added to control and increase the power of the bleach mixture. (The prefix 'per' before the names of the chemicals simply means they give off oxygen.) Emulsion bleaches have the advantage of being particularly suitable for full head bleaches because they have cooling agents added to help make the bleach feel more comfortable on the scalp. They also have an excellent consistency that helps prevent dripping or drying out and flaking. However, this type of bleach can have the disadvantage of expanding while it is working which results in the product seeping onto areas of the hair that do not require treatment. Next time this type of bleach is used in your salon, take a look at how the remaining bleach left in the bowl expands due to the release of oxygen.

Powder bleaches

Powder bleaches are also made up of three parts although you will only be mixing the powder (which contains two of the parts) with peroxide: the bulk of the powder is magnesium carbonate whose function is to form the paste when you mix the bleach powder with the peroxide. Within the powder there will also be ammonium carbonate which speeds the release of the oxygen from the peroxide. Powder bleaches are mixed to form a smooth paste and either liquid or cream peroxide can be used. It is particularly suitable to use for partial colouring techniques such as highlights because it does not expand quite as much as the emulsion bleach but it can have a tendency to dry out and flake. Powder bleach can be used with equal effect for full head bleaches but it may cause more scalp irritation than bleach which contains cooling agents.

It is interesting to compare the prices of different bleaches and look for reasons that justify varying costs. New product developments have resulted in bleaches having excellent lightening properties combined with a reduction of the ways they can flake or expand during development.

Questions
1. Why do we use bleach to remove colour?
2. What does the word bleach mean?
3. What pH do bleaching products have?
4. Why are they alkaline?
5. Why is it necessary to lighten hair to the correct depth when you apply toners?
6. What is hydrogen peroxide used for?
7. Why must great care be taken when using peroxide?
8. Why should you follow manufacturer's instructions?
9. What strengths is peroxide available in?
10. What do these strengths mean?
11. How would you dilute 40 volume peroxide to 10 volume?
12. How is peroxide available in your salon?
13. Can cream peroxide be accurately diluted?
14. Why is it kinder to the hair?
15. What are the rules to follow for storing peroxide?
16. Why is melanin described as granular while pheomelanin is described as diffuse?
17. In what order does bleaching occur?
18. What happens to the pigment in bleaching?
19. Is the pigment lost from the hair?

20. How much damage can be caused to the hair?
21. What are boosters?
22. What are the advantages and disadvantages of emulsion bleaches?
23. What two chemicals are found in powder bleach?
24. What do you use powder bleaches for in your salon?

Application techniques

There are three main application techniques for bleach which are:

- full head (all the hair, as for a first time bleach application);
- regrowth (the newly grown hair since the last application);
- partial head (highlights).

Virgin hair application (full head)

Bleaching all the hair for the first time is often time-consuming and there are different techniques to be used for long and short hair. However, it is not difficult to perform. The anxiety that many hairdressers have about carrying this out has to do with the worry that the client won't accept the drastic colour change. If you fully discuss the expected result with your client before you start, this will minimise both your client's and your own uncertainty. Also, remember that you can get an idea of what it will look like by taking a test cutting [see Chapter 2]. Remember that it is quite usual for clients to be a little apprehensive when having a colour change. You will therefore need to be reassuring and display confidence in what you are doing. Saying things like 'I think it will look all right' or 'I hope you like it' are not positive statements and will do nothing to build confidence. Be positive in what you say by saying things like 'This will look really good on you' and 'You're going to love how it will look'.

Application for hair shorter than 20 cms

When bleaching hair for the first time, the sequence for the application is always carried out so that the bleach is applied to the middle lengths and ends of the hair before the roots. This may seem a little odd, but if you consider how heat will speed up the development of bleach, you will appreciate that if the roots are treated first, they will lighten more quickly than the rest of the hair because of the warmth from the head, resulting in an uneven colour result.

Preparation

1. Gown and protect your client. Protect yourself by wearing an overall or apron and rubber or plastic gloves.
2. Mix the bleach according to the manufacturer's instructions.

3. Divide the hair into four main sections (forehead to nape and from ear to ear across the crown) and secure with clips.

Application (first stage)

4. Beginning at the base of one of the back sections, part off a horizontal mesh of hair that is no deeper than 1 cm and clip the remaining hair in the section out of your way. Lay the mesh of hair across the palm of your hand as shown in Figure 9.7 and apply the bleach to within 2–3 cms of the scalp *only*.
Place a narrow strip of cotton wool along the root area where there is no bleach and part off your next mesh. (The cotton wool stops any of the bleach touching the roots at this stage.)
5. Continue working up the head towards the crown until all of that back section is finished. Repeat this on the other back section.
6. When the back is completed, begin parting your meshes on one of the forward sections. Work towards the front hairline and take care to avoid any bleach dripping or splashing into the client's eyes. Repeat this on the other side, completing the first stage of this application at the front hairline.

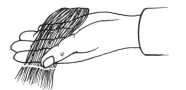

Figure 9.7 Position for applying bleach to middle lengths and ends.

Development

7. Allow the bleach to develop until you can see that half the degree of lift required is achieved. This means visually checking the hair by taking a strand test to check how much the hair has lightened. If the target colour is six shades lighter than the client's natural base colour, allow the hair to lighten only three shades before you move onto the second stage of the application.

Application (second stage)

8. *Mix fresh bleach* of the same strength and remove the cotton wool strips that were used to keep the bleach off the roots. Apply the bleach to the root area following the same pattern that you used for the initial application (i.e. starting at the nape). As you apply the bleach to the roots, also refresh bleach that is already on the middle lengths and ends by applying some of the new bleach over the top. You need to do this to ensure that the bleach on the middle lengths and ends has the necessary lightening power. Cross-check your application to ensure that all the hair is treated with the bleach.

Final development

9. Develop the bleach until the hair has lightened and check this by visually testing hair on several areas of the head.

Removal

10. Using tepid water, thoroughly flush the bleach out of the hair and then gently shampoo the hair. You may want to use a toner on the hair to achieve the desired colour or alternatively leave the hair the colour that has been achieved by the bleach.

Bleaching hair longer than 20 cms

When bleaching hair which is longer than 20 cms for the first time a different sequence has to be followed to ensure an even colour result. This is because the differing degrees of porosity along the hair's length will affect how quickly the bleach will lighten the hair. The older the hair, the more porous it will be because it has been subjected to more wear and tear. This means that the ends of the hair are the most porous (because they are the oldest) and will therefore be more receptive to the bleach than the less porous areas. Porous hair has a damaged and open cuticle which allows chemicals to penetrate the hair shaft more quickly than hair with a closed cuticle. Although the root area will not be porous because it is the newest, freshly keratinised hair, remember that the warmth of the head will mean the roots will lift quickly in comparison to the hair further away from this heat source. The middle lengths of the hair will be most resistant to bleaching so it stands to reason that this is the area that will require the longest development and is therefore where the application is begun. The order for the bleach application on this length of hair is shown in Figure 9.8.

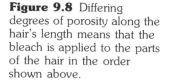
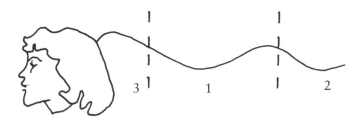

Figure 9.8 Differing degrees of porosity along the hair's length means that the bleach is applied to the parts of the hair in the order shown above.

Preparation

1. Gown and protect your client. Protect yourself by wearing an overall or apron and wear rubber or plastic gloves.
2. Mix the bleach according to the manufacturer's instructions.
3. Divide the hair into the four main sections and secure these with clips.

Application (first stage)

4. Starting at the nape as you would for shorter hair, apply the bleach to the *middle lengths* (number 1 in Figure 9.8) of the hair only to within 2 cm of the scalp.

Development

5. Allow this to develop until half the degree of lift is achieved. Remember that you will need to visually check the hair at regular intervals.

Application (second stage)

6. Apply the bleach to the ends of the hair then mix fresh bleach for the roots.
7. Apply the bleach to the root area and refresh the bleach already on the middle lengths and ends. Cross-check your application to ensure all the hair is treated with the bleach.

Development

8. Allow the hair to develop until the desired degree of lift is achieved. Before the bleach is rinsed out of the hair, do check that the hair is sufficiently lightened by taking strand tests in several areas.
9. Using tepid water, flush all traces of the bleach out of the hair. It can then be gently shampooed.
10. You may want to apply a toner to achieve the target colour or leave the hair in this pre-lightened state.

Bleaching a regrowth

This service is carried out on hair that has been bleached before and the purpose of the client's visit is to match the newly grown hair (the regrowth) to the colour of the rest of the hair. Obviously, this is not as time-consuming as a virgin application.

Preparation

1. Gown and protect your client. Protect yourself by wearing an overall or apron and plastic or rubber gloves.
2. Mix the bleach according to the manufacturer's instructions.
3. Divide the hair into the four main sections and secure with clips.

Application

4. Starting at the nape, apply the bleach to the *regrowth only* following the same pattern as you would for the applications described earlier.
5. When you finish your application at the front hairline you should cross-check your application to ensure all the hair has been treated with the bleach.

Development

6. Develop the hair until sufficient lift is achieved, visually checking at frequent intervals by doing strand tests in several areas of the head.

Removal

7. Once the roots are developed, use tepid water to flush all traces of bleach from the hair before gently shampooing.

8. You may want to apply a toner or leave the hair in this pre-lightened state.

Application of bleach for highlights

Highlighting is a method of colouring selected strands of hair (the highlights) as opposed to all the hair. This is a popular colouring technique because the client will not need to return to the salon every 4−6 weeks to have the regrowth bleached as the effect is far more natural and the new hair that grows is not so apparent as a full head bleach.

The two main techniques for highlighting are:

Figure 9.9 Easi-Meche method of highlighting. (Courtesy L'Oréal.)

- weaving out the highlights and wrapping the hair in foil or Easi-Meche;
- pulling the strands to be bleached through a rubber highlighting cap or plastic bag. These highlighting techniques are shown in Figures 9.9 to 9.12.

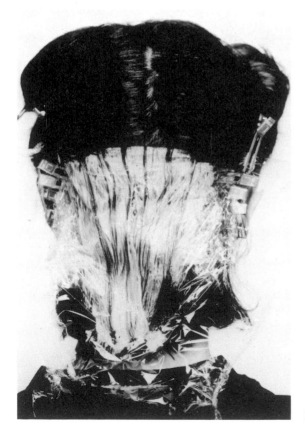

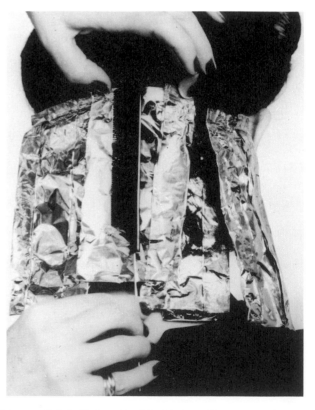

Figure 9.10 Foil method highlights. (Courtesy L'Oréal.)

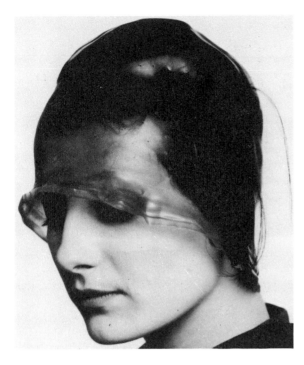

Figure 9.11 Cap method highlights. (Courtesy L'Oréal.)

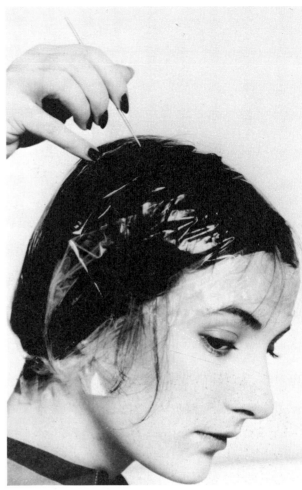

Figure 9.12 Plastic bag method highlights. (Courtesy L'Oréal.)

Questions
1. What are the three main types of application for bleaching?
2. Why is it important to talk to the client before a full head bleach?
3. Describe the method of application for short hair.
4. How do you check development?
5. How is the bleach removed?
6. Describe the application for longer hair.
7. Describe the application for a regrowth.
8. What advantage have highlights?
9. What different techniques are there for highlighting?

Colouring hair with temporary colorants

Temporary colours are colorants which have an instant result because they do not require a development time to see the resultant colour. They are available in several forms, the most common being coloured setting lotions, mousses and sprays. This type of colorant is designed to last until the hair is next shampooed so is an excellent means of introducing a colour-shy client to hair colour. What can possibly be easier than using a coloured mousse on a client's hair for an instant colour change, which might lead to a more permanent form of colouring that will boost the salon's turnover? Also, temporary colorants have proved to be a profitable retail commodity that is easy and safe for the client to use at home between salon visits.

What types of temporary colorants are available?

Temporary colours are available in the following forms:

- setting lotions;
- mousses;
- sprays;
- crayons;
- concentrated rinses;
- gels;
- liquid 'paints'.

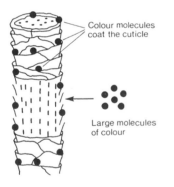

Figure 9.13 Effect of a temporary colour on the hair shaft.

Colour molecules coat the cuticle

Large molecules of colour

What are the effects of temporary colorants on the hair?

Temporary colours are ready for use and are quick and easy to apply for instant colour changes. They contain large coloured molecules which cannot penetrate the hair shaft, unless the hair is particularly porous, resulting in an open cuticle. Due to the size of the coloured molecules, they are only able to lodge themselves in the cuticle, hence they are easily removed the next time the hair is shampooed. The ingredients of temporary colours range from methylene blue to azo dyes. Figure 9.13 shows how a temporary colour adheres to the cuticle.

Temporary colorants cannot lighten the hair but can change the tone and darken the hair. However, having said they can't lighten the hair you may come across temporary colorants called 'brighteners' which will gradually lighten the hair with continuous use. These brighteners contain weak hydrogen peroxide, that have a similar effect as the sun does on the hair. They should only be used on hair which is light brown or lighter.

How are temporary colorants applied?

Temporary colorants are easy to apply and will not require mixing unless they are only available in a concentrated form, which requires the addition of water. The colorant does not need to be developed to see the colour change, but it should be applied evenly to prevent patchy results, or staining of the scalp or skin around the hairline. Most temporary colorants can be applied to the hair with good effect directly from the container, although you may need to vary this according to the type of colorant you are using, the effect you are aiming to achieve and the hair type of your client.

Porous hair is always the most difficult hair type on which to achieve even colour results because the damage, which is uneven on the hair's length, allows colorants to be absorbed at irregular rates. If you are applying a coloured setting lotion to porous hair (such as highly bleached hair) improved results can be achieved by using a tint brush to apply the lotion. The setting lotion is put into a bowl and is applied in the same manner as a tint is applied, making narrow sections and using the tint brush to ensure an even application.

When applying temporary colorants which are in the form of a lotion or mousse, the hair must be towel-dried after shampooing to ensure that the colour will not be diluted by excess moisture in the hair. Conversely, if the hair is too dry, the resultant colour might be too intense. Coloured mousse is easy to apply. The container should be given a good shake and then, pointing the nozzle downwards, the required amount is squirted into the palm of your hand. By spreading the mousse between both hands, it can then be evenly distributed through the hair. Alternatively, the mousse can be squirted onto a vent brush or comb so that by drawing the brush or comb through the hair the mousse is applied evenly.

There are temporary colorants that are only applied when the hair is styled and dry. These include coloured sprays, crayons, gels and paints. Care needs to be taken when applying colour to the finished style because it is very easy to get carried away and apply too much. If this happens, the hair will need to be shampooed to remove the colour. When applying spray colorants, do remember that it is far more difficult to control where the colour ends up because aerosols emit the colour at a wide angle. This makes it hard to confine the application to small areas and parts of the hair that do not require coloration will need to be protected by your free (gloved!) hand or a piece of tissue. Also, if the spray is held too close to the hair, the hair will become wet and separate into strands. Gels are easily applied with the fingers while paints usually have a brush for ease of application similar to that used for nail varnish. Crayons are simply stroked against the areas of hair to be coloured, allowing for maximum control of where the colour is placed.

Questions
1. What are temporary colours?
2. How long do they last?
3. Why are they a good way of introducing colour to a client?
4. In what forms are they available?
5. How do they work?

6. What chemicals are found in them?
7. How are the different types applied?
8. Why do temporary colours not work so well on porous hair?

Colouring hair using semi-permanent colorants

Semi-permanent colorants last longer than temporary colours because they are allowed to develop on the hair, during which time they partly penetrate the cortex. They last on average between six to eight shampoos (six is an average) and usually impart a shine to the hair because they contain conditioning agents.

What types of semi-permanent colorants are available?

Semi-permanent colours are available in the following forms:

- liquids;
- creams;
- mousses.

They contain chemicals such as nitro-phenylenediamine and anthraquinones, but some also contain the paraphenylenediamine found in tints. If they contain para-dyes, a skin test should be given.

What effect do semi-permanents have on the hair shaft?

Semi-permanent colorants do not give an instant colour change like temporary colours. They need to be left on the hair to develop for between 5 and 30 minutes after which they are rinsed from the hair. The colour molecules of a semi-permanent are smaller than those contained in temporary colorants and during the development time, these molecules partly penetrate the cortex via the cuticle scales. This ability to enter the hair shaft results in the colour lasting longer and it can stay on the hair for anything between four to eight shampoos. Most semi-permanent colorants have built-in conditioning agents to add shine as well as colour to the hair so are easy to sell to clients. Each time the hair is shampooed, some of the colour is lost and gradually fades with each shampoo. Therefore, this type of colouring is not permanent as it does not chemically change the internal structure of the hair. Recent developments by manufacturers have resulted in a new type of semi-permanent colorant that has a superior durability which can last up to 15 shampoos. The lasting power of semi-permanents is usually achieved by adding small quantities of para compound (the substance contained in permanent tints).

Semi-permanents cannot lighten the hair but can change the tone and make the hair darker. Usually, they can only cover up to 40 per cent white hair (this means that about 4 in 10 hairs are white) and more vibrant colour results are achieved on lighter hair. If the hair is porous, results may not be even due to the erratic way in which the hair will

Figure 9.14 How a semi-permanent colour affects the hair.

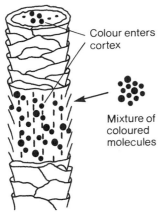

Colour enters cortex

Mixture of coloured molecules

absorb the colorant. Also, results on porous hair will last longer because the open cuticle permits easy penetration for the colour molecules. If you are in doubt of a colour result take a test cutting first.

If you look at Figure 9.14 the diagram shows how semi-permanents work on the hair.

How are semi-permanent colorants applied?

Semi-permanent colorants are either applied to dry, unwashed hair, or to shampooed, towel-dried hair, so always check the manufacturer's instructions.

Semi-permanent colorants are usually applied to hair that has been shampooed and towel-dried. Shampooing will not only remove dirt, oil and other debris from the hair but will also help to open the cuticle which enables the colorant to penetrate the hair shaft. Towel-drying the hair after it has been shampooed will remove any excess moisture that could dilute the effect of the colorant.

Many semi-permanent colorants can be applied to the hair directly from the bottle or tube while others may need to be applied with either a tint brush or sponge from a bowl, or from an applicator flask. Whichever application technique is used, it is important that you apply the colorant evenly so that the result is not patchy.

Application techniques

- Applying directly from bottle, tube or applicator flask.
- Applying colour with a brush or sponge from a bowl.

You will only be able to apply the colorant directly from the tube or bottle if there is no need to mix two shades of the colorant together. You would not achieve satisfactory results if you attempted to mix the colours together once they are on the client's hair! If it is necessary to mix the colorant, you could use an applicator flask to measure the amounts of the product you need and then, placing your finger over the opening of the nozzle, give it a shake to blend the colorants together. Most manufacturers are aware that many hairdressers prefer to apply the colorant directly from the product container so they put nozzles on the bottles and tubes to make the application easier. The application begins at the nape where the hair is least receptive, and it is evenly applied from the roots to the points. Gentle massage and combing with a wide-toothed comb will ensure the colorant is evenly distributed. The colour is then allowed to develop for the time recommended by the manufacturer. The development time can be anything between 5 and 45 minutes depending on the type of product you are using. The instructions may suggest that the client's head is covered with a plastic cap during the development to help the colour work more quickly. Some manufacturers may suggest that you place the client under a hood dryer or other form of heat, which will assist the colour molecules in penetrating the hair shaft. If you do put a plastic cap over the hair during processing, put a strip of cotton wool around the hairline to prevent any drips from staining the client's skin. A light smear of barrier cream on the hairline will help to keep the cotton wool strip in place. The cap should be secured so that it keeps in the body heat given off by the head, so it is usually necessary to take up the loose excess of the cap at the nape of the neck and secure this in a twist with a clip.

If you use a tint brush or sponge to apply the colorant, you will be applying it from a bowl. The brush or sponge is dipped into the colorant and then it is applied to the hair. Just as for other application techniques, the nape area is treated first, gradually working up towards the front hairline by making narrow partings. The hair is then combed through with a wide-toothed comb before it is left to develop.

There may be times when you need to apply a semi-permanent to certain areas of the hair only, in which case your application will need to be selective, applying the colorant only to the parts that need colouring. If, for example, a client was growing out a permanent tint and wanted her regrowth to be less noticeable, you might suggest that a semi-permanent is applied to the middle lengths and ends to disguise the obvious demarcation line between the coloured hair and the regrowth. In such an instance, the semi-permanent would not be applied to the roots. At other times you may want to colour a certain area of the head such as the front, for which the hair needing coloration is divided, and the rest of the hair secured out of the way using clips. Whichever application technique you use, always try to keep the semi-permanent off the skin and scalp to prevent unnecessary staining.

Semi-permanents can be removed by repeated shampooing or by using old-fashioned soap shampoos which are alkaline and open the cuticle more.

Questions
1. Why do semi-permanents last longer than temporary colours?
2. In what forms are they available?
3. How long do they last?
4. What chemicals are found in them?
5. Is a skin test required?
6. How do they affect the hair?
7. What coverage of white hair can be achieved?
8. How are semi-permanents applied?
9. How do you protect the client's skin?
10. When would heat be used?
11. What is a selective application?
12. How are semi-permanents removed?

Colouring hair using permanent (para) tints

Before applying a tint to a client's hair a skin test must be done to determine if the client is allergic to the para compounds contained in this type of colorant (refer to Chapter 2 for skin test procedure). There is a very wide colour choice and this type of coloration is permanent, which means that the client will need to return to the salon every four to six weeks for the regrowth to be treated.

The use of tints can lighten, darken, cover white hair and change the tone of natural hair colour, giving the client and hairdresser a wide range of colouring options. Although manufacturers may produce about thirty to fifty shades in a particular range of tints, they can be intermixed (within the range) to produce customised colours for individual clients.

What types of permanent (para) tint are available?

There are three main types of tints available today:

- oil-based (bottle);
- cream (tube);
- oil/cream emulsion (bottle/tube).

Oil-based tints come in a liquid form and when they are mixed with hydrogen peroxide they thicken to a gel-like consistency that will not run when it is applied to the hair. This type of tint tends to give a more transluscent colour result than cream tints but is sometimes unable to cover resistant white hair completely.

Cream tints come in the form of a thick cream in a tube. They are more difficult to blend with hydrogen peroxide because of their thick consistency but will usually be able to cover successfully quite resistant white hair. Cream tints have a tendency to produce a less transluscent result because of their effective covering properties but many hairdressers will claim that the tenacity of the colour means that the hair will resist fading, resulting in a more durable result.

Cream emulsions can be described as having the covering properties of cream tints combined with the translucency that oil-based tints produce. They have all the advantages of cream tints but mix into a cross between a gel and a cream, giving the hairdresser an excellent consistency of product with which to work.

Tints are chemical substances which contain ingredients such as para-phenylenediamine, para-toluenediamine or meta dyes such as meta-dihydroxybenzene. It is these chemical substances that some people will be allergic to, so a skin test must precede the application of tint to ensure it is safe to use this type of tint.

Within a particular manufacturer's range of tints, special lightening tints and concentrated shades might be included. The tints that have special lightening properties are usually only suitable for hair that is dark blonde or lighter. Trying to use one of these on hair which is darker than this will result in disappointing colours that are not light enough nor have the anticipated tone. They have a limited effect because their lightening power is capable of lifting up to only four shades on a relatively light natural base.

Concentrated colours are excellent for increasing the tonal vibrance of a tint to achieve the desired target colour. They need to be carefully and accurately measured (usually in very small amounts) and blended with the tint before the peroxide is added to the mixture. They are available in strong, vibrant tones which include concentrated ash, copper, red, gold and mauve.

What is the effect of para tints on the hair?

Although the tints we use today are superior when compared to earlier developments in terms of performance and ingredients, they still have a tendency to affect the condition of the hair, making it more porous. This is because the tint has to open the protective cuticle scales on the hair shaft to be able to penetrate the cortex, where the hair's natural pigment is found. The tint contains small colourless molecules which develop their colour when mixed with hydrogen peroxide. The small colourless molecules are oxidised to form large coloured molecules, which can be trapped in the cortex. The molecules of colour do not swell up, as many hairdressers insist, otherwise there would never be a loss of colour! Because red molecules are smallest, it is usually the red in a tint that is lost first, resulting in fade. The effect on the hair is shown Figure 9.15.

Figure 9.15 The effects of a tint on the hair.

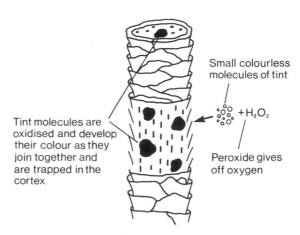

Small colourless molecules of tint

$+H_2O_2$

Tint molecules are oxidised and develop their colour as they join together and are trapped in the cortex

Peroxide gives off oxygen

How are tints mixed?

Tints are not ready for use because they have to be mixed with hydrogen peroxide. The amount and strength of the peroxide will be given in the manufacturer's instructions, and because this can vary between product ranges, always refer to the instructions if you are not familiar with a particular type of tint. However, the majority of tints are mixed with equal parts of hydrogen peroxide. That means in the ratio of 1:1. For example:

30 mls of tint + 30 mls of H_2O_2, *or*
60 mls of tint + 60 mls of H_2O_2

Sometimes the instructions may tell you to mix the tint with the hydrogen peroxide in the ratio of 2:1. For example:

30 mls of tint + 60 mls of H_2O_2

Never ignore the manufacturer's instructions telling you how their tints should be mixed. Tints are a delicate balance and combination of artificial pigments that require careful mixing to perform as intended by the manufacturers to produce the best results.

If you are using a tube of tint, you will notice that the tube is marked with a dotted or continuous line half way down to show you how much you would need to squeeze out if only half the contents of the tube was required. This is helpful to the hairdresser because you may want to mix two shades of tint together. Tubes should always be squeezed from the bottom to avoid wastage and there are special keys available that not only empty the tube more effectively but also help you to achieve accurate measurements, especially if you only want a quarter of the tube.

When mixing a full tube of tint, squeeze the entire contents into a bowl. Pour out the amount of hydrogen peroxide as recommended by the manufacturers into a measure. It is important that the amount of hydrogen peroxide is measured accurately and the best way of making sure you do this properly is to place the measure on a shelf which is level to your eyes. If this is not possible, you should hold the measure so that it is level with your eyes as shown in Figure 9.16. If you look down onto a measure to check the amount you have poured into it, you will get a false reading.

It is easier to blend tint with the hydrogen peroxide if the peroxide is added gradually rather than poured into the bowl all in one go. While the peroxide is gradually added, the mixture is blended by stirring with a tint brush. If two different shades of tint are being used, it is advisable to blend these together with your brush before the peroxide is added.

Tints that come in bottles do not usually have markings on the outside like tube tints, but the amount that the bottle contains will be printed on the label. Tint bottles are usually dark to protect the contents from becoming affected by light, so it is tricky to get an accurate measurement if you only require a half or quarter of the bottle's contents. Therefore it is advisable to pour the liquid tint into a measure when anything other than the full bottle is required. If you do need to use the whole of the bottle and the tint is to be mixed with the peroxide in a ratio of 1:1, the tint is emptied into a bowl and then the bottle refilled with peroxide to give the correct amount.

Tints should be mixed just before they are needed so that they can be left to stand for a couple of minutes to allow the mixture to stabilise.

Can tints be intermixed within a product range?

Once you are familiar with the coding system (ICC) of the tint range you are using in the salon, you will be able to intermix colours to make your colour choice wider and to help you if you discover that a particular shade is out of stock.

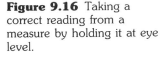

Figure 9.16 Taking a correct reading from a measure by holding it at eye level.

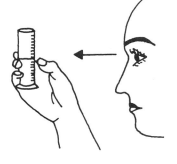

Tints which are of the same tone can be intermixed to make a different depth. For example:

Half 6/1 + half 8/1 = 7/1
Half 7/03 + half 9/03 = 8/03

What would the following mixes make?

Half 4/0 + half 6/0 =
Half 5/01 + half 7/01 =
Half 3/0 + half 5/0 =

Notice that you can only accurately mix shades which are only two depths apart. It is *not* recommended to try mixing shades that are more than two depths apart (e.g. half 4/0 + half 7/0) as results cannot be accurately estimated.

There are certain intermixes which are not suitable simply because the delicate tones contained in the tints would be lost. If an ash tint was to be mixed with a copper tint, neither tones in the tints would be shown to their best advantage in the final result. Therefore, it is advisable to read the manufacturers' literature concerning their products so that you are knowledgeable about the tint's performance and limitations. All tint manufacturers have training centres where short courses are run to help familiarise hairdressers with their particular products. Such courses are invaluable for an in-depth colour awareness, especially for those who may wish to specialise in the field of hair colouring.

Application techniques for tint

There are three main methods of application for tint which are:

- regrowth application;
- full head application (virgin hair);
- partial colouring (lowlights, block colouring, etc.).

Tint is always applied to dry, unwashed hair except when it is applied as a toner after pre-lightening with a bleach, when it is applied to towel-dried hair. The reason for omitting the shampoo before applying a tint is that the body's natural oil (sebum) helps to protect the hair and scalp from the chemicals contained in tints. Also, the action of shampooing has a tendency to stimulate the scalp, bringing the blood to the surface of the skin, making the scalp more sensitive to the tint. There might be the odd occasion when you will need to shampoo the hair before the hair is tinted but such instances will be rare. Pre-shampooing is only necessary when the hair is so heavily coated with oil or styling products (such as gel or pomade) that the tint would be unable to penetrate this barrier. A single application of shampoo, cool water and minimal massage is used if pre-shampooing is necessary. After the shampoo, the hair would need to be dried before the tint was applied.

Whichever application technique you are using, you should work in a neat, speedy and competent manner. Applying a tint for a regrowth application should not be a lengthy procedure and we would estimate that it should take no longer than twenty minutes for an average head of hair with a 1 cm regrowth.

Regrowth application

When tinting a regrowth you will be working on hair which has been tinted before, and the client will want the newly grown hair coloured to match the existing colour on the middle lengths and ends. If the client is a regular visitor to your salon, there will be a record card that tells you which tint should be applied and the length of the development time. This card should be referred to and the client should be consulted to determine whether any changes need to be made to the formula *before* the tint is mixed. If the client is new to your salon, you will need to carry out an analysis of the hair to determine which products will produce the desired target colour.

> N.B. A tint should not be applied unless the client has been given a skin test to determine whether or not they are allergic to the chemicals contained in this type of colorant.

Figure 9.17 Hair divided into four main sections in preparation for a regrowth tint application.

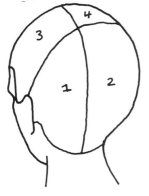

Application techniques will vary between salons due to personal preference, so we have chosen to describe one of the most commonly used methods.

Method

1. Divide the hair into four main sections from the front hairline to the nape and from ear to ear across the crown as shown in Figure 9.17. Each section is then secured with clips.
2. Beginning at the nape, apply the tint *to the regrowth area only* up to the crown where the partings form a cross.
3. Start making narrow, horizontal partings at the nape area of one of the back sections which are not deeper than 1 cm and apply the tint carefully to the regrowth. Continue taking these narrow sections, applying the tint as you progress up to the crown as shown in Figure 9.18.
4. This procedure is repeated on the other back section.
5. The two front sections can then be treated, but instead of using horizontal partings, the hair is parted so that the hair is always held back from the face, so that the chances of the tint dripping or splashing into the client's eyes are reduced.
6. After applying the tint to the regrowth, your application needs to be cross-checked to ensure that no area has been missed. This is done by taking narrow partings in an *opposite* direction to the way you parted the hair to apply the tint. In other words, where you made horizontal partings for the hair at the back, it is cross-checked by taking vertical partings. Any area you notice that has been missed is covered with the tint during the cross-checking.

Figure 9.18 Making 1 cm partings from the nape up to the crown to apply the tint to

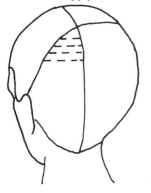

Development

The tint is then left to develop either naturally or with the aid of additional heat provided by an infra red appliance such as a Climazon. Using additional heat accelerates the development time, reducing it by 50 per cent. However, you will need to check the product instructions to ensure whether the acceleration of the development time is recommended by the manufacturer. Do not cover the hair with a plastic cap or towel because these would smudge the tint you have carefully applied onto areas of the hair other than the regrowth. If no additional heat is used, the normal development time for the roots will be about 20−30 minutes.

Once the roots are developed, the hairdresser needs to check whether the tint requires to be combed through onto the middle lengths and ends. This is only necessary when the previously tinted hair has faded and requires to be refreshed to restore lost colour. The best way to determine if combing through is necessary is to scrape off some tint from the roots using the back of a comb, and compare the newly tinted regrowth with the colour of the ends. If there is an obvious degree of colour difference, the tint will need to be taken through to the ends to achieve an even colour result.

Combing through

If tint is to be applied to the previously coloured hair that has faded, the remaining tint in the bowl is usually diluted with equal parts of warm water. The addition of the water dilutes the strength of the peroxide in the tint mixture so that it acts more as a semi-permanent than a tint, restoring the lost colour. Depending on the degree of fade, the diluted tint is left on the hair for 5 to 15 minutes before it is rinsed.

Important points to remember when tinting a regrowth

1. Apply plenty of product.
2. Narrow (1 cm) partings ensure complete coverage of the regrowth area.
3. Do not overlap the tint onto the previously coloured hair as this can cause 'banding'. A darker line appears where this has happened.
4. Avoid dabbing on the tint − lay the product onto the hair.
5. Do not apply tint unnecessarily to the neck, ears or other areas of skin. We are in the business of colouring the hair *not* the skin!

Before a tint is removed, the hairdresser should check that the colour result is even along the hair shaft. This check is made by doing a strand test which is fully explained in Chapter 2. Refer to Chapter 4 for an explanation of how tints are removed from the hair after their development.

Application of tint to a full head (virgin hair)

Virgin hair is hair that has not been treated with chemicals. This term is also used to describe hair that may have been given a perm or a semi-permanent colour but has not been subjected to a process involving colouring chemicals penetrating the hair shaft and altering the internal composition of the cortex.

It is a major decision for a client to opt for a complete colour change that will be permanent and require regular visits to the salon to maintain its appearance. Understandably, many clients will need reassurance from their hairdresser during the colouring procedure and need to have confidence about what is being done to their hair. The first-time tint application takes longer to carry out than a regrowth application because the effect of body heat needs to be taken into account, requiring a different application procedure. Heat given off by the scalp helps to speed up the development of tints. The middle lengths and ends of a head of hair do not receive this body heat because they are too far away from the heat source. It therefore stands to reason that if the tint were applied straight through the entire length of the hair from roots to points and left to develop, the hair nearest the scalp would develop more quickly than the hair which is further away from the heat. To enable the hair to develop so that the end result is evenly coloured throughout its length, the tint is applied and partly developed on the middle lengths and ends *before* it is applied to the roots.

Method

1. Divide the hair into four main sections as you would for a regrowth application.
2. Beginning at the nape, make 1 cm horizontal partings and apply the tint to the middle lengths and ends of the hair *only* within 1–2 cms of the scalp.
3. When the tint has been applied to all the hair *except* the root area, leave the hair to develop for *half* the time recommended by the product manufacturer.
4. When this time is up, *mix fresh tint* and apply to the root area, refreshing the tint that has already been applied to the middle lengths and ends.
5. Allow the hair to develop for the *full development* time.

Partial application techniques using tint

Today, there are many different ways of applying tint to specific areas of the hair to produce subtle or dramatic effects. Such techniques are used to add interest and emphasis to particular haircuts and will help to introduce the colour-shy client to experiment. For more information about these techniques please see our book, *Colouring – A Salon Handbook* for some stimulating ideas on fashion colouring techniques.

Questions

 1. What tests should be carried out prior to tinting?
 2. Why must clients who have their hair tinted return to the salon?
 3. What can be achieved using tints?
 4. In what forms are tints available?
 5. What are the advantages and disadvantages of each type?
 6. What type of hair are lightening tints most frequently used on?
 7. What are concentrated colours?
 8. How do tints affect the hair?
 9. How is tint mixed in your salon for different ranges?
10. What are the rules for mixing tint?
11. Get someone to test you on mixing tints to obtain different depths.
12. What are the main methods of application for tints?
13. Is shampooing necessary before application?
14. Describe a regrowth application in steps.
15. When is a tint combed through?
16. How is this done?
17. Describe a full head application in steps.
18. When would partial colouring be carried out?

Colour correction

There are only three corrections you can make to hair colour:

- changing the tone;
- darkening;
- lightening.

In this section we will be dealing with all of these possible changes but feel we should point out that some of the techniques described are really for the more experienced colourist and should not be attempted by a novice unless they are under close supervision. Therefore, we will not be going into each technique in depth but offer an overview of what each corrective colouring technique involves. However, it is important that all staff have a knowledge of these treatments so that they are able to converse with their clients on a professional level about colour correction and be in the position to offer sound advise. We suggest that you refer to our book *Colouring — A Salon Handbook* for an in-depth explanation of colour correction which includes several case studies.

The most limiting factor to all chemical processes carried out in the salon is the condition of the client's hair. The hair may not be strong enough to withstand further chemical treatment, in which case *do not carry out the service*. There are many hairdressers who can recall an instance when they knew that they should not have given a particular service because of the condition of the hair they were working on, but did do it because the client seemed really insistent. They will look back with a mixture of regret and guilt because they now realise they should have trusted their own professional judgement rather than end up with a head of hair that is completely out of condition and lifeless.

The analysis that precedes colour correction will take time to explain fully and discuss the options open to the client. There may be restrictions other than the condition of the hair, such as the time it will take to do, the cost of the service or the necessary after-care. It is also worth remembering that it could just be a client's personal whim and that they might want it changed back to their original colour the following day!

Colour correction is a matter of deciding:

- the problem you are faced with;
- the new target colour;
- if necessary, how to achieve that colour on the regrowth;
- how to achieve that colour on the already coloured hair.

Table 9.1 gives some common problems and their solutions.

Table 9.1	What is the problem?
Problem	Solution
Hair too light.	Restore colour.
Hair too dark.	Remove colour.
Wrong tone.	Neutralise colour or clean out.

Restoring lost colour

Pre-pigmentation is the term used to describe restoring lost pigment to pale hair that needs to be made darker or warmer. A typical example of the need to pre-pigmentate would be that of a client whose hair has been bleached and now wishes it to go darker or back to the natural colour. The bleach will have removed the warm pigments from the hair by changing them to oxymelanin and oxypheomelanin and these pigments must be restored for the hair to be successfully coloured to a darker shade. If the lost pigment is not replaced, the new colour will look flat and might even take on a greenish appearance!

Both semi-permanent colorants and tints can be used to restore lost pigment but in the case of using tint, it is *not* mixed with peroxide before it is applied. Instead, it is mixed with a little water. Only a very small amount of product is used to pre-pigmentate, as set out below:

Using cream tint as a pre-colour − 12 cms of colour + 15 mls of water
Liquid tint as a pre-colour − 2−4 capfuls of colour + 2−4 capfuls of water.

The pre-colour is applied to the faded areas *sparingly*, avoiding any regrowth. It can either be applied with a tint brush or a small damp sponge. The pre-colour must be applied carefully and combed through to distribute it evenly. The client is then placed underneath a hood dryer to dry the pre-colour, which helps it to 'lock' into the hair. The tint that has been chosen to achieve the target colour is then applied directly on top of the pre-colour, having been mixed in the normal way by adding peroxide.

If the hair you are working on is particularly porous and pale, you will notice that the pre-colour is absorbed by the hair very quickly. Do not think your application is wrong if the pre-colour gradually fades as you are working; this is the result of the colour penetrating the hair.

Removing artificial pigment from the hair

Product manufacturers have developed bleach to lighten natural hair pigment while the removal or lightening of artificial pigment (e.g. tint) requires the use of a special product called a colour stripper or colour reducer. *It is impossible to lighten already tinted hair by the application of a lighter tint over the top.* As you will have read earlier on in this chapter, bleaching is an oxidation process. Colour strippers work differently from bleach because they involve a reduction process which breaks up the tint molecules that have been deposited in the hair. The large colour molecules deposited during the tinting process are reduced in size by the stripper until they are small enough to escape through the cuticle where they are rinsed from the hair. Colour stripping is explained in Figure 9.19.

Figure 9.19 Stripping of colour by reduction.

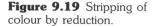
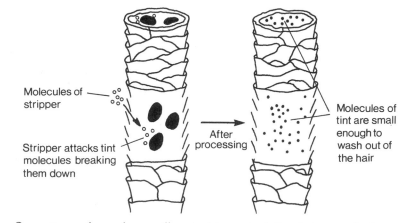

Molecules of stripper

Stripper attacks tint molecules breaking them down

After processing

Molecules of tint are small enough to wash out of the hair

Sometimes the colour will not strip out of the hair evenly because tints are a mixture of red, yellow and black molecules and the red molecules, being the smallest, may be left behind. Depending on the result the stripper leaves, you may need to make a second application to the more stubborn areas. A stripper will always work more quickly on the more porous parts of the hair because it is able to penetrate the cuticle more easily and begin to attack the tint molecules faster than in the less receptive areas. Do remember to warn your clients that the colour left after the stripper will not be the colour they will be wearing when they leave the salon. It can be alarming for a client to see their hair various shades of red, yellow or orange after the stripper is rinsed off! Obviously, a tint is applied over the stripped hair to achieve an even end result and you will need to recommend a comprehensive home hair care programme for a client that has undergone such treatment.

Neutralising hair colour

In hair colouring, 'neutralising' has nothing to do with what we do to hair after it has been permed or relaxed. Neutralising hair colour is a way of eliminating and subduing unwanted tones by the application of its colour opposite. To understand this principle, you will need to have a knowledge of the colour circle (or triangle) and how the primary and secondary colours are positioned around it. A diagram of a colour triangle was shown earlier, in Figure 9.2.

The principle of colour neutralisation is that opposite colours will cancel or subdue each other. Therefore, it can be seen from Figure 9.2 that:

> orange will be neutralised by blue;
> yellow will be neutralised by mauve;
> orange-yellow will be neutralised by bluish-mauve.

Cleaning out unwanted tone from bleached hair

It is not unusual for the repeated application of toners onto bleached hair to gradually build-up so that the result is too intense or uneven. This can be corrected by cleaning out the unwanted build-up of colour by running a weak bleach mixture (e.g. 3 per cent peroxide + powder bleach) through the affected hair. The bleach is developed until the unwanted colour is removed, which could be as quick as five minutes. This procedure is also followed should clients decide to change the toner they have been having. A new toner applied over the old colour will not achieve the desired effect.

Questions
1. What three changes can be made to hair colour?
2. Why do you need some knowledge of colour correction?
3. What governs whether correction should be carried out on a head?
4. What decisions must be made in colour correction?
5. List colour correction problems and their solutions.
6. How do you restore lost colour?
7. Get someone to ask you some questions on the problems suggested in this section.
8. How does colour stripping work?
9. What is colour neutralisation?
10. How is toner cleaned out of bleached hair?

Chapter Ten
Neutralising

Neutralising cold permanent waves

Neutralising (or normalising) is the term given to the chemical process of fixing a permanent curl into the hair. If neutralising is not carried out properly, the new curl pattern will not be fixed as firmly as it should be, resulting in the hair losing the desired curl. Loss of curl may not be apparent for several weeks, until the client notices that the curl is weaker and the hair lank. Evidence of really poor neutralising will be instantly recognisable when the hair is ready for styling, for it will simply be straight. From this, you will appreciate how important the neutralising process is to the durability and overall success of a perm.

What types of neutralisers are available?

Unlike the actual perming which is a reduction process, neutralising is an *oxidation* process. This means that the chemicals involved will provide oxygen. The most common oxidising agent used in neutraliser solutions is hydrogen peroxide, but sodium bromate is also often used. Sodium bromate is found in a lot of home perm neutralisers as well as in the neutralisers for a number of acid perms. It is less damaging to the skin because it is less irritating. Neutralisers will usually contain either a 6 per cent (20 volume) solution of peroxide or a 5 per cent solution of sodium bromate. Stronger solutions of either of these oxidising agents are to be avoided, as there is likely to be some loss of hair colour due to the oxidation (bleaching) of hair pigment. Because neutralisers may contain different oxidation agents, always use the matching one for the perm you are using to avoid disappointing results.

Many neutralisers are now available ready to use and packaged for individual client applications in applicator bottles. Others may only be available in large one litre containers which means the hairdresser has to measure the amount of neutraliser that is needed into a bowl or applicator bottle. Some neutralisers may even require that they are mixed in exact proportions with warm water or 6 per cent hydrogen peroxide. If the neutraliser has to be mixed before it is ready for use, you should read the instructions carefully and measure the exact quantities as prescribed by the manufacturer. Inaccurate measurements can result in the neutralising solution being too weak or too strong and the perm result will be unsatisfactory.

Some neutralisers are designed to be applied from a bowl with a sponge and might foam up to produce a rich lather. The lather is produced by the addition of a small amount (about 1 per cent) of soapless detergent by the manufacturer. Using a sponge to apply the solution very quickly aerates the liquid to produce a thick lather. Other neutralisers will not have soapless detergent added so consequently will not produce a foam when they are applied with a sponge. Always check how the manufacturer recommends the solution should be applied to achieve the best results.

All neutralisers are acid, having a pH of between 3.0 and 4.0 to help cancel out any residue of the perm lotion left in the hair, and to stabilise the hair structure. Mild organic acids are used in neutralisers, such as acetic, citric or tartaric acids.

How do neutralisers affect the hair?

When the neutraliser is applied to the hair the oxidation agent in the solution will release oxygen. The oxygen atoms fix the curl in the hair by joining with the two hydrogens from adjacent cysteines, thus water is formed along with a new cystine. This is discussed below in the chemistry of neutralising. Because neutralisers release oxygen they can oxidise the bonds of the hair and cause damage. This would be referred to as 'over-neutralising'.

The chemistry of neutralising

The purpose of applying the neutraliser is to stabilise the hair structure, so that it hardens to take on the shape of the curler permanently. The term neutralisation is, strictly, incorrect, because this would describe an acid and an alkali reacting together to give a neutral pH, and a salt and water. This is why you will hear terms like 'normalising' used instead. The chemical contained in the neutraliser is an *oxidising* agent, usually hydrogen peroxide, which removes the hydrogens from two cysteines to form water with the oxygen released by the neutraliser (see Figure 10.1). The disulphide bonds are reformed in a new position to hold the curl in place.

Figure 10.1 The application of neutraliser. (Key: S = Sulphur; H = Hydrogen; O = Oxygen; H_2O = water.)

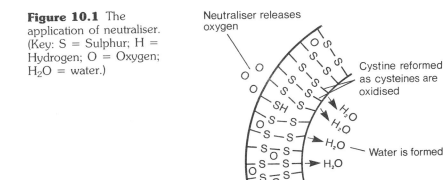

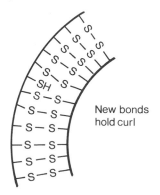

Figure 10.2 After neutralisation, hair is normal again.

New bonds hold curl

You can now see (Figure 10.2) that the hair has mostly cystines present again. Not all the disulphide bonds will rejoin in practice, however, and there will be an increase in the number of cysteines. Some cysteines are also oxidised by the neutraliser to form cysteic acid. When this happens in excess (over-neutralisation) the structure of the hair will be seriously weakened because these sulphurs are no longer available to hold the structure of the hair intact. As with all alkaline treatments, the hair is now more *porous*.

What is the procedure for neutralising?

As soon as the perm is sufficiently processed, the perm lotion must be thoroughly rinsed from the hair. It is the rinsing that stops the perm from processing any more so time should not be wasted between taking the curl test and the neutralising. Read this in conjunction with the beginning of Chapter 8.

1 Testing and controlling water temperature

The water should be adjusted so that it is tepid. It is easier to test the temperature of the water on a sensitive area of your skin such as the inside of your wrist. In some salons you may find that the water temperature changes when another person uses the basin next to you. If this happens in your salon, try to hold the hand set so that one of your fingers is always in contact with the water. By doing this, you will be instantly aware of any changes to the temperature. If the temperature does suddenly change, move the hand set away from the client's head until you have re-adjusted the temperature.

2 Controlling the flow of water during rinsing

When rinsing the perm lotion out of the hair you will find that you will need to hold the hand set fairly close to the client's head to prevent unnecessary splashing. Use your free hand to shield the client's face and ears from the water. The rods should be rinsed with tepid water for a *minimum* of 3−5 minutes. It takes at least five minutes to thoroughly rinse hair that is 15 cm (6 inches) long and an extra minute should be added to this time for every additional 2.5 cm (inch).

Rinsing is made easier if the water pressure in your salon has force because it helps to flush out the lotion. Remember to hold the hose close to the rods to prevent unnecessary splashes and shield your client's face with your other hand. There is no need to rub the rods to help flush out the lotion − all this does is to disturb the hair that is around the rods.

It is far safer to use a backwash for rinsing perm lotion out of the hair because it reduces the chance of chemicals entering the eyes. If you have no other choice than to use a forward basin, do make sure that you give clients a small towel to protect their eyes and replace this as soon as it becomes saturated.

Some salons train their staff to check that all the lotion is out of the hair by making them taste the hair! They are taught to wipe their finger along a rod and then taste their finger. If they taste salt, it tells them there is still lotion in the hair. An alternative method is to use litmus paper which will change colour when it comes into contact with alkaline solutions.

3 Blotting the rods to remove excess water

After thorough rinsing, the rods need to be blotted to remove the excess water from the hair. This is important because if there is too much water left in the hair, the neutralising solution will be diluted and this will affect its performance.

Use a towel to blot the hair by pressing it against the rods. Next, take a wad of cotton wool and press this onto every rod. You will be amazed at how much more water will be removed from the hair.

4 Mixing and measuring the neutraliser

Most neutralisers today do not require mixing but if they do need to have water (or anything else) added, do make sure you measure it in the correct proportions. If the neutraliser is ready for use but comes in a large (litre) container, you will need to measure out the quantity you will need. Check the instructions because the manufacturer will normally tell you how much to use. When using a measure, it is important that you check the readings with the measure level with your eyes. Looking downwards to check the measure will give you a false reading. It is best if the measure can be stood on a shelf which is at eye level but if this is not possible, hold the measure so that it is level with your eyes as shown earlier in Figure 9.16.

5 Application of the neutraliser

Whether you are applying the neutraliser with a sponge from a bowl or by using an applicator bottle, your application must be thorough and you should wear gloves while doing it. Every single rod must be saturated with the neutralising solution to ensure that all the hair is treated. It is usually best to begin the application at the nape, working up towards the front hairline in a systematic way. By starting at the nape, there is less chance of the solution dripping into the client's eyes or missing out a rod. We are presuming that you will be using a backwash basin for doing all neutralisers as they are safer. Sometimes, manufacturers will recommend that you apply the solution a second time to ensure that every rod has been treated and properly saturated. Usually, you need to use about two-thirds of the solution for the application onto the rods, leaving the remaining solution for when it is applied to the hair once the rods have been removed.

The manufacturer's instructions will tell you how long the solution needs to be left on the wound rods. Do check that your client is comfortable at this stage because leaning backwards into a backwash basin for about 5 minutes can be a real pain in the neck!

6 Removing the rods

After the neutralising solution has been left for the recommended time, the rods need to be removed. This has to be done very gently because any undue stress on the hair when it is in this delicate state will pull the curl out. Again, it is usually best to begin removing the rods starting at the nape. This avoids hair getting in the way while you take out the rods. Do not pull the rods out – gently unwind the hair and remove the end paper from the points of the hair as the hair is released from the rod. You must aim to keep the hair in an undistorted shape so it must not be pulled or twisted in any way. When all the rods have been taken out, you are ready to apply the remaining neutraliser solution.

7 Applying the neutraliser to the unwound hair

The remaining neutralising solution is now applied to the unwound hair. This should be done carefully so that the hair is not pulled or distorted. The reason for applying the solution to the unwound hair is to make sure the middle lengths and ends of the hair are fixed into their new curl formation. Remember that the first application may not have penetrated right through the length of hair that was wrapped around the rod, especially if the hair is long. This second application will ensure that the ends are treated. Again, the solution is left on the hair for the length of time given in the manufacturer's instructions. While the neutraliser is on the unwound hair, use this time to rinse and dry your perm rods and to clear away any equipment you will no longer be needing.

8 Rinsing the neutraliser out of the hair

After the second application of the neutraliser has been on the hair for the recommended time, the solution is thoroughly rinsed out of the hair. Again, adjust the temperature of the water so that it is tepid, testing it on the inside of your wrist before putting the water on the client's head.

Generally, you would apply a conditioner after the neutraliser because most perms tend to dry out the hair. Also, do not forget to recommend to clients how they should maintain their new perm and the products they should use between salon visits. At the end of the client's visit, do remember to write out your record card and file it away.

Summary of safety guidelines for neutralising

- Always use a backwash for neutralising to minimise the chance of chemicals entering the client's eyes.
- If you need to measure or mix the neutralising solution do so carefully in the exact quantities as stated by the manufacturer.
- Test the water temperature before you put it on the client's head by testing it on the inside of your wrist.
- During rinsing, shield the client's face with your free hand to protect the face from splashes.
- Wear gloves when applying the neutralising solution to the hair.

Questions

1. What is neutralising?
2. What can happen if it is done incorrectly?
3. Chemically, what is neutralising?
4. What are the main ingredients of neutralisers?
5. If neutralisers are too strong, what effect can they have on the hair?
6. How are neutralisers made ready for use in the salon?
7. Why are exact measurements important when mixing neutralisers?
8. Why do some neutralisers produce a foam?
9. What is the pH of neutralisers?
10. Draw some simple diagrams to illustrate how neutralising works chemically.
11. What is over-neutralisation?
12. How do you keep a check on water temperature during rinsing?
13. How do you protect the client during rinsing?
14. What are the rules for calculating rinsing time of perm lotion from the hair?
15. Why are backwashes preferred?
16. How can you tell if the hair is properly rinsed?
17. How is the hair blotted dry?
18. How can you check measurements of liquids accurately?
19. Describe the application of neutraliser.
20. Why must great care be used when removing the rods?
21. Describe the removal of the rods.
22. Why is neutraliser applied to the unwound hair?
23. What can you be getting on with while the hair is processing?
24. What advice can you give clients about their hair?
25. Are there any products from your salon that you would recommend?

Chapter Eleven
Client Communication and Selling

The most successful salons are the ones which attract clients *and* keep them. But what is it that attracts a client to a particular salon in the first place and why do they regularly return? Before we attempt to answer this question we need to first look at *why* people go to the hairdressers:

- To make them feel good.
- To get out of the house.
- To relax in pleasant surroundings.
- As a special treat.
- To look more fashionable, youthful or healthy.
- As a break from the children.
- For company and a sympathetic ear.
- To have a manageable hairstyle.

You can probably think of more reasons than we have listed above, which are worth discussing with your colleagues to establish what you need to be offering your clients in terms of their reasons (needs) for visiting the salon. For example, is your salon a sanctuary for the stressed housewife or business woman, or does very loud music make it imposs-ible for clients to relax? Are the staff friendly, making people feel welcome or are clients treated as if they are doing the salon a favour by stepping through its door? Do the clients feel really looked after when they visit your salon, because of the service you offer? Do the clients that have saved up for their visit to the salon get value for money?

Once clients are in the salon they will have certain expectations for their visit. They are likely to expect the following:

- A high standard of hygiene.
- A good cut.
- A manageable style.
- Prompt and attentive personal service.
- Pleasant surroundings.
- A consultation before the service is begun.
- Advice about their hair.
- A courteous service.
- Professionalism.
- The chance to buy from a professional range of products.

Below is a questionnaire that will give you an indication of the quality of the service your salon offers. You should circle the number that you think is closest to your feeling about each statement. It is not a quiz and there is no perfect final score, but it will help you to evaluate your service.

Self evaluation for salons

Our clients rarely complain.	5 4 3 2 1	Our clients are always complaining.
We provide a very special service.	5 4 3 2 1	Our service is the same as the other salons.
Our clients are mainly regulars.	5 4 3 2 1	We are always trying to attract new ones as we lose them.
We are the busiest salon in the area.	5 4 3 2 1	Other salons are more successful.
The salon makes a profit on all its services.	5 4 3 2 1	We lose money on some of our services.
All our clients are given a consultation before their hair is started.	5 4 3 2 1	We only talk to those who ask to be seen first.
All the staff have been given special training in selling techniques.	5 4 3 2 1	The staff sell without any special training.
We make a point of using a client's name.	5 4 3 2 1	We only know the names of our regular clients.
Our salon is kept very clean and tidy.	5 4 3 2 1	We are too busy to keep tidying up.
All the staff have nice hairstyles.	5 4 3 2 1	We are too busy to get our hair done.
We offer our clients a cup of tea or coffee as part of the service.	5 4 3 2 1	We make a drink if the client asks for one.
We have a good selection of recent magazines for our clients to read.	5 4 3 2 1	All our magazines are old and tatty.
The salon has a sales area for clients to buy a range of products and commodities.	5 4 3 2 1	We don't have a sales area.
All the staff have regular training sessions.	5 4 3 2 1	Only the juniors have any training.
The work our salon does is of a high standard.	5 4 3 2 1	Our standard of work could be better.

As we said, there is no perfect score for the questionnaire but it will help you to assess the quality of service you offer. If you have completed the questionnaire and feel that you need to take action to improve your service, don't drop this book and rush off to try and make changes! Your first line of action is to do your research and find out *who* your clients are and *why* they come to you. The maximum score was 75 and the minimum 15; most salons will be somewhere midway.

Who are my clients? (Place a tick.)

1. Professional people ____   2. Senior Citizens ____
3. Manual workers ____   4. Unemployed ____
5. Students ____   6. Housewives ____
7. Children ____   8. Fashionable & young ____
9. European ____   10. Afro-Caribbean ____
11. Asian ____   12. Oriental ____
13. Middle-aged mums ____   14. Tourists ____
15. Other ____

Now that you have an idea of the composition of your clientele, you can move onto the next question.

Why do they come to us?

The best way of answering this is to get together with some of the other trainees (and possibly other staff) and have a brain-storming session. You will probably find it useful to use a flip chart to write down and display the reasons that are given by the staff as shown in Figure 11.1. Once you have the reasons listed, ask the others to identify what they consider to be the main reasons.

Once the main reasons for your clients coming to the salon are identified you can then go about analysing how you compare with the competition in your area. For example, if the majority of your clients come because you offer a special type of service, does this positive aspect feature in the way the salon is publicised and promoted? Looking at the main reasons identified by the staff of the salon given in the example above, how would you go about promoting these positive aspects? As an exercise, try to design an advertisement (for a local paper) that will promote the positive aspects of your salon.

Figure 11.1 Examples of reasons given by one London salon for clients going to them. The main reasons are marked *.

* We do Afro-Caribbean and European hair.
  We don't keep clients waiting.
* We offer free consultations.
  We provide free refreshments.
* The salon is modern and air-conditioned.
* Our standard of hairdressing is high.
  We belong to a large organisation.
  We are a well-known salon.
  The salon is well situated.
* We have a high standard of hygiene.
* The staff are established (not much turnover).

Ways of promoting your salon

The most important thing about promotion, is that you need to monitor the success of the idea. By doing this successful ideas can be repeated.

The promotion ideas must be changed regularly so that clients (and staff) do not get bored. Here is a short list of promotional ideas. It is by no means exhaustive — try to add your own ideas to this list.

Promotional ideas:

- Special offers on particular services.
- Leaflets to local hospitals, doctor's surgeries, schools, social clubs, etc.
- Putting on a show and giving any proceeds to a local or national charity.
- Offering regular clients a free hair-do on their birthday.
- Special carrier bags printed that advertise the salon.

One of the most effective ways of evaluating how satisfied your clients are is by doing a client survey. You can use the information offered in a

---

Client questionnaire

We would appreciate your cooperation in completing this questionnaire before you leave the salon. We endeavour continually to improve the quality of the service we offer and value your opinions which will help us to identify areas that could be improved. Your comments, will of course, be treated in confidence.

Please circle a number from 1–5 that represents how you feel about each particular aspect as indicated below.

	score (1 = Poor − 5 = Excellent)
(a) Comfort and salon surroundings	1 2 3 4 5
(b) Cleanliness of salon	1 2 3 4 5
(c) Type and volume of music	1 2 3 4 5
(d) Refreshments	1 2 3 4 5
(e) Friendliness of staff	1 2 3 4 5
(f) Reception and waiting area	1 2 3 4 5
(g) Efficiency of service	1 2 3 4 5
(h) Quality of service	1 2 3 4 5
(i) Satisfaction of service (hair)	1 2 3 4 5
(j) Courtesy of staff	1 2 3 4 5

Were you happy with your consultation?   Yes/No

Were you given enough information about our services and products?   Yes/No

What things did you like about the salon?

_____

_____

What do you think we could improve? _____

_____

_____

Which stylist did your hair? _____

What did you have done? _____

How long did this take? _____

THANK YOU FOR TAKING THE TIME TO COMPLETE THIS
QUESTIONNAIRE

number of ways:

- Evaluating present service;
- Identifying areas that could be improved;
- As a basis for staff appraisal;
- As a promotion: incentives can be offered to staff that provide the best service and prizes to clients who provide the best suggestions.

How can I keep my clients?

Once you have attracted any clients to your salon you must work equally hard at keeping them. The main reason for clients not remaining loyal to a particular salon is that they feel their custom is taken for granted.

All salons should keep client records as a system of keeping information about the frequency and types of services that are given to particular clients. Many of the points made below are for when you have your own salon so that client records are used to good effect to make each client feel special:

- Send your clients a birthday card.
- Send appointment 'reminders'.
- After a period of loyalty (e.g. one year) send a leaflet or letter which thanks them for their custom. You could even include a voucher or small gift.
- Send out leaflets which advertise special promotions to new and 'lost' clients.

Questions

1. For what reasons do people go to the hairdressers?
2. Can you think of any other reasons not included on the list?
3. Why do you think the majority of clients come into your salon?
4. What do you think they expect from a visit to your salon?
5. Fill in the 'self evaluation for salons' questionnaire on a piece of paper and total up the score.
6. What group do the majority of your clients come from?
7. Does this reflect the area the salon is in?
8. Why do you think your salon attracts the clients it does?
9. Design a poster or advert to attract clients for your salon.
10. Why should a promotion be monitored?
11. Try to add to the promotional ideas given.
12. What do you think can be found out from clients using surveys?
13. The questionnaire is an example. Get someone who knows your salon to fill it in, but only ask a client with the salon owner's permission.
14. What can you do so that new clients become regulars?

Dealing with people

All clients need to be made to feel special, whether it is their first or tenth visit, and the quality of service given should be consistent from the moment they walk into the salon. This level of service does not just happen. Staff have to be well trained in dealing with people as well as in hairdressing skills.

Hairdressing is an occupation which revolves around the skill of being able to communicate effectively with colleagues and, of course, clients. Hairdressers need to be good communicators, patient listeners, always cheerful, pleasant, polite *and* good at their work. It seems a lot to ask of anybody especially on the morning you go to work feeling under the weather with a busy day ahead of you. It can take a great deal of effort to smile and cheerfully welcome the client you dread coming into the salon (and look sincere!), but the professional hairdresser will always treat clients equally, and value their loyalty.

We communicate with each other in two ways; verbally and non-verbally. We do this by speech, our appearance and the movements we make with our bodies.

Communication between client and hairdresser is without doubt as important to success as a thorough knowledge of all the practical and theoretical aspects of a hairdresser's work.

Verbal communication

Speech is a very complex human communication and there are many different uses for speech:

- to ask questions;
- to convey information;
- to give orders, instructions, etc.;
- informal conversation (chatting, gossiping, joke-telling, etc.)
- social routines and rituals (greetings, farewells, apologies, etc.).

In the salon, hairdressers are expected not only to be expert at interpreting what clients are communicating, but also to be good conversationalists. Good conversationalists are simply people who have the ability to convey what they are saying in a clear, precise and interesting manner. We can all become experts, because it is often our own laziness that prevents us from developing this talent. By following a few basic guidelines anyone can become a good conversationalist:

- Learn everything you can about hairdressing. This includes the products and services your salon offers. You can't talk about something if you don't know what it is, or what it is for.
- Develop your knowledge on a wide range of subjects, even if only by watching television or reading a newspaper.
- Learn to be a good listener. By listening to your clients you will know what interests them so that you can develop the conversation accordingly.

- Avoid discussing issues that could cause offence or anger your clients. Topics to avoid discussing in the salon are sex, religion, politics and race.

It is often quite difficult for a sixteen-year-old to talk easily to much older clients, because the young person has less in common with someone older than they do with a person from their own age group. Suitable conversation topics might include television programmes, recent holidays, Christmas or Easter activities, local area news, and of course, the client's hair and latest products. Clients will be very impressed if you ask how they enjoyed that wedding they were going to last time they came to the salon, or how the shampoo they bought from you was performing. You don't need to have a magnificent memory to be able to do this. Your clients need never know that you jotted down a note to remind yourself to ask about something next time they came in!

Each salon will have its own rules regarding what can and can't be said. Swearing is not normally permitted in salons, neither are racist remarks nor too familiar comments or remarks. Joke-telling can be fun but be careful that you select your material carefully!

Non-verbal communication

Non-verbal communication is the way we transmit information without the use of speech. There are several ways in which we do this; our appearance, our posture and stance, the gestures we use and our facial expressions.

Appearance

Hairdressing involves helping others to create their image — a very responsible task. Our appearance is the initial way in which we tell others the sort of person we are. We wear particular clothes and hairstyles that reveal a great deal to others. For example, sub-culture groups such as punks, hippies and skinheads present themselves in a particular way to tell others they belong to a certain group. This leads us to presume that they behave in a particular way, and hold certain attitudes, because we stereotype them. Stereotyping is a way that human beings categorise people, to help us make sense of all the information which bombards us when we meet people. At a party when you first walk through that door not knowing anybody, you look at the other guests and make assumptions about what they are like before you even speak to them! These assumptions are made purely on the way a person looks.

The moment a client enters the salon you will read the non-verbal information they are transmitting by their appearance. What they are wearing will tell you quite a lot about them, especially if they are wearing a 'uniform' for their work, as in the case of nurses, traffic wardens, lawyers, etc.

Posture and stance

The ways in which people 'arrange their bodies' as they stand or sit can also be extremely communicative. As a general rule, the body frame is more widely spaced, whether seated or standing, when we are feeling at ease. A person feeling nervous, uncomfortable or tense, will occupy less space, with the arms and legs being held closer together. The ability to be able to read what people are 'saying' through the way their bodies are arranged is very useful to hairdressers. For example, recognising a client who is feeling nervous can enable you to respond with the necessary reassurance that all is well.

Gestures

As we speak, we use our hands, head and body as part of the total communication we are making. These gestures are often co-ordinated with our speech to emphasise or explain certain things we are saying, or made without sound when speech is superfluous. Some gestures are made consciously while at other times we are not always aware of the gestures we are making. A car driver who points his finger to his head with a screwing motion is demonstrating what he thinks about the quality of someone's driving, and it is a gesture that does not have be supported with speech. However, in hairdressing, we use gestures to add an extra dimension to what we are trying to communicate by using our hands to help us describe shape, line and form that would be difficult to describe with words alone.

When people become emotionally aroused, they tend to use gestures that reflect their emotional state, which may appear to be pointless. People often touch themselves when experiencing certain emotions and examples include:

- fist clenching − aggression;
- face touching − anxiety;
- scratching − self-blame;
- forehead wiping − tiredness.

Head nods are a rather special kind of gesture, and have a distinct role. They act as reinforcers; that is, they reward and encourage what is being said. They can also be used to encourage a person to talk more. A single nod usually means that the speaker is encouraged to continue by the listener, whereas a rapid succession of nods may mean that the listener wants to speak himself. Tilting the head to one side and holding eye contact tells the other person that you are actively listening to what they are saying.

Eye contact

Eyes are an important means of feedback. Eyes can express friendliness or hostility, and people regard them as an important communicator of character. We have all heard the expression that someone 'has shifty eyes'. If you feel this to be true about someone you will not trust him.

Basically, if we hold eye contact with people, it indicates that we are interested in them or what they are saying. This can be used to show general interest, love, lust, anger or sympathy. Gazing upwards expresses lack of interest and total avoidance of eye contact can show total lack of interest, dislike, dissatisfaction or shyness.

If a client avoids eye contact with herself in the mirror while you are doing her hair, it could mean that she does not like what she sees and what you are doing with her hair!

Selling

Stylists will often miss golden opportunities of persuading a client to have a particular service or to buy a specific product. Why does this happen? Perhaps the best way of analysing this situation is to understand a little of the psychology of selling. Imagine that a client has made an appointment with you for a cut and blow-dry. While looking at her hair and discussing what she wants, your judgement tells you that her hair would benefit from having a special treatment because it is out of condition. We can look at that example in the form of the diagram shown in Figure 11.2.

Figure 11.2 The possible responses of a client to extra services. (Courtesy L'Oréal.)

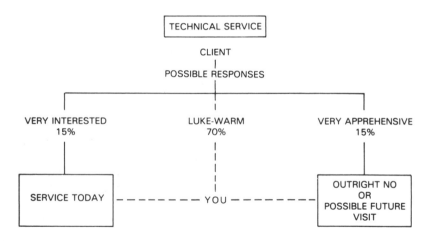

As you can see from the diagram, most clients fall into the 'lukewarm' category, and it is your influence on such clients which could be defined as selling. However, never push a client into a service she neither wants, needs or can afford – this is bad selling and is ultimately bad for business. Clients must always feel at ease or they will not return. If it is a good product that will benefit their hair and appearance, they will appreciate your interest. The process of selling can be divided into three steps:

(1) analysing the client's needs;
(2) giving advice (introducing the service or product);
(3) gaining agreement on how to meet these needs, if required.

Let us look at these three steps in more detail.

Step (1) (analysing the client's needs) can be done by:

- establishing a relationship by developing interest and trust;
- asking questions which begin with How? When? Where? Why? and Which?;
- demonstrating understanding by using visual aids such as style books or product leaflets;
- formulating an opinion which will rely on your technical knowledge.

Step (2) (giving advice) is introduced by:

- explaining the service in terms of what it will do for the client;
- convincing the client of these benefits;
- being enthusiastic and having a positive belief in the service that you are recommending.

Step (3) (gaining agreement) is achieved when your client is interested by:

- suggesting the service is given at that moment;
- reassuring the client if she is still apprehensive and perhaps suggesting lesser alternatives.

Salon retailing

It is true to say that most clients buy their shampoo, hair spray, mousse, and conditioners from supermarkets with the weekly shopping, or from the chemist. Why? Because salons don't appear to be the place where they should buy them. Millions of pounds' worth of haircare products are being sold through a vast number of retail outlets. Currently this is a £400 million a year market. If salons could take just 5 per cent of this market it would generate an extra £20 million of turnover each year! Just an extra £25 worth of retail profit per week generates £1300 additional profit a year.

Here are some quotes from those who really know about retailing:

'Selling should be included in *every* normal training programme' – Wella.
'With more and more clients visiting the salon less and less often, the only growth area in salon business is through retailing' – Redken.
'Recommendation from a professional is something you don't get at the local chemist' – Schwarzkopf.
'We are getting daily phone calls from people whose total business has trebled' – L'Oréal.

Research shows that clients want more advice from their hairdressers about what products they should be using on their hair. Usually, they do not get it. To be professional, stylists need to analyse the clients' needs and give them advice. As a stylist, you have the undivided attention of your client during each appointment, but do you take advantage of it? How much better it would make your service if you spent time talking to the client about what she thinks of her hair and what products she uses at home. A careful lowering of the eyebrows will have the client asking you what you would recommend. Sadly, clients usually learn more about hair-care from women's magazines and television commercials than from the person who knows her hair personally – her hairdresser.

Salon retailing can be a very profitable business. Not only is your standard of service improved by analysing your clients' needs and recommending the appropriate home products but you may also draw prospective clients into your salon through an attractive product display. Another advantage of retailing is giving the client a bag bearing the salon name to take their products home. It is an advertisement wherever it is carried. These are some simple guidelines for displaying goods in the salon:

Do's	Don'ts
Do display all of your stock as a large amount attracts more interest.	*Don't* leave most of your stock in the stockroom where it can't be seen.
Do mark every product clearly with its price.	*Don't* leave products unpriced; clients may be reluctant to ask you the price.
Do make sure that the goods are easy to see and accessible.	*Don't* have goods under lock and key as clients will be reluctant to ask you to take them out.
Do make displays large to attract attention.	*Don't* set up too many small displays as they have less impact.
Do use your salon window and entrance area to let passers-by know that you sell retail goods.	*Don't* miss the opportunity to exploit your salon frontage to its full extent.
Do make displays attractive and change them regularly.	*Don't* leave items in the window until they are faded, or use damaged items.

One of the most important factors of all in retail selling is to get your staff interested in selling products. This can be done in a variety of ways, including commission, profit-sharing for the whole salon, and simply using the products in the salon.

Questions
1. Make up a single sentence that describes how you should treat your clients.
2. What reasons are there for speech in the normal working day?
3. How can you become a good conversationalist?
4. What rules are there for conversation?

5. How can you show interest in particular clients?
6. How does appearance communicate information about somebody?
7. What can posture and stance tell you about the way somebody is feeling?
8. What kinds of gesture can you think of that do not need speech to support their meaning?
9. Why do people nod their heads?
10. How can the head nod have different meanings?
11. What can eye contact tell you?
12. What opportunities for selling have you lost in the last week?
13. How is the process of selling broken up into steps?
14. Go through these steps and give examples of how you would use them.
15. Why do you think salons miss out on the retail market?
16. How can you show clients that you have retail sales?
17. Make a list of do's and don'ts for displaying goods.
18. What do you intend to do as a stylist to improve *your* service to clients?

We hope you have enjoyed the book and have seen it as a worthwhile investment in your career. Just like you, we will not miss this opportunity for selling. You now know the basics; the Salon Handbooks will be the icing on your cake! You will find them as useful as any hairdressing tool. Have a good career!

Glossary

If you have forgotten the meaning of a term used in hairdressing, this glossary will be a quick reference for you. If you still do not understand, look it up in the book itself.

Accelerator: a device that produces infra red radiation as a source of heat to speed up chemical processing of hair. Accelerators can also be used to 'natural-dry' the hair.

Acetic acid: the weak organic acid found in vinegar and used in acid rinses.

Acid: a chemical compound that contains hydrogen ions and has a pH of less than 7.0. Acids close the cuticle layer of the hair.

Acid conditioner: a conditioner which has an acidic pH and helps to restore the hair's natural pH.

Acid mantle: the layer of acidity maintained on the skin's surface. Gives the skin a slight antiseptic property.

Acid rinse: a rinse containing a weak organic acid used to close the cuticle and to neutralise alkalinity.

Acne: the term used to describe 'spotty' skin usually seen in adolescents.

Activator: any agent that induces activity. In acid perms an activator is mixed with the perm lotion immediately before application to make it work properly.

Aerosol: a container (usually a cannister) in which the contents are kept under pressure and released by propellants. See *CFCs*.

Aescalup: alternative name for thinning scissors.

Afro: the term used to describe negroid hair, which has a tight curl formation.

AIDS: stands for 'acquired immune deficiency syndrome', a viral disease which destroys the immune system so that the sufferer eventually dies of a variety of illnesses to which she or he has no resistance. Can be spread in blood.

Albino: a person whose hair and skin lack pigment due to a genetic defect.

Alkaline: chemicals with a pH of more than 7.0; they contain hydroxide ions and open the cuticle of the hair.

Allergy: a reaction to contact with something, usually seen as a dermatitis on the skin. Not everyone has an allergy, but some hairdressing products recommend a skin test before use on the client to avoid allergic reactions. Asthma and hay fever are allergies.

Alopecia: the medical term for baldness.

Alpha-keratin: hair in its unstretched state.

Amino acids: the small molecules that proteins are made of; in the cortex they help maintain moisture balance.

Ammonium carbonate: the active part of a powder bleach; causes rapid release of oxygen from peroxide.

Ammonium hydroxide: the alkaline chemical that combines with thioglycollic acid to make ammonium thioglycollate. It is added by manufacturers to cold wave lotions to make them alkaline. Also found in bleaches as a catalyst.

Ammonium thioglycollate: the salt which is the active ingredient of most cold wave perm lotions.

Anagen: the part of the hair growth cycle in which the hair is actively growing. It lasts between 1−7 years.

Analysis: the examination of the client and the client's hair before any hairdressing procedure is carried out. It enables clients to express their desires and the hairdresser to carry them out without unnecessary damage to the hair.

Androgens: the name given to male hormones which control the growth of underarm and pubic hair. They cause male pattern baldness and acne in sensitive individuals.

Aniline dyes: colorants made from coal derivatives.

Anthraquinones: dyes contained in some semi-permanents.

Antibiotics: chemicals that are capable of attacking and destroying bacteria.

Antibodies: the name of the particles produced by the immune system in response to an infection.

Anti-clockwise: an expression used to describe curl formation in a direction opposite to that travelled by the hands of a clock.

Anticoagulant: a substance that prevents the blood from clotting.

Anti-dandruff treatment: a lotion or shampoo that is used in the treatment of dandruff; they contain substances which inhibit the production of epidermal cells − the cause of dandruff. Please refer to *selenium sulphide* and *zinc pyrithione*.

Anti-oxidant rinse: a rinse containing an acid which is also a reducing agent (such as ascorbic acid); helps to reduces oxidation damage in hair.

Anti-perspirant: an agent that reduces the amount of sweat secreted. Used in the control of body odour.

Antiseptic: a chemical that will inhibit the growth of bacteria without necessarily destroying them.

Apocrine gland: the type of sweat gland found attached to hair follicles in the armpits, pubic regions and nipples. The decomposition of this sweat by bacteria leads to body odour.

Applicators: the attachments which can be fitted to a vibro machine.

Arrector pili: the muscle attached to the hair follicle that causes the hair to stand on end on contraction.

Artery: a large blood vessel which carries (oxygenated) blood from the heart to all areas of the body.

Ash: shades containing blue or violet; opposite to warm.

Asymmetrical: not evenly balanced.

Athlete's foot: the common name for ringworm of the feet, *tinea pedis*, the most common type of ringworm.

Atoms: small particles, not visible to the naked eye, that make up all matter.

Azo dyes: dyes contained in some temporary colorants.

Bacilli: a type of bacteria which are rod-shaped.

Backbrushing: brushing back from points to roots to add volume to the hair; hairs entangle because the cuticle is roughened.

Backcombing: a method of achieving support and fullness; the shorter hairs are pushed down towards the roots with the aid of a comb.

Backwash: a basin in which the client's hair is shampooed by reclining so that the back of the neck rests into the basin. It is much safer to use a backwash than a frontwash when rinsing out strong chemicals.

Bacteria: a type of micro-organism that can be seen with a microscope. Bacteria can be either harmful, harmless or useful.

Baldness: lack of hair in a place where it would be considered normal to have hair; the medical term to describe baldness is alopecia of which there are many types.

Banding: a dark line that appears on hair when tint is allowed to overlap the regrowth onto the previously coloured hair.

Barber's itch: see *sycosis barbae*.

Barrel curl: an open centred pincurl.

Barrier cream: a waterproof cream used to protect the skin from chemicals.

Basal layer: the bottom layer of the epidermis where cells are actively dividing.

Base: the area of the scalp from which a mesh of hair is taken for setting and perming.

Benzyl alcohol: used in some semi-permanent colorants to help the colour molecules penetrate the hair shaft.

Beta-keratin: keratin in its stretched condition.

Blackhead: (also known as a comedone) a plug of oxidised sebum which blocks the opening of a pore. Often seen in acne.

Bleach: a product capable of lightening the hair.

Blonde: a light hair colour.

Blow-drying: using a hand-held hairdryer in unison with a brush or the hands to dry and style the hair.

Blow-waving: using a hand-held hairdryer in unison with a comb to dry and shape the hair into wave movements.

Blunt cut: alternative name for club cutting.

Boil: (also known as a furuncle) a septic condition of a hair follicle with a characteristic single large head. Scars from boils are often seen on men's necks.

Booster: chemicals (persulphates) which release extra oxygen in bleaching.

Bottle trap: a trap often fitted underneath shampoo basins to prevent smells and airborne infections entering the salon. It is also easy to open if the sink becomes blocked.

Braid: plaiting of hair.

Breaking point (of hair): see *tensile strength*.

Brightening shampoo: a weak oxidant mixture in a shampoo base which lightens the hair.

Bristle: animal hairs used in brushes.

Bromidrosis: body odour due to sweating. It is usually caused by the decomposition of apocrine sweat, but the same term is often used to describe the smell of sweaty feet which is due to eccrine sweat.

Buckled end: distorted points of hair caused by incorrect winding when setting, perming or styling the hair.

Bunions: the term used to describe the deformity of the bone at the side of the big toe, usually caused by tight shoes.

Calamine lotion: a lotion which helps to reduce irritation and soreness of the skin; often used for treating sunburn. Can be used to soothe a positive skin test.

Calcium stearate: the scum that is formed when soap reacts with hard water.

Camomile: a vegetable colorant derived from the flowers of the camomile plant. Used to lighten fair and blonde hair.

Canities: hair that grows without colour; white hair.

Cap: usually made of plastic or polythene, it is used as an insulator during some hairdressing services, e.g. perming.

Cape: a wrap-around protective garment used to protect the clothes of your client.

Capillary: small blood vessel found between arteries and veins; supplies the hair follicles with oxygen and nutrients.

Carbuncle: a group of boils.

Catagen: the breakdown period of the hair growth cycle which usually lasts about two weeks.

Catalyst: agent which speeds up a chemical reaction while itself remaining unchanged in the process.

Cationic conditioners: positively charged conditioners which are attracted to the negative charges in hair.

Caustic: a strong alkali, e.g. sodium hydroxide, capable of attacking and damaging other substances; used in relaxers and to clean drains; can damage the hair and skin.

Cell: the basic unit of life; the skin and hair are made up of a collection of cells.

Cell division: the way in which a cell grows; a parent cell divides into two smaller copies of itself. This process is called mitosis.

Cetrimide: a chemical which can act as a conditioner, a soapless detergent, a disinfectant and an antiseptic.

CFCs: abbreviation for chlorofluorocarbons. CFCs are propellants found in aerosols. They are damaging to the ozone layer that surrounds the earth and helps shield it from harmful ultra violet radiation. Banned in many countries.

Charge card: a means of credit that allows the user to pay for goods using a plastic card e.g. American Express. The card holder settles *all* payments made by using the card at the end of each month. Unlike *credit cards*, no extra credit is permitted.

Cheque: an official bank document that enables the account holder to make a payment without using cash.

Cheque card: a card issued to the holder of a cheque book, which is used to support a payment by cheque up to the value of £50.00 (sometimes £100).

Chignon: type of long hair dressing.

Chipping: a method of thinning the hair.

Citric acid: an organic acid found in citrus fruits, used in acidic rinses to neutralise alkalinity and close the cuticle of the hair.

Clip: a clamp-like device used to secure the hair.

Clippers: hair-cutting tools which can be either electric or mechanical.

Clockwise: in hairdressing, the movement of hair in the same direction as the hands of a clock.

Club cutting: cutting the hair straight across to achieve blunt cut ends.

Coal tar: the tar extracted from coal used to treat a number of scaling conditions of the scalp.

Coarse hair: a hair fibre with a large diameter.

Cocci: round-shaped bacteria.

Cohesive set: wetting, moulding and drying hair in a stretched position – e.g. setting and blow-drying.

Cold sore: the common name for herpes simplex, a skin infection caused by a virus.

Collodion: flexible plastic covering for the skin applied as a liquid which sets hard; e.g. 'Nuskin'. Can be used in skin tests.

Colour circle: shows the primary and secondary colours. Used for the selection of correct colours when subduing unwanted tones in hair.

Colour reducer: product which strips unwanted artificial colour from the hair.

Comb: an instrument used to part, dress and arrange the hair.

Comb-out: the use of a hair brush or comb to dress hair into the finished style.

Compatible: able to mix without an unwanted reaction.

Compound colorant: mixture of vegetable and mineral. For example, compound henna which is henna and a metallic salt.

Concentrated: condensed, usually by the removal of water. Increasing the strength of a chemical solution by decreasing the bulk.

Condensation: water produced when warm moist air meets a cold surface.

Conditioner: any product applied to the hair to improve its condition.

Conditioning: the application of special chemicals to the hair to help restore its strength and moisture.

Conduction: the transfer of heat or electricity in solids by movement of atoms.

Conjunctivitis: inflammation of the eyeball. Can be caused by bacteria or as a reaction to ultra violet radiation.

Contact dermatitis: skin inflammation caused by contact with a chemical to which a person is allergic.

Contra-indication: indication against performing a service.

Convection: the movement of heat in gases or liquids; warm air rises, cools and falls again, setting up a convection current.

Convex: used to describe a surface that curves outwards.

Corrective colouring: rectifying unwanted colour results.

Cortex: the central layer of the hair, consisting of bundles of fibres. The natural pigment of the hair is found here.

Counterclockwise: the movement of hair in the opposite direction to the hands of a clock.

Cowlick: strong area of hair growth in the opposite or an unusual direction on the front hairline.

Cranium: the bones of the skull which protect the brain.

Credit card: a plastic card which permits the holder to make payments which are paid off at a later date, e.g. Access. Interest is charged by the credit company for any outstanding or overdue payments.

Credit limit: the maximum amount that can be 'spent' using a credit card. The limit is set by the credit company but it might be possible to negotiate a new limit if your record of settling accounts is good.

Crest: the raised part of a wave.

Croquignole: winding of the hair from the points to the roots.

Cross linkages: bonds in the hair between cortical fibres.

Crown: the top part of the head from where the hair takes its direction of growth.

Curler: an alternative word to describe a roller used for setting or perming the hair.

Current account: the account used to draw cheques on and for everyday bank transactions.

Cuticle: the outer layer of the hair, consisting of several layers of overlapping scales.

Cyst: a fluid-filled sac that may be found on the head.

Cysteine: an amino acid containing one sulphur atom. Two cysteines are oxidised to form one cystine molecule during the neutralising of a perm.

Cystine: an amino acid containing a disulphide bond, which is reduced by perm lotion to form two cysteine molecules.

Damaged hair: hair which is either porous, brittle, split, dry, or has little elasticity.

Dandruff: overproduction of skin scales, which are seen on the scalp. Also called pityriasis.

Decompose: to disintegrate, become broken down into constituent parts. For example, hydrogen peroxide decomposes into water and oxygen if it is exposed to the air.

Delivery note: a piece of paper received with an order that details what has been delivered by the manufacturer or supplier.

Dense: thick, heavy, abundant.

Depilatory: a substance that has a high pH value and is capable of completely destroying the structure of the hair so that it dissolves.

Depth: how light or how dark the hair is.

Dermal papilla: the collection of cells at the base of the follicle which is the source of hair growth.

Dermatitis: inflammation of the skin as the result of being in contact with some external agent, such as perm lotion.

Dermis: the second layer of the skin, containing nerves, blood vessels and connective tissue.

Detergent: an agent that cleanses, a synthetic soap.

Development: the process of forming a colour.

Development time: the time that a colorant is left on the hair to enable the colour molecules to form the colour.

Disentangling: method of removing tangles and combing the hair smooth, usually carried out with a wide-toothed comb.

Disinfectant: a chemical substance that destroys bacteria.

Distilled water: water that has been purified to remove dissolved salts.

Disulphide bonds: the strong cross linkage in hair formed between two sulphurs.

Dry hair: hair that lacks natural oils (sebum).

Earth wire: wire that does not normally carry electricity, but does if an appliance develops a fault. Protects the user from electrocution.

Eccrine glands: the type of sweat gland that is found all over the body. The sweat consists of water and a little salt.

Ectoparasite: a parasite found on the outside of the body.

Eczema: inflammation of the skin with itching, caused by an internal agent such as allergy to food.

Effleurage: a stroking massage movement.

Egyptian privet: a plant whose leaves are used to produce henna. The leaves of this plant are ground into a fine powder to produce lawsone.

Elasticity: the ability of a hair to be stretched and return to its original length.

Elasticity test: a test performed by the hairdresser to assess the strength of the hair's internal structure, i.e. the cortex.

Electrode: attachment for high frequency machine.

Electronic Funds Transfer Card: type of cheque card which can be used to debit a current account at the point of sale without writing a cheque.

Emulsify: in colouring, the process of adding water to the hair and massaging to loosen the colorant from the hair and skin.

Emulsion bleach: a type of bleach that is used to lighten the hair.

Endoparasite: a parasite that is found inside the body.

End papers: papers used to prevent buckled and distorted points when winding perms.

Ends: the last few centimetres (one inch) of hair, furthest away from the scalp.

Epidermis: the very top layer of the skin; protects the body from physical damage and water loss.

Epileptic fit: a fit involving uncontrollable convulsions of the muscles.

European hair: type of hair found on people originating from Europe; hair of Caucasians.

Evaporation: the process in which a liquid turns into a gas.

Expansion: when something increases in size, usually on heating.

Fading: when the intensity of a colour diminishes.

Fainting: passing out due to an insufficient supply of oxygen to the brain.

Fat: a type of foodstuff made up of fatty acids combined chemically with glycerol. All animal fats and plant oils are fats; their main role is to store energy.

Feathering: alternative name for taper cutting.

Filler: a chemical preparation that equalises porosity by filling in the more porous areas.

Fine hair: a hair fibre that is relatively small in diameter.

Finger wave: the process of moulding the hair in a pattern of waves by using the fingers and comb.

First aid: the first action that should be taken in the event of an emergency in order to minimise or lessen any harmful consequences.

Flammable: a substance that will ignite or burn.

Fluorescent lighting: strip lighting; some tubes (warm white) give out light which is similar to daylight.

Foil: thin sheet of metal (usually aluminium) which is used in some hairdressing services, e.g. weave highlights.

Follicle: a downgrowth of the epidermis from which hair grows.

Folliculitis: infection of the hair follicle by bacteria. Usually, a hair is protruding from the pustule at the skin's surface.

Formaldehyde: the name of the vapour given off by formalin which is used to sterilise tools.

Formalin: liquid heated in some older sterilising cabinets.

Fragilitis crinium: alternative name for split ends, a condition caused by harsh treatment of the hair. The only remedy is to remove the split ends by cutting.

French pleat: a hairstyle which is dressed so that the back hair is made into a fold.

Frizz: hair having too much curl.

Fungi: these are a group of plant micro-organisms, which contain no chlorophyl and cause several types of ringworm and other diseases such as thrush.

Furuncle: another word to describe a boil.

Fuse: a protective device in plugs which should blow in the event of an overload.

Gel: a thick oil-in-water emulsion used to style hair.

Gland: tissue which produces a secretion, e.g. eccrine and sebaceous glands.

Grab: a term used in hair colouring to describe a colorant having a more intense or durable result than anticipated.

Graduation: a method of cutting which blends longer meshes of hair into shorter hair lengths.

Grey hair: a mixture of white and coloured hairs that gives the overall impression that the hair is grey.

Guide line: the first cutting line which is made and followed throughout the entire haircut.

Hair: form of keratin which grows from a follicle.

Hair growth cycle: the three-part cycle which describes the stages of a hair's growth.

Hairline: the edge of the scalp where the hair begins.

Hair shaft: that part of the hair that projects from the skin.

Hair spray: a spray used on dry hair to keep the hair in position.

Hard water: water that contains calcium and magnesium salts, which will not easily form a lather with soap.

Head louse: correct name is *Pediculus capitis*; an insect that infests the human hair and lays eggs called nits.

Heart attack: the condition that arises when cardiac tissue is deprived of oxygen, usually because of a blood clot. Will result in the death of all, or some, of the heart muscle.

Henna: a natural hair dye that can coat the hair and join with sulphur bonds in the cortex, so much so, that perming may be affected. See *Egyptian privet*.

Herpes simplex: the scientific name for cold sores.

High frequency: an alternating current used to stimulate the scalp.

Hirsute: term used to describe a person that has an abnormal growth of hair in areas that do not usually have such a dense growth.

Horny layer: the top layer of the epidermis, which consists of a lot of dead cells. The main function is to protect the cells underneath from physical injury and water loss.

Humidity: moisture in the air.

Hydrogen ions: hydrogen atoms which have a positive charge because they have lost an electron. Found in acids.

Hydrogen peroxide: an oxidising agent used in hairdressing, found in many neutralisers and bleaches and mixed with tints.

Hydrometer: instrument used to measure the density and strengths of liquids and solids.

Hydrophilic: something which is water-loving.

Hydrophobic: something which is water-hating.

Hygrometer: instrument used to measure amount of atmospheric moisture or relative humidity.

Hygroscopic: the tendency of something (e.g. hair) to absorb moisture from the atmosphere.

Hyperaemia: reddening of the skin caused by the blood coming to the surface due to stimulation by massage or friction.

Hyperidrosis: the overproduction of sweat, most often sweating of the hands and feet. Usually a nervous condition.

Imbrications of hair: the point where cuticle scales overlap.

Impetigo: a bacterial skin infection where there are yellow, crusty blisters. May also arise as a secondary infection caused by head lice infestation.

Incompatible: a chemical reaction that causes damage to the hair.

Incompatibility test: a test to determine whether damage would be caused by the use of a hairdressing product containing hydrogen peroxide.

Infectious: describes a disease or condition that can be caught, or passed from one person to another. Can be spread by direct or indirect contact, depending on the disease.

Infestation: describes something or someone having living creatures in or on them. A building can be infested by rats while a person can be infested by lice.

Inflammation: the reaction of the body to irritation, usually seen as an area of redness.

Infra red: a type of radiation, which is invisible and provides heat.

Insulation: the process of helping to reduce the passage and loss of heat; in hairdressing a perm cap acts as an insulator.

Inversion: a term used to describe the cutting of hair so that it is shaped inwards to form a concave or 'V'.

Invoice: a piece of paper from the manufacturer or supplier that details the individual prices and total cost of an order.

Itch mite: the mite that causes scabies. The scientific name is *Sarcoptes scabiei.*

Keratin: the protein from which hair, skin and nails are made. It differs from other proteins because it contains sulphur.

Keratinisation: the hardening process of keratin during its growth and development.

Kilowatt: a unit for measuring electrical power (i.e. the rate of supplying electrical energy) which is equivalent to 1000 watts.

Kinky: very curly hair.

Lacquer: originally derived from shellac; today made from water-soluble substances that 'stick' and hold the hair in place after styling.

Lanolin: purified sheep's sebum.

Lanugo: the hair found on a foetus.

Lawsone: extract from Egyptian privet leaves; the active ingredient of henna.

Layering: a method of cutting hair which reduces its length.

Lead acetate: a metallic salt found in some hair colour restorers.

Lice: the name of three different types of insect that live on human blood. One variety is found on the body and is called *Pediculus corporis*. The type that infests the hair is called *Pediculus capitis* and the one which infests the hair of the pubic region is called *Phthirus pubis*, commonly referred to as 'crabs'. Lice are killed with insecticides.

Lime scale: a hard crusty deposit which is caused by calcium bicarbonate decomposing into calcium carbonate. Commonly referred to as 'fur'.

Litmus: a dye that is used to indicate whether something is acid or alkaline by a change in colour (acid = red; alkali = blue).

Live wire: wire which carries electric current, coloured brown.

Lowlights: the colouring of selected hair strands so that they are generally darker than the overall colour of the hair.

Lymphocytes: the type of white blood cell which produces antibodies to help fight infection.

Mains (electricity supply): the electrical power supplied to the consumer. In the UK, it is supplied at 240 volts.

Male pattern baldness: type of alopecia caused by a sensitivity to androgens. Can affect both men and women although it is more common in males.

Mandible: the lower jaw.

Marcel waving: a technique of forming waves in the hair by means of heated irons.

Massage: manipulation of the scalp or body by rubbing, kneading, stroking or tapping, to increase circulation.

Medulla: the name given to the hollow air spaces that form the centre of the hair. It may not be present in some hairs.

Melanin: the black or brown pigment found in both hair and skin.

Melanocytes: the cells which produce the pigment melanin, found in the germinating layer of the epidermis.

Membrane: the semi-permeable outer covering of cells.

Menopause: the time in a woman's life when menstruation ceases due to hormonal changes.

Mesh: generally a small, manageable amount of hair taken to make the work of the hairdresser more efficient.

Metallic dye: a hair colorant which contains metallic salts.

Micro-organisms: living animals or plants that are too small to be seen with the naked eye.

Minerals: chemical elements that are an essential part of the diet because of their function. Mineral deficiency can cause serious conditions of ill health.

ml: millilitre; a metric unit for measuring which is one-thousandth of a litre.

Mitosis: type of cell division where one cell divides to give two smaller copies of itself.

Molton Browners/Permers: flexible foam- or cloth-covered 'rollers' used for setting or perming hair.

Monilethrix: the production of beaded hair which breaks off easily.

Mousse: an aerosol foam hairdressing product. Most often in the form of styling or colouring foams applied to damp hair.

Nape: the name used to describe the back of the head.

Neutral: having neither an acid nor an alkaline pH reading. Having a pH of 7.0.

Neutralisation: the correct chemical definition refers to the reaction between an acid and an alkali to give a salt and water and a neutral pH.

Neutralise: (in colouring) to apply the opposite colour to eliminate unwanted tones in hair.

Neutralise: (in perming) the fixing of a curl put into the hair by means of a chemical process.

Neutralising shampoo: a special shampoo used after relaxer has been rinsed from the hair to restore the natural pH.

Nerve impulses: electrical 'messages' sent to the brain along the nerves.

Nervous system: the network of nerves in the body that control the other body systems under the overall control of the brain.

Nit: the egg of a louse. In a head louse infestation nits will be found attached to the hairs, close to the scalp.

Nitro dye: chemicals used in semi-permanent colorants.

Normaliser: an alternative name for a neutraliser used in the fixing of a chemically induced (permed) hair curl.

Nucleus: the part of a living cell that contains all the genetic information.

Occipital: the name of the bone which forms the back of the head.

On-base: the placing of a roller so that it sits squarely on its own base. This is the most commonly used method for putting in rollers.

Oil bleach: a type of hair lightener which is in the form of an oil.

Opaque: allows no light to pass through.

Opposite colours: colours which are opposite to each other on the colour circle.

Organic: a substance which contains carbon, derived from living or once living sources.

Over-directed: the placing of a roller so that it sits on the upper part of its base to produce maximum volume.

Overlapping: incorrectly applying a tint, bleach or relaxer so that the previously treated hair is covered instead of restricting it to the regrowth.

Over-processed: over-exposure of hair to chemicals; usually caused by chemicals which are too strong or that have been in contact with the hair longer than was necessary.

Oxidant: a chemical which releases oxygen, e.g. hydrogen peroxide.

Oxidation: the process of adding oxygen or taking away hydrogen.

Ozone: a form of oxygen which is given off during a high frequency treatment.

Ozone layer: a layer of ozone in the upper atmosphere of the earth which filters out harmful ultra violet radiation.

Papilla: the source of hair growth, found at the base of the hair follicle.

Para dye: a synthetic hair colorant containing chemicals called para-phenylenediamine or para-toluenediamine which can cause dermatitis; mixed with hydrogen peroxide to develop the colour molecules in the cortex of the hair.

Parasite: a living creature that lives in or on another creature, causing it harm.

Patch test: an alternative name for skin test.

Pathogenic: micro-organisms that cause disease.

Pediculosis capitis: the scientific name for a head lice infestation.

Pediculus capitis: the scientific name for the head louse.

Pediculus corporis: the scientific name for the body louse.

Permanent wave: a chemically produced hair curl which alters the internal hair structure; achieved by breaking the disulphide bonds in the cortex and then fixing them into a new formation.

Permanent colour: a colorant that produces a regrowth, e.g. bleach and tint; the colour is not removed by shampooing.

Peroxometer: an instrument used to measure the strength of hydrogen peroxide.

Persulphates: chemicals which give off oxygen; used as boosters to give off extra oxygen in bleaching.

Petrissage: a deep, penetrating massage movement that is used on the scalp.

pH (potential of hydrogen): the symbol for hydrogen ion concentration; a scale of numbers tells you exactly how acid or alkaline something is.

Phagocyte: a cell that ingests foreign bodies such as bacteria in the blood.

Pheomelanin: the natural hair pigment responsible for the yellow and red tones in hair; found in the cortex.

Phthirus pubis: scientific name for the louse that infests the pubic hair; commonly called 'crabs'.

Pin curl: a strand of hairs organised into a flat ribbon form, and wound into a series of continuous untwisted circles.

Pityriasis: the correct name for dandruff, the overproduction of epidermal scales.

Plait: intertwining of hair strands to form a braid.

Plane mirror: flat mirror.

Plantar wart: wart on the foot.

Plastic cap: a cap used to cover the hair to help retain moisture and body heat, and so speed up processing.

Pli: originates from 'mise en pli' the French term used to describe the setting of hair with rollers, pincurls and finger waves.

Pointing: a method of thinning the hair that is restricted to the ends of the hair.

Porosity: the ability of the hair to absorb liquids.

Porosity test: a test to check the porosity of the hair and therefore the condition of the cuticle.

Porous: full of pores, an open cuticle, able to absorb liquids.

Post-damping: applying perm lotion to the rods when the whole head is wound.

Posture: the way in which people arrange their bodies whether they are standing or sitting.

Powder bleach: a type of bleach that is a powder and mixed with hydrogen peroxide to form a paste.

Pre-damping: the application of perm lotion to the hair during the winding of the rods.

Pre-disposition test: an alternative word for a skin test.

Pre-lighten: to bleach the hair in preparation for the application of a toner.

Pre-perm treatment: a lotion that is applied to the hair before it is permed to equalise its porosity.

Pre-pigmentation: the process of replacing lost pigment caused by bleaching or colour fade.

Pre-softening: the process of applying hydrogen peroxide to resistant hair to lift the cuticle scales and make it more receptive to hair colorants.

Primary colours: colours from which all other colours are made; red, yellow and blue.

Primary irritant: something which causes dermatitis.

Processing time: the period of time required for a chemical action upon the hair to achieve the desired result.

Progressive colorant: the colour result is gradual as in the case of colour restorers.

Propellant: a gas which is contained in aerosols to force the contents out through a nozzle. See *CFCs*.

Protein: a type of foodstuff that is made up of amino acids linked chemically together. Found in meat, fish, and various vegetable sources. Needed for growth and repair of cells.

Psoriasis: a non-infectious skin condition that is sometimes seen on the scalp, characterised by thick silvery scales. Caused by the cells of the epidermis multiplying too quickly. Treatments containing coal tar can prove useful in controlling the scaling.

Pus: yellowish-white matter that collects at the site of an infection; a mixture of bacteria and dead white blood cells.

Pustule: the 'head' or raised part of a spot containing pus.

Quasi: a term used to describe a colorant that is between being semi-permanent and permanent; will give a regrowth but the colour will gradually fade each time it is shampooed.

Quaternary ammonium compounds: a group of chemicals with germicidal properties which can be used as detergents and conditioners. They have a positive charge and cetrimide is a good example.

Radiation: the transmission of energy in the form of rays.

Reagent: a substance that is used to bring about a chemical reaction; e.g. perm lotion.

Receipt: a statement that shows that payment has been received.

Receptive: hair that responds quickly to the application of chemicals; opposite to resistant.

Record card: a means of recording information about clients and the services they are given.

Recovery position: the name given to the position in which any unconscious casualties should be placed to make sure they don't choke or smother on vomit.

Reducer: a product used to remove unwanted artificial colour from the hair; also called a colour stripper.

Reducing agent: a chemical that adds hydrogen or takes away oxygen; e.g. perm lotion.

Reflection: occurs when heat or light hits a surface and bounces off. The image that is seen in a mirror is reflected.

Refraction: the bending of light rays as they pass from one medium to another.

Regrowth: newly grown hair after hairdressing treatments that has the client's natural colour and wave pattern.

Rehabilitating rinse: an alternative way of describing pH-balanced conditioning rinses; have a pH reading of between 4.5 and 5.5.

Relaxer: a chemical applied to hair to reduce unwanted curl and wave movements.

Resistant: opposite to receptive; the hair does not respond easily or quickly to the penetration of hairdressing chemicals.

Restructurant: a hairdressing lotion that helps to strengthen the internal structure of the hair.

Retouch: term used to describe the application of a chemical treatment to the newly grown hair only.

Reverse pincurling: the placing of open pincurls in alternate rows, in clockwise and anticlockwise directions; produces a wave pattern.

Ring main: a common type of electrical power supply circuit used in homes and salons.

Ringworm: also called *tinea*: name given to a group of fungal skin infections.

Rod: alternative name for a perm curler.

Root sheath: the cells which hold the hair in a follicle.

Roughage: the name given to the part of the diet that provides bulk but no nutritional value. It helps to prevent constipation and certain intestinal diseases.

Sabourand-Rousseau test: a test to determine whether a person is allergic to the chemicals contained in para-tints; named after the two people who invented the test. See *skin test*.

Salt linkages: type of linkage found in the hair.

Saponification: the scientific term used to describe the production of soap.

Scrunch: a technique which involves grasping meshes of hair during drying to achieve curl and movement; ideal for increasing natural movement during blow-drying.

Scurf: layman's term often used to describe dandruff. See *pityriasis*.

Sebaceous glands: the oil glands attached to the hair follicle; they secrete sebum directly into the hair follicle.

Seborrhoea: over-activity of the sebaceous glands that results in greasy hair and skin.

Seborrhoeic dermatitis: type of scaling condition.

Sebum: the oily secretion of the sebaceous gland; helps lubricate and waterproof the skin.

Secondary colour: colours which are produced by mixing two primary colours together; e.g. orange, green, mauve.

Sectioning: dividing the hair into separate parts, or panels.

Sectioning clip: a clip used to secure sections of hair.

Selenium sulphide: an ingredient found in some anti-dandruff treatments; slows down cell division.

Sensitivity: being easily affected by chemicals, resulting in a skin reaction.

Shade chart: a book or folder made by manufacturers of hair colorants to display the various shades in any given range.

Shampoo: to wash the hair with detergent and water or the name given to a soapless detergent used to clean the hair. Shampoo is a Hindu word, which means 'to clean'.

Shingling: using the scissors or clippers over comb technique to cut hair short in the neck region.

Skin test: a test that should be carried out 24–48 hours before the application of a para-tint; determines whether a person is allergic to the chemicals contained in para-tints.

Soap scum: calcium stearate, produced by the reaction between soap and hard water.

Soapless shampoo: a shampoo that contains a synthetic detergent rather than a soap. Almost every shampoo used today is soapless.

Sodium hydroxide: a caustic chemical, commonly called lye, used in a number of hair relaxers. It can also be used to dissolve hair in blocked basins and drains.

Spectrum: the seven colours that make up white light; red, orange, yellow, green, blue, indigo, violet. (Can be remembered by using the mnemonic 'Richard of York gave battle in vain' – the first letter of each word tells you the colours that make up the spectrum.)

Spiral winding: winding the hair from roots to points.

Spirochaetes: bacteria cells which are in a spiral shape.

Split ends: damage to the ends of the hair which results in splitting along the length of the hair; the correct term is *Fragilitis crinium*.

Spongy: porous.

Stabiliser: an acid added to hydrogen peroxide to stop it from losing its strength.

Stand-up curl: an open pincurl which stands up from its base producing volume at the roots.

Staphlyococci: round bacteria in bunches which are responsible for skin infections such as acne.

Static electricity: the term used to describe the build-up of a charge on the hair, caused by friction when brushing or combing hair, especially when newly dried.

Steamer: a machine used to produce moist, moving heat.

Stem direction: the part of the hair that determines its root direction in setting.

Straightener: alternative name for relaxer; please refer to relaxer.

Strand test: a test used to monitor the development of hair colorants and bleaches.

Streptococci: round bacteria in chains which cause impetigo and sore throats.

Sterilisation: the complete destruction of all living organisms on an object.

Stripper: alternative name for colour reducer.

Strop: a flat piece of leather used to maintain the edge of a razor.

Substantive: describes a substance which is attracted to hair; e.g. cetrimide.

Sulphide dye: a metallic salt used in hair colour restorers.

Sulphur bonds: bonds found in the cortex which are broken down during perming and relaxing treatments.

Surface tension: the force exerted at the surface of a liquid.

Surfactant: a chemical which lowers surface tension; e.g. a soapless detergent.

Suspension: small particles of grease and dirt 'floating' in water after removal from the hair during the shampooing process.

Sweat: the liquid produced by sweat glands in the skin, composed mainly of water with a small amount of salt. Its function is to maintain the body's temperature by cooling the skin.

Sweat gland: a gland which produces sweat.

Sycosis barbae: the medical term for 'barber's rash'; a skin infection caused by bacteria.

Symmetrical: evenly balanced and proportioned.

Symptoms: the indicators and signs of a condition.

Synthetic: something which is man-made; produced by artificial synthesis in a laboratory or factory.

Tail comb: a comb, half of which is shaped into a slender, tail-like end.

Tapering: removing length and bulk from the hair using either scissors or a razor on wet hair.

Target colour: the hair colour you are aiming for.

Technique: a method of accomplishing a desired aim.

Telogen: the resting part of the hair growth cycle which usually lasts between 3–4 months.

Temporary colour: a form of hair colorant that will last until the hair is next shampooed.

Tensile strength: the amount of tension that is put on a hair, by means of a weight, that will cause the hair to break. (A hair in good condition could support about 120–150 g before breaking.)

Tension: the stress put on the hair by stretching and holding tightly.

Tepid: slightly warm; lukewarm.

Terminal hair: the coarse hair found on the scalp and other areas of the body after puberty (beard, underarms and pubic region).

Test curl: a test performed before a permanent wave to determine strength of lotion, rod size and approximate processing time.

Test cutting: a test performed before colouring the hair to see the result before it is applied to all the hair.

Texture: the 'feel' of hair; the quality of hair as being coarse, fine, etc.

Thermostat: an automatic device which controls and regulates temperature.

Thinning: a method of cutting which removes bulk, without affecting the overall length of the hair, e.g. pointing.

Thio: a shortened term for the chemical ammonium thioglycollate.

Thrush: the name of a fungal infection of the genital tract (usually female) which causes a thick discharge and irritation. Caused by a yeast, the condition is usually treated with antibiotics in tablet, cream or pessary form.

Tinea: the scientific name for ringworm.

Tint: a permanent hair colorant containing para compounds.

Tissue: a group of cells and their intercellular substance that forms one of the structural materials of the body.

Tone: the type and intensity of a colour; the colour we actually see in the hair, e.g. copper, red, ash, etc.

Toner: a colorant used to add colour to the hair or mask unwanted tones after bleaching (sometimes referred to as pastel toners).

Toxins: poisonous substances (toxaemia is blood poisoning).

Traction alopecia: baldness due to placing tension on the hair, causing it to loosen in the follicle and fall out.

Translucent: something that allows some, but not all, light to pass through it.

Transparent: something that allows all light to pass through it.

Trichonodosis: a hair condition; abnormal growth of hair resulting in knots forming along the hair shaft.

Trichorrhexis nodosa: name given to a hair condition recognised by swelling on the hair shaft caused by physical or chemical abuse.

Trichotillomania: name given to pulling out one's own hair; usually caused by an obsessional or nervous disorder.

Triethanolamine lauryl sulphate: the main detergent base used in soapless shampoo.

Trough: the dip or hollow of a wave.

Tungsten: a metal used to make light filaments; the light emitted is yellowish. Most light bulbs have tungsten filaments.

Ultra violet: the invisible rays present in sunlight that promote tanning of the skin. Can damage the eyes and burn the skin. Used in UV sterilising units.

Under-development: insufficient development of a hair colorant. If hair colorant is not left on the hair for the time that is required or recommended by the manufacturers, the result is unsatisfactory.

Under-directed: the placing of a roller so that it sits on the lower part of its base to produce less volume at the roots.

Under-processed: hair that is not sufficiently processed during the perming process; insufficient bonds have been broken down in the cortex to achieve satisfactory curl results.

Uneven colour: a colour result which is not uniform along the hair length or in specific areas; caused by incorrect application or the irregularity of the hair's porosity.

Varicose vein: surface veins of the legs in which failure of some valves has caused slower circulation and swelling.

Vegetable colorants: hair colorants derived from plants and vegetables; e.g. camomile, henna.

Vellus hair: the soft downy hair found on the body.

Ventilation: the changing of air in a room. Should take place 3−4 times an hour without the production of draughts.

Verruca: the medical term for wart; a viral infection of the epidermis which shows as a raised circular mound of skin.

Vertex: the top, or crown, of the head.

Vibrance: the brightness and intensity of colour.

Vibrio: a comma-shaped bacteria.

Vibro: an electrical machine used to give mechanical massage.

Virgin hair: refers to hair which has not been previously chemically processed.

Virus: the smallest of micro-organisms that cause infectious diseases. e.g. warts, cold sores.

Viscous: thick and sticky (liquids).

Vitamins: accessory food factors needed in extremely small quantities by the body; without them, the body would be unable to function properly.

Volatile: a liquid which has a low boiling point and so evaporates easily and quickly; e.g. setting lotion.

Volt: a unit of electrical pressure.

Volume strength: a means of describing the strength of hydrogen peroxide; the number of parts of free oxygen that can be given off by one part of hydrogen peroxide if it completely decomposes.

Vulcanite: a material that is produced by treating rubber with sulphur to increase resistance to heat.

Warm colour: a colour that appears to be golden, red, copper, etc.; opposite to ash.

Wart: see verruca.

Water vapour: water in the form of a gas.

Wattage: a unit measurement of the rate of supply of electrical energy; 1,000 watts = 1 kilowatt (kW).

Weave colouring: a method of selecting strands of hair to be coloured; e.g. foil highlights.

Weave cutting: a method of selecting strands of hair for cutting; a method of thinning.

Wetting agent: a substance which lowers the surface tension of water allowing more thorough wetting of hair; e.g. shampoo.

White hair: hair which contains no pigment.

Whiteheads: scientific name is *milia*; small, hard, whitish spots that form at the opening of a follicle, usually associated with greasy skin.

White light: the result of mixing the seven colours of the spectrum together.

Wind: term used to describe the wrapping of hair around rollers, perm rods and the barrel of curling tongs.

Wood's light: a type of ultra violet radiation which causes ringworm to fluoresce and is used in the diagnosis of this condition.

Yeast: a single-celled fungus which is found on the scalp. A yeast also causes thrush.

Zinc pyrithione: chemical used to treat dandruff; found in some anti-dandruff treatments.

Index

If there is a topic that you wish to look up, do so by checking under the main heading for a particular topic. For example, if you want to know about tints or semi-permanents, look under colouring. If you want a definition of a word, check the glossary.